# Women's Midlife Health and Wellness

Edited by Bridget Lucas

hayle
medical

New York

Hayle Medical,
750 Third Avenue, 9ᵗʰ Floor,
New York, NY 10017, USA

Visit us on the World Wide Web at:
www.haylemedical.com

ISBN: 978-1-63241-903-3

**Cataloging-in-Publication Data**

Women's midlife health and wellness / edited by Bridget Lucas.
   p. cm.
Includes bibliographical references and index.
ISBN 978-1-63241-903-3
1. Middle-aged women--Health and hygiene. 2. Women--Health and hygiene.
3. Women--Diseases. I. Lucas, Bridget.
RA564.85 .W66 2020
613.042 44--dc23

# Table of Contents

# Preface

The world is advancing at a fast pace like never before. Therefore, the need is to keep up with the latest developments. This book was an idea that came to fruition when the specialists in the area realized the need to coordinate together and document essential themes in the subject. That's when I was requested to be the editor. Editing this book has been an honour as it brings together diverse authors researching on different streams of the field. The book collates essential materials contributed by veterans in the area which can be utilized by students and researchers alike.

Midlife is the stage in the life of a human being between young adulthood and the onset of old age. It is generally assumed to fall in the bracket of 45 to 65 years of age. This period is characterized by the slowing down of the body, sensitivity to diet, stress and substance abuse. During midlife, several health conditions may develop like fibroids, migraine and systemic lupus erythematosus. This makes midlife a period warranting attention for gynecologic and hormone-sensitive conditions. Women further experience menopause around the age of 50, which ends their fertility. Over the past decades, studies have advanced the understanding of ovarian aging and its relationship to cardiovascular, bone, cognitive and musculoskeletal health. Signs of aging may become prominent and more rapid in women with osteoporosis. Decline in physical fitness such as reduction in aerobic performance and decrease in maximal heart rate, as well as changes in the skin occur in midlife. Healthy behavior, in particular the maintenance of healthy body weight and physical activity can moderate certain negative changes. Therefore, this period constitutes a critical period for optimizing health and functioning, and preventing chronic diseases. This book is compiled in such a manner, that it will provide in-depth knowledge about women's midlife health and wellness. It presents researches and studies performed by experts across the globe. It is a vital tool for all researching or studying women's health as it gives incredible insights into emerging trends and concepts.

Each chapter is a sole-standing publication that reflects each author´s interpretation. Thus, the book displays a multi-facetted picture of our current understanding of application, resources and aspects of the field. I would like to thank the contributors of this book and my family for their endless support.

**Editor**

# Depression in the menopause transition: risks in the changing hormone milieu as observed in the general population

Ellen W. Freeman

## Abstract

There is accumulating evidence but no definitive answers about the incidence of depressed mood in the menopause transition and its association with the changing hormonal milieu. While a changing hormonal milieu is the natural condition for all women, only a minority of mid-life women experience debilitating depressive symptoms or clinical depression. This review focuses on associations between depressed mood and the menopause transition, primarily as identified in longitudinal, population-based studies in the past decade. Further aims were to present reported associations between depressed mood and reproductive hormones in the menopause transition as evaluated in the general population and associations of depressive symptoms or clinical depression with menopausal hot flashes or poor sleep in perimenopausal women. There is evidence to support the role of the changing endocrine milieu in the development of depressed mood in the menopause transition, but the contribution of hormones as measured is small. Disentangling the numerous factors that are associated with depression in midlife women is a major challenge for research and for clinical care, where treatments are needed to improve the most distressing menopausal symptoms.

**Keywords:** Depression, Menopause, Transition to menopause, Menopausal symptoms, Perimenopause, Reproductive hormones, Estradiol

## Introduction

Changes in menstrual bleeding patterns signal the approach of menopause in mid-life women, and many women report hot flashes, poor sleep, depressed mood and other symptoms along with these menstrual changes. The extent to which symptoms that arise around menopause are directly associated with the hormone changes of ovarian aging is not well understood. There is accumulating evidence but no definitive answers about many potential risk factors and the role of the changing hormone milieu associated with depressed mood around menopause. Further information is clinically important, because of the diminished functioning and significant disability that accompany depression [1, 2], the exacerbation of disorders associated with

Correspondence: freemane@mail.med.upenn.edu
Department of Obstetrics/Gynecology and Department of Psychiatry, Perelman School of Medicine, University of Pennsylvania, 3701 Market Street, Suite 820 (Mudd Suite), Philadelphia, PA 19104, USA

the neuroendocrine system [3], and the associations of depression with other major health problems, including cardiovascular disease [4–6], metabolic syndrome [7–9] and osteoporosis [10, 11], that complicate treatments and contribute substantially to disability and the high costs of health care.

Depressive symptoms are common in all populations but appear to increase among women in the transition to menopause. Major depression is more common in women than in men in all age groups until late life, with a lifetime prevalence of 21 % compared to 12 % for men in the National Comorbidity Survey [12]. Depression in women also appears to increase around reproductive events. Postpartum depression following childbirth, premenstrual dysphoric disorder linked to the menstrual cycle, and depression around menopause may possibly share a sensitivity to normal shifts in reproductive hormones, which in turn modulate neuroregulatory systems associated with mood and behavior [13, 14]. However, definitive answers about these associations, the etiology of depression, and the role of reproductive hormone changes in depressive disorders have been elusive.

Reports pertaining to depression around menopause have changed over the years. In 2005, the National Institutes of Health (NIH) issued a State-of-Science review of the management of menopause-related symptoms, which concluded that evidence for associations between depressed mood and menopausal status was poor or mixed [15]. Another review of prospective cohort studies that assessed mood symptoms of mid-life women around menopause similarly concluded that there was no clear evidence of an independent effect of the menopause transition on depression [16]. These conclusions stimulated further research leading to more precise definitions of menopausal status and the use of standard measures of depressive symptoms or depressive disorders. Subsequently, multiple, but not all, population-based studies reported an increased prevalence of depressive symptoms in the menopause transition compared to premenopausal women [17]. Some studies differentiated a first-onset depression from a history of depression in perimenopausal women. The studies overall showed that both women with a history of depression and women with no history of depression had an increased risk of depressive symptoms and possibly an increased risk of depressive illness around menopause, but the prevalence was significantly greater among women with a history of depression [18–20].

The aims of this review were to examine associations between depressed mood and the menopause transition, focusing on longitudinal studies in the general population. Further aims were to present reported associations of reproductive hormones with depression in the menopause transition, observed associations between depressive symptoms and menopausal hot flashes or poor sleep, which have been identified as risk factors for depressive symptoms or clinical depression in perimenopausal women. The review did not include intervention studies, neuroendocrine studies, animal models, or studies of postmenopausal women. These domains are clearly important for understanding the development of depression around menopause but are beyond the range of this review and are examined elsewhere [14, 21–29].

## Review

### Common menopausal symptoms

More than 80 % of women experience physical or psychological symptoms around menopause, with varying degrees of severity and disruption in their lives [30, 31]. Depression and other mood changes, hot flashes and sleep difficulties are among the most frequently reported menopausal symptoms [32, 33], although reports of their prevalence and duration can vary widely, due in part to differences in symptom measures, definitions

of menopausal status, retrospective or prospective observations in relation to menopause, cross-sectional study designs, sample sizes, and adjustments for confounding factors.

### The menopause transition (perimenopause)

Menopause is defined post hoc after no menstrual bleeding for at least 12 months [34]. In the classic longitudinal study of Treloar, the mean age at menopause was 50.7 years, with a 95 % range of 44–56 years [34]. In the Massachusetts Health Study of the normal menopause transition, the *median* age at menopause was 51.3 years [35]. The transition to menopause is marked by progressively expanding variability in menstrual bleeding, which results from the increasing frequency of anovulation as the number of oocytes declines. The data of Treloar show that this reproductive transition extends for 2 to 8 years before menopause, and that the age at onset of the menopause transition ranges from 39 to 51 years for 95 % of women [34]. Thus, the mean duration of the menopause transition is about 5 years, although both the age at onset and the duration vary widely among individuals, and factors such as smoking, obesity and mood disorders may alter the timing or the duration of the transition period [36–39].

The development of a staging system for reproductive aging by the Stages of Reproductive Aging Workshops (STRAW) led to considerable increases in information about the rise of symptoms in relation to menstrual status and potential associations between symptoms and hormone changes of ovarian aging. The STRAW definitions of stages of reproductive aging were based primarily on observed bleeding patterns. The definitions were further refined as data accumulated, with revised definitions presented in STRAW + 10 [40]. The STRAW-defined stages in the menopause transition are early transition (persistent difference of 7 days or more in the length of consecutive menstrual cycle) and late transition (amenorrhea of 60 days or longer). Postmenopause is divided into early (2 years: +1a, +1b; and 3–6 years: +1c after the final menstrual period) and late (the remaining lifespan) stages. Perimenopause indicates the time around menopause and extends from the early transition stage through 12 months after the final menstrual period [40].

### Prevalence of depression

The National Comorbidity Study reported 30- day estimates of major depression for women aged 45–54 years of 5.0 % and lifetime estimates of 21.8 % [41]. Depression tends to wax and wane with repeated episodes or persist in a chronic state, which occurs in up to 35 % of depressed patients as reported by Nierenberg [42]; a prior depression is the strongest predictor of a subsequent depression [43]. The rates of *recurrent* depression for women are highest in the 45–54 year age-group [41], which are the years proximal to menopause. Consequently, recurrent depression may coincide with the perimenopausal years, contributing to reports of increased prevalence of depression around menopause.

## Depression and the menopause transition

An association between depression and menopausal status is one of the most controversial issues in the menopause transition. Epidemiologic studies based on self-report of menopausal status and depressed mood consistently indicated that most respondents did not report high rates of depressive symptoms, and that reported depressive symptoms were not associated with menopause per se but with other health problems [16, 43–46]. Bosworth et al. reported that 28.9 % of women aged 45–54 years had a high level of depressive symptoms based on an abbreviated CES-D scale but found no association between the depressive symptoms and menopausal status as defined by the women's perceptions [47]. In the Massachusetts Women's Health Study, there was an increased risk of depression in the menopause transition but no significant association between the increased risk of depression (CES-D scores) and the onset of menopause [43]. A subgroup of women with a long transition period had an increased risk of depression, but the causal direction could not be determined; the researchers speculated that the increased risk could be explained by increased menopausal symptoms.

Early data from the large Study of Women's Health Across the Nation (SWAN) indicated that rates of persistent mood symptoms were higher in early perimenopausal women than among premenopausal women (18.4 versus 14.9 and 12 % versus 8 %, respectively) [48]. Dennerstein et al. defined perimenopause status from bleeding patterns and reported that more late perimenopausal women reported depressive symptoms in the previous 2 weeks (38 %) compared to premenopausal (26 %) and postmenopausal women (28 %) [49]. In contrast to community-based samples, evaluation of women attending a menopause clinic identified higher rates of depressive disorders. Soares et al. reported that 28.7 % of women ages 40–58 years in a menopause clinic met DSM-IV criteria for depressive disorders [50]. These studies all suggested an increased prevalence of depressive symptoms and possibly depressive illness in the transition to menopause.

As studies more specifically defined a menopause transition period and systematically assessed depression status, associations between depressive symptoms and menopausal status were consistently observed in longitudinal cohort studies.

The Harvard Study of Moods and cycles found that women with no history of depression were nearly twice as likely to experience depression in the menopause transition compared with premenopausal women (OR 1.8, 95 % CI:1.0 – 3.2) [36]. When adjusted for a history of adverse life events and vasomotor symptoms, the risk of depressive symptoms further increased to 2.5 times for women in the menopause transition compared with premenopausal women (OR 2.5; 95 % CI: 1.2 – 5.2).

In a series of studies in the Penn Ovarian Aging cohort (POAS), the risk of depressive symptoms (CES-D scores) was nearly three times greater in women in the menopausal transition compared with premenopausal women, after adjusting for other predictors of depression including a history of depression, hot flashes, poor sleep, and severe premenstrual syndrome (early transition OR 1.55, 95 % CI: 1.04 – 2.32 and late transition OR 2.89, 95 % CI: 1.29 – 6.45) [51]. In a further study of women with no history of depression, the risk of CES-D depression was more than four times greater in the menopause transition compared with when the same women were premenopausal (OR 5.44; 95 % CI: 2.56 – 11.59 in adjusted analysis) [19]. When only women who had a DSM-IV clinical diagnosis of depression were evaluated, the odds of the onset of a diagnosed depressive disorder were significantly greater in the menopause transition compared with the woman's own premenopausal period (OR 1.60; 95 % CI: 1.25 – 5.02 in adjusted analysis) [19]. When depressive symptoms (high CES-D) were evaluated across 14 years of follow-up relative to the final menstrual period (FMP), the findings demonstrated a pivotal role of the FMP in the risk of depressive symptoms: there was a higher risk of high depressive symptoms before and a lower risk after the FMP [18].

A series of SWAN studies evaluated menopausal status in relation to outcomes of dysphoric mood [48, 52], depressive symptoms (CES-D) [53–55] and depressive disorder [56, 57]. These studies overall showed that depressive symptoms and dysphoric mood varied by menopausal status and were independent of other known risk factors for depression. Women were more likely to report depressed mood (CES-D scores) in the menopause transition and early postmenopausal years compared with premenopause after adjusting for other demographic psychosocial, behavioral, and health factors [54]. The likelihood of depressive symptoms was significantly higher in the early transition (OR 1.30; 95 % CI: 1.09 – 1.55), the late transition (OR 1.71; 95 % CI:1.27 – 2.30), and postmenopause (OR1.57; 95 % CI: 1.15 – 2.15) compared with premenopausal women [54]. Perimenopausal women were nearly twice as likely to experience a major depressive episode after adjusting for a history of depression, vasomotor symptoms, BMI, age, race, upsetting life events and medication use (OR 1.98; 95 % CI: 1.00 – 3.92) [56]. The likelihood of experiencing an episode of major depression during a 10 year follow-up did not differ between African American and Caucasian women [56]. When African American women were hypothesized to have greater persistence or recurrence of mood disorders compared to Caucasian women, no significant difference in recurrence of depression was found between African American and Caucasian women in 11 years of follow-up [58].

The Seattle Midlife Women's Health Study (SMWHS) showed that depressive symptoms (CES-D scores) significantly increased in the late menopause transition stage after adjusting for multiple risk factors (beta 1.56, SE 0.73, $P = 0.032$) [59]. Menopausal stage increased depression scores more than age and the late transition stage remained an independent factor after adjustment for age, life stress, body mass index, history of postpartum blues, and use of antidepressants, each of which remained significantly associated with depressed mood in the final adjusted model.

In the Melbourne study, depressive symptoms (a shortened version of CES-D) were higher in women who were in the early and late stages of the menopause transition compared to postmenopausal women [60]. CES-D correlated with negative mood measured concurrently with Affectometer ($r = 0.63$) and baseline negative mood ($r = 0.37$). Prior negative mood, history of premenstrual complaints, negative attitudes toward aging or menopause, poor health, and daily hassles significantly predicted depressed mood.

The Norway HUNT-II study added further support to evidence of increased depressive symptoms in the menopause transition. Based on the Hospital Anxiety and Depression Scale (HADS), a widely-published, brief self-report measure that is validated to detect the presence and severity of depression and anxiety in non-psychiatric populations) [61], scores for depression and anxiety were significantly higher for perimenopausal women compared to premenopausal women [62].

Several studies evaluated the risk of *clinical depression* in the menopause transition but had conflicting results. In a study of 29 women who met clinical criteria for depression, the risk of a depression onset was significantly greater in the 2 years surrounding the final menstrual period than in the preceding premenopausal years [63]. Two population-based studies extended these findings [19, 36], although conclusions are limited by different definitions of new onset depression in these studies.

A third community-based study utilized a standard psychiatric interview to identify current major depression over a 7-year time period; 42 cases of first-onset major depression were identified, but no significant associations were found between first-onset major depression and

menopausal status or reproductive hormone levels [57]. The identification of major depression is a strength of the study. However, the small number of identified cases may have yielded less reliable estimates, and interpretation of the results must consider the possibility of type 11 error.

The Harvard Study of Moods and Cycles enrolled a second cohort to continue studies of new-onset depression in late reproductive-age women. Unexpectedly, the rates of new-onset depression were extremely low in the second cohort [64]. The risk of incident major depression or dysthymia over a 3-year period was 5.7 % in cohort 1, but only 1.2 % in cohort 2, yielding a highly significant difference (4.5 %, 95 % CI: 2.2, 6.8). An in-depth analysis to determine possible sources of bias for these disparate findings identified selection bias associated with self-referral of the participants and elements of the study design as the likely reasons for the very disparate rates of depression identified in the two cohorts. These findings underscore the importance of considering the possible impact of selection biases, particularly in populations with differing racial and economic conditions.

In summary, these longitudinal studies in the general population consistently showed that depressive symptoms were greater in the menopause transition compared to premenopause. However, the use of standard diagnostic criteria for *depressive illness* was limited, and evidence for an increased risk of diagnosed depressive illness (rather than depressive symptoms) in the menopause transition was less clear. This was emphasized in another review of relationships between menopause and depression, where the researchers concurred that "the change in menopausal status over time was associated with an increased risk of elevated depressive symptoms, independent of demographic, psychosocial, behavioral and health factors" [65]. However, when menopause-associated depressions were distinguished from depressive disorders, the more limited data from women with depressive disorders were insufficient to conclude that depressive illnesses occurred as a biological response to hormonal changes in the menopause transition.

## Hormone associations with depression in the menopause transition

Associations of reproductive hormones with mood are difficult to measure in large epidemiologic studies. Differences in frequency and timing of measurements, assay sensitivities and different statistical models in analysis of the data contribute to the limited and inconsistent findings of hormone associations with depression in the menopause transition.

Accumulating data suggest that perimenopausal depression is not simply due to low hormone levels, but that fluctuations or changes in hormone levels, which characterize the transition to menopause, may be endocrine triggers for perimenopausal depression is some women [14]. Evidence from clinical research and animal models was reviewed by Gordon et al. as a basis for a theoretical model for perimenopausal depression [21]. In the conceptual model, ovarian hormone fluctuations, particularly progesterone-derived neurosteroids, were modulators of the GABA-ergic modulation of the hypothalamic-pituitary-adrenal (HPA) axis. This may sensitize vulnerable women to psychosocial stress and potentially lead to increased vulnerability to depression in some women. The researchers concluded that "this proposed model provided a basis for understanding the mechanisms by which the changing hormonal environment of the menopause transition may interact with the psychosocial environment of midlife to contribute to risk of perimenopausal depression".

Another review considered the role of allopregnanolone, a stress-responsive regulator of neuronal function, in triggering affective dysregulation in susceptible women [66]. They concluded that the source of susceptibility to affective disorder remains unclear, but evidence in multiple animal models suggests that allopregnanolone may trigger mood symptoms, possibly as a function of alterations in central neurotransmitter systems, possibly y-aminobutyric acid (GABA), consequent to allopregnanolone withdrawal combined with stress.

Several epidemiologic studies have evaluated hormone variability in relation to mood in the menopause transition with conflicting results. In an 8-year follow-up of the SWAN cohort, testosterone levels and increased testosterone from baseline were associated with an increased likelihood of high depressive symptoms (CES-D scores) (OR 1.15; 95 % CI: 1.01 – 1.31 and OR 1.23; 95 % CI: 1.04 – 1.45, respectively) [55]. There were no associations with depressive symptoms of either levels or changes in estradiol or FSH. A subsequent study of the SWAN mental health sample evaluated these hormones in relation to major depressive episode but found no significant associations in the menopause transition [56].

In contrast, depressive symptoms adjusted for history of depression, race, and age were significantly associated with subject aggregate profiles of increased estradiol levels in the menopause transition in the POAS cohort (OR 1.27; 95 % CI: 1.00 – 1.60) [51]. In a subsequent longitudinal study of women with no history of depression, significant hormone associations with the onset of depressed mood included levels of follicle-stimulating hormone (FSH), decreased levels of inhibin b, decreased levels of luteinizing hormone (LH), and increased variability of estradiol, FSH and LH around the woman's own mean level of each hormone [19]. Among women who met clinical diagnostic criteria for depressive

disorder, increased levels of FSH and LH, decreased levels of inhibin b, and increased variability of estradiol and FSH were significant associated with the first occurrence of depression in the menopause transition (estradiol variability: OR 2.45; 95 % CI: 1.54 – 3.89). Possibly differences in the frequency and timing of hormone measures contributed to differing results between these studies.

Findings differed in other community-based studies. In the Melbourne study, a 2-year decline in estradiol levels was the strongest risk factor for depressive symptoms, adjusted for baseline depression, age and BMI (OR 3.41; 95 % CI: 1.24 – 9.36) [67]. While the findings suggested a role for declining estradiol in depression, the participants were postmenopausal, aged 56–67 years, and the assessments did not describe hormone associations with depression in the menopause transition. In contrast, the SMWHS found no significant association of urinary measures of estrone, FSH, testosterone and cortisol with depressed mood [33, 59]. A community-based, cross-sectional study of women ages 45–54 years found that 25 % experienced depressed mood (CES-D > =16), but there were no significant associations of depressed mood with estradiol or androgens [68].

The association between depressive symptoms and androgens of both adrenal and ovarian origin has also been studied. Two cross-sectional studies showed an inverse relationship between serum levels of dihydroepiandrosterone sulfate (DHEAS) and depression [69, 70], while longitudinal studies found either no significant association [55] or a positive association between DHEAS levels and depressive symptoms during the menopause transition [71].

The association between testosterone levels and depressive symptoms across the menopause transition is also controversial. In the 10-year SMWHS, there was no association between urinary testosterone levels and depressive symptoms [59]. However, in the early SWAN cohort, where the women were premenopausal or in the early menopause transition, there was a significant inverse association between testosterone and high depressive symptoms [72]. The association reversed in an 8-year follow-up, where testosterone levels were positively associated with depressive symptoms [55]. Further evidence from the Multiethnic Study of Atherosclerosis (MeSA) showed a significant inverse relationship between free testosterone levels and high depressive symptoms among women who were in the first 10 years postmenopause [73].

While these studies suggest possible associations of hormone fluctuations or changes with depression in the menopause transition, there are no definitive conclusions. It can be emphasized again that differences in the frequency and timing of hormone measurements, differences in measures of depressed mood, different comparisons of menopausal stages, and differing approaches and models in data analysis contribute to conflicting results.

### History of depression

A history of depression is one of the strongest predictors of depressive symptoms and depressive disorders in the menopause transition [18, 20, 51, 59, 74], with consistent findings in a number of large cohort studies.

An early report in the Massachusetts Women's Health Study indicated that prior depression was the strongest predictor of subsequent depression (CES-D), with an odds ratio of 9.62 (95 % CI: 6.78– 13.70) [43]. In the Harvard Study of Moods and Cycles, women with a history of depression had a 20 % increased rate of entering the menopause transition sooner than women with no history of depression [74]. In the SWAN mental health study, the risk of MDD was three times greater for women with a history of MDD compared to women with no history of MDD (OR 2.98; 95 % CI: 1.55 – 5.72) [56]. In a follow-up of this study, twice as many women with a history of major depression (MDD) developed MDD compared to women with no history of MDD (59 and 28 %, respectively) [20]. Women with a history of depression in the POAS cohort had a 13 times greater risk of depressive symptoms in the menopause transition compared to women with no history of depression (OR 13.62; 95 % CI: 7.20 – 25.80, $P < 0.001$) [51]. In a longitudinal study of the pattern of depressive symptoms around menopause, approximately 50 to 65 % of women with a history of depression had high CES-D scores in the years before the FMP compared to 10 to 30 % of women with no history of depression [18]. In another large community-based, prospective study, women with prior depression were two times more likely to report increased depressive symptoms in the transition from pre- to perimenopause (OR 1.98; 95 % CI: 1.47 – 2.67) [75].

### Depression and vasomotor symptoms

Vasomotor symptoms (hot flashes and/or night sweats) are the most frequently reported menopausal symptoms across all races/ethnicities [76]. Many studies confirm their prevalence, which peaks around menopause, when more than 70 % of women report experiencing this symptom [32, 77]. In spite of their common occurrence, the etiology remains poorly understood, with diverse hypotheses and many associations with other behavioral, psychological and physical factors. A leading hypothesis is that hot flashes are triggered centrally by noradrenergic activation in association with changes in estrogen, which is known to influence thermoregulatory functioning [78]. While it is known that vasomotor symptoms are associated with changes in estradiol and other reproductive hormones, including follicle-stimulating

hormone (FSH) and inhibin b, the associations are complex and do not clearly explain their occurrence [79, 80].

Although vasomotor symptoms (VMS) are highly correlated with depressive symptoms, evidence for the causal direction is conflicting. There are many differences in study designs, sample sizes and assessments of both VMS and depression, as delineated in an extensive review of the directional associations between VMS and depressive symptoms or major depressive disorder (MDD) [81]. The review included 17 cross-sectional studies that examined associations between VMS and depressive *symptoms* and 7 studies that examined the association between VMS and major depressive disorder (MDD); another 10 studies assessed the risk of women with VMS developing depressive symptoms, and 2 studies examined the reverse direction, i.e., the risk of women with high depressive symptoms developing VMS.

A statistically significant, positive association between VMS and depressive symptoms was identified in 9 of 17 cross-sectional studies, with odds ratios ranging from 1.27 (95 % CI: 1.08 – 1.51) to 8.1 (95 % CI: 2.5 – 26.4) [82, 83]. The researchers concluded that the evidence consistently supported *a positive association between VMS and depressive symptoms*, but the direction of association remained unclear. Of the 7 studies that examined the association between VMS and major depression, only 2 studies reported a significant association [63, 81], while 5 studies found no statistically significant association. However, the researchers determined that most of the 7 studies had moderate to high risk of bias due to small samples, convenience sampling and missing information, which strongly limited conclusions about the association between VMS and major depression.

Ten studies evaluated the risk of women with VMS developing depressive symptoms, and 8 of these indicated that VMS increased the risk of developing depressive symptoms, with odds ratios ranging from 1.62 (95 % CI: 1.43 – 1.84) to 8.88 (95 % CI: 2.57 – 30.68) [55, 84]. These studies were determined to be methodologically sound with adjustments for numerous covariates and low risk of bias, consequently providing consistent evidence for VMS increasing the risk of depressive symptoms. Further evidence was reported in a SWAN study, which investigated a very narrow time interval to show that VMS predicted next-day negative mood (OR 1.27; 95 % CI: 1.03 – 1.58); however, negative mood did not predict next-day VMS [85].

Two studies evaluated the risk of women with high depressive symptoms developing VMS, and both reported a positive association to suggest that depressive symptoms were more likely to precede hot flashes in women with no previous experience of either symptom [86, 79]. Women with consistently high depressive symptoms in the SMWHS were more likely to experience subsequent VMS [86]. Of women who had no high depressive symptoms or hot flashes at baseline in the POAS, 24 % reported depressive symptoms (high CES-D scores) before reporting hot flashes in a 10-year follow-up [79]. In contrast, only 8 % of the women reported hot flashes before reporting depressed mood.

Aims of this review did not include intervention studies, although they are clearly important for evaluating changes in hormone levels and associations of these changes with depressed mood and VMS. For example, estradiol administered to women with a diagnosis of depressive disorder in the menopause transition showed that estradiol improved depression independent of the presence of hot flashes [87]. In another study, estradiol was administered to women who had depressive disorders, hot flashes and disturbed sleep in the menopause transition. Results indicated that increased estradiol levels and improved sleep quality predicted improvement in depressed mood, while reduction of hot flashes did not improve depressed mood [88]. This evidence suggested that in spite of high correlations between depressive symptoms and VMS, these variables may have distinct pathways, and hot flashes alone are not a likely cause of depression around menopause.

These findings overall indicate that depressive symptoms and vasomotor symptoms frequently co-occur around the menopause transition. Endocrine events are a shared component of these symptoms but are not the only factor in their development. Numerous studies suggest that women with VMS have an increased risk of developing depressive symptoms, but the reverse direction is also observed. Data further indicate that menopausal depression can occur in the absence of VMS and that the cause of depression is not likely due to VMS alone. The studies suggest that VMS and depressive symptoms may have different underlying pathways and/or are modulated by different exogenous or endogenous factors. Further studies that are designed to unravel components of these complex associations are needed.

**Depression and poor sleep**
Sleep difficulties are a common problem in the menopause transition. About 30 % of adults have one or more symptoms of insomnia, according to the American Academy of Sleep Medicine [89], and these symptoms are more prevalent in women, particularly in mid-life [90–93]. While a high prevalence of poor sleep quality in mid-life women is well-documented, several well-designed studies concluded that influences of both age and menopausal status on poor sleep were modest [92, 93]. In addition, while there is considerable evidence that sleep difficulties are correlated with depressive symptoms, poor sleep is a core symptom of

clinical depression [94, 95], which frequently makes it difficult to determine whether sleep difficulties are a component of or independent of depressed mood or clinical depression.

The causal direction of poor sleep and depressed mood is particularly difficult to disentangle, in part due to the chronic nature of sleep problems, the episodic nature of depression and the many definitions of both disorders. The long-held domino hypothesis, i.e., that the association between sleep problems and depressed mood was driven by vasomotor symptoms has only partial support. For example, sleep problems predicted next-day negative mood, but an association with vasomotor symptoms was found only in women who had depression at the study baseline [96]. In an intervention study of women who had depressive disorders, increasing levels of estradiol and improved sleep quality predicted improvement in depressed mood in perimenopausal women, but improved hot flashes did not improve depressed mood [88]. The researchers concluded that changes in estradiol and sleep quality, rather than hot flashes, may mediate depression during the menopause transition.

A recent study of the association of poor sleep, mood and reproductive status found a significant association between depressive symptoms and sleep impairment in peri- and postmenopausal women but no consistent association in younger premenopausal women [97].

Reports from the SWAN cohort indicated that 31 % of the participants reported at least one of three evaluated sleep difficulties and identified significant associations between sleep difficulties and progression through the menopause transition [98].

In contrast, other studies found no significant association between depressed mood and poor sleep in perimenopausal women in adjusted analysis [99, 100]. In the study of Cheng et al. [100], anxiety was related to all assessed sleep problems but may have obscured an association with depressed mood due to high correlation of these variables. In an evaluation of poor sleep in relation to the final menstrual period, *premenopausal* sleep status was the strongest predictor of poor sleep in the menopause transition, and there was no further increase in poor sleep around the final menstrual period [101]. Again, methodological differences may contribute to conflicting findings, as for example, in the latter study, where most participants were not clinically depressed and poor sleep was reported at a premenopausal baseline. Measures of depression and anxiety were highly correlated, and anxiety rather than depression had the stronger association with poor sleep in these studies.

In summary, the findings show a high prevalence of sleep difficulties in mid-life women, but associations between increased risk of poor sleep in relation to menopause are complex with conflicting reports at this time. Depressive symptoms and sleep difficulties are common, the symptoms are correlated and both may increase around menopause. The causal directions and associations between these variables and the hormonal changes of ovarian aging as well as other psychosocial factors remain unclear.

### Other factors associated with menopausal depression

Numerous studies have identified significant associations of health, psychosocial and demographic variables with depressed mood around menopause, but evidence for the extent to which these factors are confounding or independently associated with depressed mood or clinical depression in perimenopausal women is inconsistent or lacking. Associations with depressive symptoms around menopause have been reported for health problems [54, 102], anxiety [57, 103], poor sleep and vasomotor symptoms [49, 79, 104–106], behavioral factors such as smoking and obesity [51, 54, 107], stress and negative life events [49, 53, 54, 57, 63, 107, 108], physical activity [109, 110], marital and relationship issues [59, 102], financial problems [54, 59], and demographic variables including race/ethnicity and education [19, 51, 54, 58]. Overall, the data support the possibility that depressed mood in the menopause transition is multifactorial and not simply due to menopausal status alone. It is possible that psychosocial and lifestyle factors, together with health experience, have more effect on depressed mood than endocrine changes. Although endocrine changes may be a trigger, the causal pathways remain unclear [31, 102].

Another important question that remains open is whether a first-onset depression in the menopause transition is etiologically or qualitatively different from recurrent depression. Several studies evaluated risk factors for a first-onset depression in the menopause transition for women with no history of depression. The risk of a first depression was significantly greater for women who reported vasomotor symptoms and for women who had a history of adverse life events in the Harvard Study of Moods and Cycles [36]. Vasomotor symptoms, high BMI and smoking were independent contributors to first onset of depressive symptoms in the POAS study [19]. Vasomotor symptoms at a trend level, prior health conditions and negative perceptions of functioning were risk factors for first onset of major depression in midlife women in the SWAN mental health study [20]. Steinberg et al. compared women with first-onset versus recurrent clinical depression and found that depressive symptom scores and measures of FSH did not differ between the two groups [111]. In the SWAN mental health study, the only risk factor uniquely associated with onset of major depression among women with no

history of major depression was vasomotor symptoms (OR 2.09; 95 % CI: 1.26 – 3.47) [20].

Again, methodological differences may contribute to disparate findings. Different risk factors were evaluated and comparisons of menopausal status were not consistent across the studies. Furthermore, the risk factors identified for first-onset depression were also identified in studies that included women with recurrent depression, thus limiting conclusions. At present, there is no definitive evidence of distinct risks of a first-onset depression versus recurrent depression around menopause.

### Limitations and future directions

The majority of studies of depressed mood in the menopause transition reviewed here evaluated depressive symptoms, which are important for screening depression in the population and in clinical settings. Depressive symptoms are highly correlated with clinical diagnosis of depression but are not equivalent. Some studies evaluated samples with a diagnosis of depression, but reports of association between clinical depression and menopausal status are conflicting, and further studies are needed to determine whether the risk of diagnosed depression is increased around menopause. Studies of depression cross many domains, and this review did not include intervention or neuroendocrine studies, or in-depth consideration of the many of the identified psychosocial, behavioral and physical health factors that are important for understanding depression in midlife women. Other reviews are needed to address these areas. The reviewed studies were from different cohorts and population samples, and conclusions should be considered cautiously, particularly in comparing studies that differ in racial and social economic distributions, as recently demonstrated by Harlow et al. [64].

The greatest challenges for further research are to identify endocrine and genetic elements that may underlie depression and disentangle psychosocial factors that are associated with this disorder. Epidemiologic and clinical questions for further study include identifying the pattern and associated risk factors of depression following the final menstrual period; increasing information about associations between reproductive hormone changes and mood; further clarifying effects of hormone treatments on mood in perimenopausal women; determining confounding factors and causal directions of vasomotor symptoms and sleep difficulties in relation to depression and the extent to which these variables are associated with hormonal changes of menopause; disentangling depression and its associations with other major health problems of mid-life women such as cardiovascular disease, metabolic syndrome and osteoporosis. Longitudinal studies that clearly define menopausal stages, hormone measurements that are adequate for the questions and repeated measures of standard mood and behavioral assessments are important for increased understanding of women's health in relation to menopause.

## Conclusions

While the changing hormonal milieu is experienced by all women around menopause, only a minority experience debilitating depressive symptoms in this transition period. Accumulating evidence indicates that depressive symptoms, and possibly clinical depression, increase in the menopause transition compared to premenopause. There is also evidence that the changing endocrine milieu is associated with increased depressive symptoms, but hormones are clearly not the only factor. Further studies are needed to understand the development of depression in women around menopause.

### Abbreviations

CES-D: Center for Epidemiologic Studies - Depression; DSM-IV: Diagnostic and Statistical Manual - IV; FMP: Final menstrual period; BMI: Body mass index; HADS: Hospital Anxiety and Depression Scale; HPA: Hypothalamic-pituitary-adrenal; OR: Odds ratio; CI: Confidence interval; RR: Relative risk; FSH: Follicle stimulating hormone; LH: Luteinizing hormone; MDD: Major depressive disorder; NIH: National Institutes of Health; STRAW: Stages of Reproductive Aging Workshop; SWAN: Study of Women's Health Across the Nation; POAS: Penn Ovarian Aging Study; SMWHS: Seattle Midlife Women's Health Study.

### Competing interests

The author has no competing interests for this review.

### References

1. Lopez AD, Murray CC. The global burden of disease, 1990–2020. Nat Med. 1998;4:1241–3.
2. Bromberger JT, di Scalea TL. Longitudinal associations between depression and functioning in midlife women. Maturitas. 2009;64:145–59. Epub 2009 Oct 23.
3. Pinkerton JV, Guico-Pabia CJ, Taylor HS. Menstrual cycle-related exacerbation of disease. Am J Obstet Gynecol. 2010;202(3):221–31.
4. Perez-Lopez FR, Chedraui P, Gilbert JJ, Perez-Roncero G. Cardiovascular risk in menopausal women and prevalent related co-morbid conditions. Facing the post-Women's Health Initiative era. Fertil Steril. 2009;92:1171–86. Epub 2009 Aug 22.
5. Whipple MO, Lewis TT, Sutton-Tyrrell K, Matthews KA, Barinas-Mitchell E, Powell LH, et al. Hopelessness, depressive symptoms and carotid atherosclerosis in women: the Study of Women's Health Across the Nation (SWAN) heart study. Stroke. 2009;40:3166–72. Epub 2009 Aug 27.
6. Llaneza P, Garcia-Portilla MP, Llaneza-Suarez D, Armott B, Perez-Lopez FR. Depressive disorders and the menopause transition. Maturitas. 2012;71:120–30.
7. Goldbacher EM, Bromberger J, Matthews KA. Lifetime history of major depression predicts the development of the metabolic syndrome in middle-aged women. Psychosom Med. 2009;71:266–72.
8. Heiskanen TH, Niskanen LK, Hintikka JJ, Koivumaa-Honkanen HT, Haatainen KM. Metabolic syndrome and depression: a cross-sectional analysis. J Clin Psychiatry. 2006;67(9):1422–7.
9. Richter N, Juckel G, Assion HJ. Metabolic syndrome: a follow-up study of acute depressive inpatients. Eur Arch Psychiatry Clin Neurosci. 2010;260(1):41–9. Epub 2009 Apr 28.
10. Cizza G, Primma S, Csako G. Depression as a risk factor for osteoporosis. Trends Endocrinol Metab. 2009;20(8):367–73. Epub 2009 Sep 9.
11. Yirmiya R, Bab I. Major depression is a risk factor for low bone mineral density: a meta-analysis. Biol Psychiatry. 2009;66(5):423–32. Epub 2009 May 15.
12. Kessler RC, McGonagle KA, Zhao S, Nelson CB, Hughes M, Eshleman S, et al. Lifetime and 12-month prevalence of DSM-III-R psychiatric disorders in the United States. Results from the National Comorbidity Survey. Arch Gen Psychiatry. 1994;51(1):8–19.
13. Rubinow DR, Schmidt PJ, Roca CA. Estrogen-serotonin interactions: implications for affective regulation. Biol Psychiatry. 1998;44(9):839–50.
14. Schmidt PJ, Rubinow DR. Sex hormones and mood in the perimenopause. Ann N Y Acad Sci. 2009;1179:70–85.
15. National Institutes of Health. National Institutes of Health State-of-the-Science. Conference statement: management of menopausal-related symptoms. Ann Intern Med. 2005;142:1003–13.
16. Vesco KK, Haney EM, Humphrey L, Fu R, Nelson HD. Influence of menopause on mood: a systematic review of cohort studies. Climacteric. 2007;10(6):448–65.
17. Freeman EW. Associations of depression with the transition to menopause. Menopause. 2010;17(4):823–7.
18. Freeman EW, Sammel MD, Boorman DW, Zhang R. Longitudinal pattern of depressive symptoms around natural menopause. JAMA Psychiatry. 2014;71(1):36–43. Epub: 2013 Nov 13.
19. Freeman EW, Sammel MD, Lin H, Nelson DB. Associations of hormones and menopausal status with depressed mood in women with no history of depression. Arch Gen Psychiatry. 2006;63:375–82.
20. Bromberger JT, Schott L, Kravitz HM, Joffe H. Risk factors for major depression during midlife among a community sample of women with and without prior major depression: are they the same or different? Psychol Med. Epub 2014 Nov 24.
21. Gordon JL, Girdler SS, Meltzer-Brody SE, Stika CS, Thurston RC, Clark CT, et al. Ovarian hormone fluctuation, neurosteroids, and HPA axis dysregulation in perimenopausal depression: a novel heuristic model. Am J Psychiatry. Epub 2015 Jan 13.
22. Hale GE, Robertson DM, Burger HG. The perimenopausal women: endocrinology and management. J Steroid Biochem Mol Biol. 2014;142:121–31. Epub 2013 Oct 14.
23. Wharton W, Gleason CE, Olson SRMS, Carlsson CM, Asthana S. Neurobiological underpinnings of the estrogen-mood relationship. Curr Psychiatry Rev. 2012;8(3):247–56.
24. Deecher D, Andree TH, Sloan D, Schechter LE. From menarche to menopause: exploring the underlying biology of depression ion women experiencing hormonal changes. Psychoneuroendocrinology. 2008;33:3–17. Epub 2007 Dec 3.
25. Burger H. The menopausal transition - endocrinology. J Sex Med. 2008;5(10):2266–73. Epub 2008 Jul 1.
26. Gyllstrom ME. Perimenopause and depression: strength of association, causal mechanisms and treatment recommendations. Best Pract Res Clin Obstet Gynecol. 2007;21(2):275–92.
27. Gordon JL, Girdler SS. Hormone replacement therapy in the treatment of perimenopausal depression. Curr Psychiatry Rep. 2014;16(12):517.
28. Green SM, Key BL, McCabe RE. Cognitive-behavioral, behavioral, and mindfulness-based therapies for menopausal depression: a review. Maturitas. 2015;80(1):37–47. Epub 2014 Oct 18.
29. Weber MT, Maki PM, McDermott MP. Cognition and mood in perimenopause: a systematic review and meta-analysis. J Steroid Biochem Mol Biol. 2014;142:90–8. Epub 2013 Jun 14.
30. McKinlay SM, Jefferys M. The menopausal syndrome. Br J Prev Soc Med. 1974;28:108–15.
31. Gracia CR, Freeman EW. Acute consequences of the menopausal transition: the rise of common menopausal symptoms. Endocrinol Metab Clin N Am. 2004;33:675–89.
32. Freeman EW, Sammel MD, Lin H, Gracia CR, Pien GW, Nelson DB. Symptoms associated in menopause transition and reproductive hormones in mid-life women. Obstet Gynecol. 2007;110:230–40.
33. Woods NF, Smith-Dijulio K, Percival DB, Tao EY, Taylor HJ, Mitchell ES. Symptoms during the menopausal transition and early postmenopause and their relation to endocrine levels over time: observations from the Seattle Midlife Women's Health Study. J Women's Health. 2007;16(5):667–77.
34. Treloar AE. Menstrual cyclicity and the pre-menopause. Maturitas. 1981;3:249–64.

35. McKinlay SM, Brambilla DJ, Posner JG. The normal menopause transition. Maturitas. 2008;61(1–2):4–16.

36. Cohen LS, Soares CN, Vitonis AF, Otto MW, Harlow BL. Risk for new onset of depression during the menopausal transition. Arch Gen Psychiatry. 2006;63:385–90.

37. Freeman EW, Sammel MD, Lin H, Gracia CR. Obesity and reproductive hormone levels in the transition to menopause. Menopause. 2010;17(4):718–26.

38. Al-Safi ZA, Polotsky AJ. Obesity and menopause. Best Pract Res Clin Obstet Gynecol. Epub 23 Dec 2014.

39. Midgette AS, Baron JA. Cigarette smoking and the risk of natural menopause. Epidemiology. 1990;1(6):474–80.

40. Harlow SD, Gass M, Hall JE, ,Lobo R, Maki P, Rebar RW et al. STRAW 10 Collaborative Group. Executive summary of the Stages of Reproductive Aging Workshop +10: addressing the unfinished agenda of staging reproductive aging. Menopause. 2012;19(4):387–95.

41. Blazer DG, Kessler RC, McGonagle KA, Swartz MS. The prevalence and distribution of major depression in a national community sample: the national comorbidity survey. Am J Psychiatry. 1994;151:979–86.

42. Nierenberg AA. Long-term management of chronic depression. J Clin Psychiatry. 2001;62(Supple 6):17–21.

43. Avis NE, Brambilla D, McKinlay SM, Vass K. A longitudinal analysis of the association between menopause and depression. Ann Epidemiol. 1994;4:214–20.

44. Kaufert PA, Gilbert P, Tate R. The Manitoba Project: a re-examination of the link betwen menopause and depression. Maturitas. 1992;14:157–60.

45. Matthews KA, Wing RR, Kuller LJ, Meilahn EN, Kelsey SF. Influences of natural menopause on psychological characteristics and symptoms of middle-aged healthy women. J Consult Clin Psychol. 1990;48:345–51.

46. Nicol-Smith L. Causality, menopause and depression: a critical review of the literature. BMI. 1996;313:1229–32.

47. Bosworth HB, Bastian LA, Kuchibhatla MN, ,Steffens DC, McBride CM, Skinner CS, et al. Depressive symptoms, menopausal status, and climacteric symptoms in women at midlife. Psychosom Med. 2001;63:603–8.

48. Bromberger JT, Assmann SF, Avis NE, Schocken M, Kravitz HM, Cordal A. Persistent mood symptoms in a multiethnic community cohort of pre- and perimenopausal women. Am J Epidemiol. 2003;158(4):347–56.

49. Dennerstein L, Dudley EC, Hopper JL, Guthrie JR, Burger HG. A prospective population-based study of menopausal symptoms. Obstet Gynecol. 2000;96:351–8.

50. Soares CN, Almeida OP. Depression during the perimenopause. Arch Gen Psychiatry. 2001;58:306.

51. Freeman EW, Sammel MD, Liu L, Gracia CR, Nelson DB, Hollander L. Hormones and menopausal status as predictors of depression in women in transition to menopause. Arch Gen Psychiatry. 2004;61:62–70.

52. Bromberger JT, Meyer PM, Kravitz HM, ,Sommer B, Cordal A, Powell L et al. Psychologic distress and natural menopause: a multiethnic community study. Am J Public Health. 2001;91:1435–42.

53. Bromberger JT, Harlow S, Avis N, Kravitz HM, Cordal A. Racial/ethnic differences in the prevalence of depressive symptoms among middle-aged women: the Study of women's Health Across the Nation (SWAN). Am J Pub Health. 2004;94:1378–85.

54. Bromberger JT, Matthews KA, Schott LL, Brockwell S, Avis NE, Kravitz HM, et al. Depressive symptoms during the menopausal transition: the Study of Women's Health Across the Nation (SWAN). J Affect Disord. 2007;103:267–72.

55. Bromberger JT, Schott LL, Kravitz HM, Sowers M, Avis NE, Gold EB, et al. Longitudinal change in reproductive hormones and depressive symptoms across the menopausal transition: results from the Study of Women's Health Across the Nation (SWAN). Arch Gen Psychiatry. 2010;67:598–607.

56. Bromberger JT, Kravitz HM, Chang YF, Cyranowski JM, Brown C, Matthews KA et al. Major depression during and after the menopausal transition: Study of women's Health Across the Nation (SWAN). Psychol Med. 2011;9:1–10.

57. Bromberger JT, Kravitz HM, Matthews K, Youk A, Brown C, Feng W, et al. Predictors of first lifetime episodes of major depression in midlife women. Psychol Med. 2009;39:55–64.

58. Brown C, Bromberger JR, Schott LL, Crawford S, Matthews KA. Persistence of depression in African American and Caucasian women at midlife: findings from the Study of Women Across the Nation (SWAN). Arch Womens Ment Health. 2014;17:549–57. Epub: 2014 Jul 5.

59. Woods NF, Smith-DiJulio K, Percival DB, Tao EY, Mariella A, Mitchell S. Depressed mood during the menopausal transition and early postmenopause:

observations from the Seattle Midlife Women's Health Study. Menopause. 2008;15:223–32.

60. Dennerstein L, Guthrie JR, Clark M, Lehert P, Henderson VW. A population-based study of depressed mood in middle-aged, Australian-born women. Menopause. 2004;11:563–8.

61. Bjelland I, Dahl AA, Huag TT, Neckelmann D. The validity of the Hospital Anxiety and Depression Scale. An updated literature review. J Psychosom Res. 2002;52(2):69–77.

62. Tangen T, Mykletun A. Depression and anxiety through the climacteric period: an epidemiologic study (HUNT-II). J Psychosom Obstet Gynecol. 2008;29(2):125–31.

63. Schmidt PJ, Haq N, Rubinow DR. A longitudinal evaluation of the relationship between reproductive status and mood in perimenopausal women. Am J Psychiatry. 2004;161(12):2238–44.

64. Harlow BL, MacLehose RF, Smolenski DJ, Soares CN, Otto MW, Joffe H, et al. Disparate rates of new-onset depression during the menopausal transition in 2 community-based populations: real or really wrong? Am J Epidemiol. 2013;177(10):1148–56. Epub: 2013 Apr 14.

65. Judd FK, Hickey M, Bryant C. Depression and midlife: are we overpathologizing the menopause? J Affect Disord. 2012;136:199–211. Epub 2011 Jan 26.

66. Schiller CE, Schmidt PJ, Rubinow DR. Allopregnanolone as a mediator of affective switching in reproductive mood disorders. Psychopharmacology. 2014;231(17):3557–67.

67. Ryan J, Burger HG, Szoeke C, Lehert P, Ancelin ML, Henderson WW, et al. A prospective study of the association between endogenous hormones and depressive symptoms in postmenopausal women. Menopause. 2009;16:509–17.

68. Gallicchio L, Schilling C, Miller SR, Zacur H, Flaws JA. Correlations of depressive symptoms among women undergoing the menopausal transition. J Psychosom Res. 2007;63:263–8.

69. Schmidt PJ, Murphy JH, Haq N, Danaceau MA, St CL. Basal plasma hormone levels in depresssed perimenopause women. Psychoneuroendocrinology. 2002;27:907–20.

70. Morsink LF, Vogelzangs N, Nicklas BJ, Beekman AT, Satterfield S, Rubin SM, et al. Associations between sex steroid hormone levels and depressive symptoms in elderly men and women: results from the Health ABC study. Psychoneuroendocrinology. 2007;32:874–83.

71. Morrison MF, Freeman EW, Lin H, Sammel MD. Higher DHEAS (dehydroepiandrostrone sulfate) levels are assoiated with depressive symptoms during the menoapusal transition: results from the Penn Ovarian Aging Study. Arch Women's Ment Health. 2011;14:375–82.

72. Santoro N, Torrens J, Crawford S, Allsworth JE, Finkelstain JS, Gold EB, et al. Correlates of circulating androgens in mid-life women: the study of women's health across the nation. J Clin Endocrinol Metab. 2005;90:4836–45.

73. Colangelo LA, Craft LL, Ouyand P, Liu K, Schreiner PJ, Michos ED, et al. Association of sex hormones and sex hormone-binding globulin with depressive symptoms in postmenopausal women: the Multiethnic Study of Athrosclerosis. Menopause. 2012;19:877–85.

74. Harlow BL, Wise LA, Otto MW, Soares CN, Cohen LS. Depression and its influence on reproductive endocrine and menstrual cycle markers associated with perimenopause. Arch Gen Psychiatry. 2003;60:29–36.

75. Maartens LW, Knottnerus JA, Pop VJ. Menopausal transition and increased depressive symptomatology: a community based prospective study. Maturitas. 2002;42:195–200.

76. Williams RE, Kalilani L, DeBenedetti DB, Zhou X, Fehnel SE, Clark RV. Healthcare seeking and treatment for menopausal symptoms in the United States. Maturitas. 2007;58(4):348–58. Epub: 2007 Oct 25.

77. Whiteman MK, Staropoli CA, Benedict JC, Borgeest C, Flaws JA. Risk factors for hot flashes in midlife women. J Womens Health. 2003;12:459–72.

78. Freedman RR. Pathophysiology and treatment of menopausal hot flashes. Semin Reprod Med. 2005;23:117–25.

79. Freeman EW, Sammel MD, Lin H. Temporal associations of hot flashes and depression in the transition to menopause. Menopause. 2009;16(4):728–34.

80. Randolph JF Jr, Sowers M, Bondarenko I, Gold EB. Greendale GA, Bromberger JT, et al. The relationship of longitudinal chantge in reproductive hormones and vasomotor symptoms during the menopausal transition. J Clin Endocrinol Metab. 2005;90:6106–12.

81. Worsley R, Bell R, Kulkarni J, David SE. The association between vasomotor symptoms and depression during perimenopause: a systematic review. Maturitas. 2014;77:111–7.

Depression in the menopause transition: risks in the changing hormone milieu as observed in the general...					11

82. Thurston RC, Bromberger JT, Joffe H, Avis NE, Hess R, Crandall CJ, et al. Beyond frequency: who is most bothered by vasomotor symptoms? Menopause. 2008;15(5):841–7.

83. Blumel JE, Castelo-Branco C, Cancelo MJ, Cordova AT, Binfa LE, Bonilla HG, et al. Relationship between psychological complaints and vasomotor symptoms during climacteric. Maturitas. 2004;49(3):205–10.

84. Brown JP, Gallicchio L, Flaws JA, Tracy J. Relations among menopausal symptoms, sleep disturbance and depressive symptoms in midlife. Maturitas. 2009;62:184–9.

85. Gibson CJ, Thurston RC, Bromberger JT, Kamarck T, Matthews KA. Negative affect and vasomotor symptoms in the Study of Women's Health Across the Nation daily hormone study. Menopause. 2011;18(12):1270–7.

86. Woods NF, Mitchell ES. Patterns of depressed mood in midlife women; observations from the Seattle Midlife Women's Health Study. Res Nurs Health. 1996;19(2):111–23.

87. Schmidt PJ, Nieman L, Danaceau MA, Tobin MB, Roca CA, Murphy JH, et al. Estrogen replacement in perimenopause-related depression: a preliminary report. Am J Obstet Gynecol. 2000;183(2):414–20.

88. Joffe H, Petrillo LF, Koukopoulos A, Viguera AC, Hirschberg A, Nonacs R, et al. Increased estradiol and improved sleep, but not hot flashes, predict enhanced mood during the menopausal transition. J Clin Endocrinol Metab. 2011;96(7):E1044–54. Epub: 2011 Apr 27.

89. American Academy of Sleep Medicine. Insomnia. 2008. Available at: http://www.aasmnet.org. Accessed April 14, 2014.

90. Johnson EO, Roth T, Schultz L, Breslau N. Epidemiology of DSM-IV insomnia in adolescent: lifetime prevalence, chronicity, and an emergent gender difference. Pediatrics. 2006;117:e247–56.

91. Kravitz HM, Ganz PA, Bromberger J, Powell LH, Sutton-Tyrrell K, Meyer PM. Sleep difficulty in women at midlife: a community survey of sleep and the menopausal transition. Menopause. 2003;10:19–28.

92. Blumel JE, Cano A, Mezones-Holguin E, Baron G, Bencosme A, Benitez Z, et al. A multinational study of sleep disorders during female mid-life. Maturitas. 2012;72:359–66.

93. Tom SE, Kuh D, Guralnik JM, Mishra GD. Self-reported sleep difficulty during the menopause transition: results from a prospective cohort study. Menopause. 2010;17:1128–35.

94. Nutt D, Wilson S, Paterson L. Sleep disorders as core symptoms of depression. Dialogues Clin Neurosci. 2008;10:329–36.

95. Riemann D. Insomnia and comorbid psychiatric disorders. Sleep Med. 2007;8:S15–20.

96. Burleson MH, Todd M, Trevathan WR. Daily vasomotor symptoms, sleep problems and mood: using daily data to evaluate the domino hypothesis in middle-aged women. Menopause. 2010;17(1):87–95.

97. Toffol E, Kalleinen N, Urrila AS, Himanen SL, Porkka-Heiskanen T, Partonen T, et al. The relationship between mood and sleep in different female reproductive states. BMC Psychiatry. 2014;14:177.

98. Kravitz HM, Zhao X, Bromberger JT, Gold EB, Hall MH, Matthews KA, et al. Sleep disturbance during the menopausal transition in a multi-ethnic community sample of women. Sleep. 2008;31(7):979–89.

99. Freedman RR, Roehrs TA. Sleep disturbance in menopause. Menopause. 2007;14:1–4.

100. Cheng MH, Hsu CY, Wang SJ, Lee SJ, Wang PH, Fuh JL. The relationship of self-reported sleep disturbance, mood and menopause in a community study. Menopause. 2008;15:958–62.

101. Freeman EW, Sammel MD, Gross SA, Pien GW. Poor sleep in relation to natural menopause: a population-based 14-year follow-up of midlife women. Menopause. 2015; 22(7). Epub: 2014 Dec 29.

102. Dennerstein L, Lehert P, Burger H, Dudley E. Mood and the menopausal transition. J Nerv Ment Dis. 1999;187(11):685–91.

103. Kravitz HM, Schott LL, Joffe H, Cyranowski JM, Bromberger JT. Do anxiety symptoms predict major depressive disorder in midlife women? The Study of Women's Health Across the Nation (SWAN) Mental Health Study (MHS). Psychol Med. 2014;44(12):2593–602. Epub: 2014 Jan 27.

104. Joffe H, Soares CN, Thurston RC, White DP, Cohen LS, Hall JE. Depression is associated with worse objectively and subjectively measured sleep, but not more frequent awakenings, in women with vasomotor symptoms. Menopause. 2009;16:671–9.

105. Joffe H, Hall JE, Soares CN, Hennen J, Reilly CJ, Carlson K, et al. Vasomotor symptoms are associated with depression in perimenopausal women seeking primary care. Menopause. 2002;9:392–8.

106. Harlow BL, Cohen L, Otto MW, Spiegelman D, Cramer DW. Prevalence and predictors of depressive symptoms in older premenopausal women. Arch Gen Psychiatry. 1999;56:418–24.

107. Woods NF, Mitchell ES, Percival DB, Smith-DiJulio K. Is the menopausal transition stressful? Observations of perceived stress from the Seattle Midlife Women's Health Study. Menopause. 2009;16:90–7.

108. Schmidt PJ, Murphy JH, Haq N, Rubinow DR, Danaceau MA. Stressful life events, personal losses, and perimenopausal-related depression. Arch Womens Ment Health. 2003;7(1):19–26. Epub 2003 Dec 15.

109. Sternfeld B, Guthrie KA, Ensrud KE. et. Efficacy of exercise for menopausal symptoms: a randomized controlled trial. Menopause. 2014;21(4):330–8.

110. Wang HL, Booth-LaForce C, Tang SM, Wu WR, Chen CH. Depressive symptoms in Taiwanese women during the peri- and postmenopause years: associations with demographic, health, and psychosocial characteristics. Maturitas. 2013;75(4):355–60. Epub 2013 May 29.

111. Steinberg EM, Rubinow DR, Bartko JJ, Fortinsky PM, Haq N, Thompson K, et al. A cross-sectional evaluation of perimenopausal depression. J Clin Psychiatry. 2008;69(6):973–90.

# 2

# The importance of disability as a health issue for mid-life women

Carrie A. Karvonen-Gutierrez

## Abstract

Data suggest that disability prevalence among mid-aged populations is increasing in recent years; current prevalence estimates for mid-aged adults range from 20 to 40 %. The World Health Organization's International Classification of Functioning (ICF) has provided a multi-dimensional biopsychosocial model to understand disability that is highly relevant to mid-aged populations. Under the ICF framework, mid-aged women experience high levels of work, non-work, and mobility-associated disability but very little difficulty with self care. Despite the high prevalence, evidence suggests that there is a large proportion of non-chronic disability and that mid-aged women can both worsen and improve their functioning. Thus, the mid-life period may represent a critical window during which interventions to improve disability may be most efficacious for the improvement of current and future functioning. Interventions that are initiated during the mid-life are highly relevant as a strategy to reduce disability during this life stage and prevent or forestall the onset of late life disability. Targets for intervention include improvement of depressive symptoms and increasing physical activity levels, both of which have shown to be efficacious in older populations and are correlates of mid-life functioning and disability.

**Keywords:** Women, Mid-life, Middle age, Physical functioning, Functional limitations, Disability

## Introduction

Our world is in the midst of an epidemiologic transition whereby the burden of non-communicable diseases has now surpassed communicable diseases and injury as the leading cause of death and illness worldwide [1]. Globally, the rise in prevalence of obesity and adverse health behaviors including smoking, poor diet, and physical inactivity in concert with the overall rise in life expectancy has led to the exponential increase in chronic disease prevalence and multi-morbidity. Individuals are being diagnosed with chronic conditions earlier and have a greater number and more severe chronic conditions than ever before [2, 3]. In the United States, the average number of chronic conditions among midlife adults is increasing; the number of midlife adults with three or more chronic conditions increased by 9.7 % between 1996 and 2005 [4]. Thus, the burden of chronic disease and its effects on functioning and health is the major public health challenge of the 21st century.

Correspondence: ckarvone@umich.edu
Department of Epidemiology, University of Michigan School of Public Health, 1415 Washington Heights, Room 6618, Ann Arbor, MI 48109, USA

The increase in chronic disease prevalence and severity is concerning because chronic diseases are the leading cause of disability in the United States [5] and globally [6], so it is expected that there will be a concomitant rise in disability. Current estimates from the World Health Survey and the Global Burden of Disease indicate that more than 1 billion people in the world (based upon 2010 world population estimates) live with some form of disability [7]. While different methodologies in the World Health Study and the Global Burden of Disease suggest slightly different prevalence estimates for adult disability, 15.6 and 19.4 %, respectively [7], both suggest that the global burden of disability is substantial. Similarly, in the United States, based upon data from the Survey of Income and Program Participation (SIPP), 18.7 % of non-institutionalized persons are living with a disability [8]. This number is expected to rise given the aging of the population [9, 10] and the high burden of chronic conditions including ischemic heart disease, stroke and HIV/AIDS [11].

Globally, women represent a rapidly growing proportion of the aging population given the projected increase in the life expectancy gender gap (reaching a gap of

4.4 years by 2050) in less developed countries [12]. The focus on contextual factors and their relevance for disability may be particularly important for the initiation of disability among women. The reported Male–female Health-Survival Paradox, whereby men have higher death rates but women fare worse in terms of disability and functioning [13–15] demonstrate that women are a particularly vulnerable group for disability problems as they age. The root causes of this paradox are unknown, but may include greater total disability burden among older women as compared to men [15], decreased likelihood of mortality among women with moderate to severe disability as compared to similarly-disabled men [15] or sex and gender differences in biological, behavioral and social factors across the lifespan. For example, research demonstrates that socioeconomic disadvantage is more strongly associated with disability risk among women as compared to men [16], and sex differences in body composition (higher total and subcutaneous fat mass and lower lean mass, muscle area and muscle density) translate to worse physical performance among women [17, 18] than among men. Among elderly populations, women experience more severe disability than men but it has been hypothesized that the combined impact of various social disadvantages such as lower income, less education, and higher prevalence of widowhood among older women may make them at greater risk for disability [19]. The male-to-female advantage in functioning is not, however, limited to elderly populations. Among mid-aged adults, women have 40 % lower levels of strength [20, 21], 20 % poorer balance times [20] and nearly twice the prevalence of self-reported difficulties with stair climbing activities [20] as compared to age-matched men. Further, women experience a more rapid decline in strength commencing in mid-life than do men; accelerations in strength loss begin between ages 40 and 55 in women whereas the loss of strength in men is linear across the lifespan [22–24]. The timing of this loss in strength has been noted to coincide with the timing of the menopausal transition [24–26] and some studies suggest that strength is preserved following menopause among women using exogenous hormone therapy [24, 25]. In addition to strength changes following menopause, data from cross-sectional studies show that postmenopausal women have 3.5 times higher odds of reporting substantial physical functioning limitations [26] and 17 % poorer balance times as compared to premenopausal women [27]. Given differences in functioning among pre- and post-menopausal women as well as among mid-aged men and women it has been hypothesized that ovarian function and the consequent decrease in estrogen levels during the menopausal transition may be associated with poor functioning.

## What is disability and how do we measure it?

The traditional model of disability and the disablement process was first described by Nagi [28] and then updated by Verbrugge & Jette [29]. As shown in Fig. 1, this traditional disablement model contributed substantially to our understanding by conceptualizing disability as a *process* during which one may experience impairments and limitations before reaching a disabled state. However, utilization of this model was limited by the focus on medical pathologies as the initiating factor in the cascade toward disablement. Although underlying medical conditions are known to be a risk factor for disability, a growing appreciation for the complexities underlying disability including the contextual and environmental factors prompted an international collaboration to revise and restructure this model.

In 2001, the World Health Organization (WHO) officially endorsed the International Classification of Functioning (ICF), Disability and Health as the prevailing framework for measuring health and disability within individuals and populations. The ICF conceptualizes disability as a general construct not only defined by underlying pathology but by the interaction of individuals with their environment and the mediation of that relationship by underlying contextual factors including genetic, biological, behavioral, social and economic factors. This biopsychosocial model, shown in Fig. 2, is structured on three levels of functioning: body functions and structure, activity, and participation. Importantly, disability is not a condition of an individual but one that occurs for a given individual in certain contexts. Unlike earlier disability models, the ICF model includes both disease-related and non-disease-related disability, the latter of which may be particularly relevant among middle-aged populations who may or may not yet have manifested overt disease. Scientific interest in functional limitations and disability as health outcomes are motivated by the fact that declines in physical performance and the presence of disability are associated with

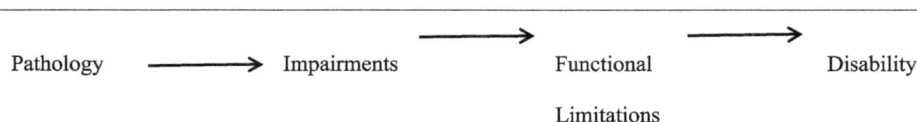

Pathology ⟶ Impairments ⟶ Functional Limitations ⟶ Disability

**Fig. 1** The disablement process by Verbrugge & Jette [17], adapted from Nagi [16]

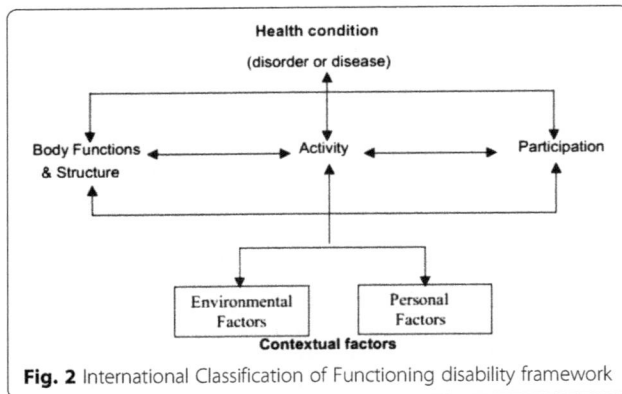

**Fig. 2** International Classification of Functioning disability framework

increased risk of death, morbidity, and reduced quality of life [12, 16, 30]. Preservation of functioning and prevention of disability is critical so that individuals can maintain independence and remain autonomous as they age.

## Disability is an increasingly relevant mid-life health issue

While there has been a large focus on the impending "silver tsunami" given the known relationship between age and disability [8], evidence from five national studies suggests that activities of daily living (ADL) or instrumental activities of daily living (IADL) disability rates among elderly individuals have remained constant in recent years [31] and even show 0.61–0.90 % improvement per year in ADLs and 0.3–1.41 % improvement per year in IADLs among the oldest old (85+ years) [31].

Among mid-aged adults, however, an emerging body of literature suggests a remarkably high prevalence of disability during this life stage. The prevalence of mid-life disability has been reported to range from 20 to 40 % [5, 11, 32, 33] and most common types of disability are mobility-based [5, 32]. Most concerning, however, are the growing number of studies reporting temporal increases in disability among middle-aged populations, suggesting that this problem is becoming more exacerbated. Odds of ADL, IADL, and mobility disability were 1.3–1.7 times higher among 60–64 year olds in the 1999–2004 National Health and Nutrition Examination Survey (NHANES) as compared to the 1988–1994 NHANES [34], independent of obesity and chronic health conditions. Similarly, among 50–64 year olds in the National Health Interview Survey (NHIS), there was a 6.8–12.1 % increase in the number of individuals reporting difficulty with lower extremity mobility including difficulty stooping, standing for 2 h, walking a quarter-mile, and climbing ten steps without resting from the 1997–99 versus 2005–07 data collection cycles [33]. Among 40–64 years old in NHIS, the odds for physical functioning limitations, ADLs and IADLs increased annually by 0.9, 0.9, and 2.7 %, respectively; the

increase in ADLs was independent of increases in obesity and was greater for women as compared to men [35]. In the Health and Retirement Survey (HRS), 15 % of adults aged 55–64 years in 2000 reported having difficulty with ADLs and there was a 0.1–0.2 percentage point increase per year [31]. However, the prevalence of ADL or IADL-assessed disability in mid-aged populations is relatively quite low as compared to older adults, and so more evidence is needed to confirm temporal trends and individual trajectories in disability.

With respect to physical functioning, the mid-life period is well accepted as a critical window for the onset of self-reported functional limitations [26, 36, 37] and diseases which ultimately lead to poor functioning and disability. In the Study of Women's Health Across the Nation (SWAN), a longitudinal study of midlife women, nearly one third of women (aged 45–57 years) reported moderate functional limitations and 11 % reported severe limitations based upon the SF-36 physical functioning questionnaire [26]. Similarly, in a British cohort of middle-aged adults, the prevalence of upper (difficulty gripping or reaching) and lower (difficulty walking or stair climbing) body limitations was 21–28 %, respectively [37]; the majority of these limitations began during the mid-life. Findings from NHIS show that deficits in functioning, defined as restricted activity resulting from illness, injury, or impairment begin during the mid-life [38] and that the most common conditions causing the need for help with ADLs or IADLs later in life, including back or neck problems, arthritis or rheumatism, diabetes, depression, anxiety, or emotional problems, hypertension, and nervous system conditions most commonly onset between 30 and 49 years of age [33].

Issues of functional limitations and disability are particularly salient among mid-aged individuals who are still in the work force and often caring for both dependent children and grandchildren as well as aging parents. Data from SIPP suggest that more than 10 % of mid-aged adults reported having limitation in their ability to work at a job [5]. Lack of employment during the midlife years may further compound health status and quality of life, as one's health insurance and ability to pay for medical care is often tightly linked to their employment.

## Challenges to studying disability

While there is substantial interest in measuring and understanding functional limitations and disability, efforts are complicated by the multi-faceted nature of disability and the substantial diversity in the assessment methods used. To illustrate this point, please refer to Table 1 which was summarizes the variability in disability prevalence estimates and definitions used among studies reporting on mid-life disability. There is no consensus in the field as to how disability should be assessed or defined,

**Table 1** Midlife disability prevalence and disability definitions

| Reference | Study, year, geographic location | Midlife sample | Disability definition | Disability prevalence (95 % CI) |
|---|---|---|---|---|
| **United States studies, national samples** | | | | |
| Altman & Gulley 2009 [45] | Joint Canada/United States Survey of Health, 2002–2003, United States and Canada national samples | 40–64 years | Disability in 4 question domains: Restriction of Activities Screener (reduction of activities at home, school, work); Health Utilities Index (functional abilities including vision, hearing, speech, mobility, dexterity, emotional well being, cognition, pain); Activity and Participation Screener (restriction caused by physical, mental or emotional problem); and Physical Functioning Limitation | |
| | | Men & women | • 40–49 years, Canada | 19.82 % (14.16, 25.48) |
| | | | • 50–64 years, Canada | 25.32 % (19.17, 31.47) |
| | | | • 40–49 years, United States | 16.80 % (12.47, 21.13) |
| | | | • 50–64 years, United States | 28.59 % (23.67, 33.51) |
| Mitra et al. 2009 [46] | Medical Expenditure Panel Survey, 2004, United States national sample | 40–61 years | At least one of the following: limitations in work, housework, or school; walking limitations; cognitive limitation; limitations in seeing or hearing | |
| | | Men and women | • 40–49 years | 29.7 % |
| | | | • 50–61 years | 45.4 % |
| Hottman et al. 2005 [5] | Survey of Income and Program Participation, 2005, United States national sample | 45–64 years | At least one of the following: (women only) | 25.9 % |
| | | Men & women | • Use of an assistive aid | 4.6 % (4.2, 5.0) |
| | | | • Difficulty performing ADLs | 4.1 % (3.7, 4.5) |
| | | | • Difficulty performing IADLs | 6.0 % (5.5, 6.5) |
| | | | • Difficulty performing specified functional activities | 19.4 % (18.6, 20.2) |
| | | | • Reported of selected impairments | 6.9 % (6.4, 7.4) |
| | | | • Limitation in ability to work around house | 10.7 % (10.1, 11.3) |
| | | | • Limitation in ability to work at Job/business | 11.3 % (10.7, 11.9) |
| Martin et al. 2010 [33] | National Health Interview Survey, 2005–2007, United States national sample | 50–64 years | Difficulty with physical functions due to a health problem | 42.0 % |
| | | Men & women | • Needing help with IADLs | 6.7 % |
| | | | • Needing help with ADLs | 6.0 % |
| Zhao et al. 2009 [47] | Behavioral Risk Factor Surveillance System, 2005, United States national sample | 50–65 years | Self-reported limitations in participation in activities because of physical, mental, or emotional problems or whether health problems required use of special equipment | |
| | | Men & women | • 50–54 years | 22.9 % (21.3, 24.5) |
| | | | • 55–59 years | 28.8 % (27.8, 29.8) |
| | | | • 60–65 years | 28.8 % (27.8, 29.8) |

**Table 1** Midlife disability prevalence and disability definitions *(Continued)*

| United States studies, local samples | | | | |
|---|---|---|---|---|
| Khoury *et al.* 2013 [69] | Female Medicaid beneficiaries, 2001–2005, Florida | 36–64 years | Presence of at least one physically disabling conditions but no use of a mobility assistive device | |
| | | Women | • 36–45 years | 35.79 % |
| | | | • 46–55 years | 47.22 % |
| | | | • 56–64 years | 53.30 % |
| | | | Presence of at least one physically disabling conditions and use of a mobility assistive device | |
| | | | • 36–45 years | 2.92 % |
| | | | • 46–55 years | 5.59 % |
| | | | • 56–64 years | 9.17 % |
| Brown *et al.* 2014 [41] | Patients admitted to San Francisco General Hospital, 2010–2011, San Francisco, California | 55–59 years | Needing help with at least one ADL 2 weeks before hospital admission | 28.9 % |
| | | Men & women | • Needing help with bathing | 21.1 % |
| | | | • Needing help with dressing | 20.5 % |
| | | | • Needing help with transferring | 14.5 % |
| | | | • Needing help with eating | 9.0 % |
| | | | • Needing help with toileting | 9.6 % |
| | | | Needing help with at least 2 IADLs 2 weeks before hospital admission | 36.1 % |
| | | | • Needing help with shopping | 32.5 % |
| | | | • Needing help with light housework | 30.6 % |
| | | | • Needing help with meal preparation | 30.1 % |
| | | | • Needing help with transportation | 21.1 % |
| | | | • Needing help with medication management | 20.7 % |
| | | | • Needing help with money management | 16.9 % |
| | | | • Needing help with using the telephone | 7.2 % |
| Mann *et al.* 2015 [48] | Behavioral Risk Factor Surveillance System (BRFSS), 2011, South Carolina | 45–64 years | Affirmative response to standard BRFSS disability questions: | |
| | | Men & women | Self-reported limitation in "activities because of physical, mental, or emotional problems" | |
| | | | Or | |
| | | | Self-reported health problem that requires use of special equipment such as a cane, wheelchair, special bed, or special telephone. | |
| | | | • 45–54 years | 22.1 % (20.0, 24.3) |
| | | | • 55–64 years | 23.3 % (21.4, 25.2) |
| Karvonen-Gutierrez & Ylitalo 2013 [32] | Michigan Study of Women's Health Across the Nation, 2011, Michigan | 55.9–67.7 years | 36-item World Health Organization Disability Assessment Schedule, severe-extreme disability: | |
| | | Women only | • Global score | 5.05 % (2.84, 7.26) |
| | | | • Understanding and communicating | 5.05 % (2.84, 7.23) |
| | | | • Getting around | 19.31 % (15.41, 23.41) |
| | | | • Self-care | 4.26 % (2.22, 6.30) |
| | | | • Getting along with people | 6.12 % (3.70, 8.54) |

**Table 1** Midlife disability prevalence and disability definitions *(Continued)*

| | | | | |
|---|---|---|---|---|
| | | | • Engaging in life activities, non-work | 43.16 %<br>(35.07, 51.25) |
| | | | • Engaging in life activities, work | 8.62 %<br>(5.00, 12.23) |
| | | | • Participation in society | 8.78 %<br>(3.92, 11.64) |
| Arterburn *et al.* 2012 [52] | Group Health Plan enrollees, Washington | 40–65 years | Modified World Health Organization Disability Assessment Schedule, any disability: | |
| | | Women only | • Global score | Not reported |
| | | | • Understanding and communicating | 26 % |
| | | | • Getting around | 27 % |
| | | | • Self-care | 7 % |
| | | | • Getting along with people | 17 % |
| | | | • Engaging in life activities, non-work | 46 % |
| | | | • Engaging in life activities, work | 45 % |
| | | | • Participation in society | 24 % |

International studies

| | | | | |
|---|---|---|---|---|
| Hosseinpoor *et al.* 2012 [16] | World Health Survey, 2002–2004, 57 countries | 50–59 years | World Health Organization Report on Disability definition, based upon Item Response Theory model using data from questions in multiple domains. | |
| | | Men & women | • 50–54 year old women | 27.3 %<br>(25.1, 29.5) |
| | | | • 55–59 year old women | 30.5 %<br>(28.0, 33.0) |

Europe

| | | | | |
|---|---|---|---|---|
| Kattainen *et al.* 2004 [39] | Finland Health 2000 Survey, 2000–2001, Finland | 45–64 years | Blindness or being unable to perform without help or having marked difficulty at least one of | 7.8 % |
| | | Women | the following: moving about in the house, getting in/out of bed, dressing, carrying a 5-kg shopping bag, walking 500 m without rest, climbing a flight of stairs without rest, managing grocery shopping | |
| Krishnan *et al.* 2004 [40] | Cross-sectional study in Central Finland District, 2000, Finland | 36–65 | Health Assessment Questionnaire (HAQ) disability index score >0. HAQ assesses difficulty with performing activities in 8 functional categories: dressing/grooming, arising, eating, walking, hygiene, reach, grip, and common daily activities. | |
| | | Women | • 36–40 years | 14.7 %<br>(7.9, 21.4) |
| | | | • 41–45 years | 17.4 %<br>(10.4, 24.4) |
| | | | • 46–50 years | 25.0 %<br>(17.4, 32.6) |
| | | | • 51–55 years | 25.6 %<br>(17.7, 33.5) |
| | | | • 56–60 years | 36.7 %<br>(27.0, 46.4) |
| | | | • 61–65 years | 33.1 %<br>(24.4, 41.7) |
| Klijs *et al.* 2011 [81] | Dutch PLOS-survey (Permanent Onderzoek Leefsituatie), 2001–2007, the Netherlands | 55–59 years<br><br>Women | Major difficulty doing or only able to do with help at least one of the following: walk up and down the stairs, walk outside, enter/leave the house, sit down/get up from a chair, move around on the same floor, get in/out of bed, eat/drink, get dressed/undressed, wash face/hands, wash completely | 6 % |

**Table 1** Midlife disability prevalence and disability definitions *(Continued)*

| | | | | |
|---|---|---|---|---|
| Almazan-Isla et al. 2014 [60] | Residents from Cinco Villas, Spain, 2008–2009, Spain | 50–59 years | 36-item World Health Organization Disability Assessment Schedule, severe-extreme disability, women only | |
| | | Men & women | • Global score | 1.27 % |
| | | | • Understanding and communicating | 1.27 % |
| | | | • Getting around | 8.28 % |
| | | | • Self-care | 2.55 % |
| | | | • Getting along with people | 1.27 % |
| | | | • Engaging in life activities, non-work | 12.74 % |
| | | | • Engaging in life activities, work | 4.46 % |
| | | | • Participation in society | 6.00 % |
| **Africa** | | | | |
| Miszkurka et al. 2012 [54] | World Health Organization World Health Study, 2002–2003, Burkina Faso, Mali, and Senegal | 35–64 years | Mobility disability, defined as self-reported mild, moderate, severe or extreme difficulty or unable to move around. | |
| | | Men and women | • 35–44 years, Burkina Faso, women | 21 % (16, 28) |
| | | | • 35–44 years, Mali, women | 22 % (19, 26) |
| | | | • 35–44 years, Senegal, women | 36 % (28, 44) |
| | | | • 45–54 years, Burkina Faso, women | 25 % (19, 32) |
| | | | • 45–54 years, Mali, women | 31 % (24, 39) |
| | | | • 45–54 years, Senegal, women | 41 % (23, 63) |
| | | | • 55–64 years, Burkina Faso, women | 52 % (40, 64) |
| | | | • 55–64 years, Mali, women | 48 % (38, 58) |
| | | | • 55–64 years, Senegal, women | 56 % (38, 72) |
| Payne et al. 2013 [55] | Malawi Longitudinal Study of Families and Health, 2010, Malawi | 45–64 years | Having any health problem that limits ability to carry out culturally-relevant moderate activities or strenuous activities. | |
| | | Men & women | • Moderately disabled ('somewhat limited' in either moderate or strenuous activities) | 22.4 % |
| | | | • Severely disabled ('limited a lot' in either moderate or strenuous activities) | 5.3 % |
| Wandera et al. 2014 [56] | Uganda National Household Survey, 2010, Uganda | 50–59 years  Women | Having a lot of difficulty or being unable to perform at least one of the following OR having some difficulty with at least two of the following: difficulty seeing, even if wearing glasses; difficulty hearing, even if wearing a hearing aid; difficulty walking or climbing steps; difficulty remembering or concentrating; difficulty washing all over or dressing, feeding and toileting; difficulty communicating because of a physical, mental or emotional health condition. | 24.8 % |
| **Asia** | | | | |
| Zheng et al. 2011 [57] | China National Survey, 2006, China | 45–64 years | Doctor-diagnosed disability following positive screen for self-reported visual, hearing, speech, physical, intellectual or mental disability | |
| | | Men and women | • 45–54 years | 11.0 % |
| | | | • 55–64 years | 13.2 % |
| Peng et al. 2010 [58] | China National Sample Survey on Disability, 2006 | 35–64 years | Visual, intellectual, mental or physical disability assessed from an impairment-based examination | |

**Table 1** Midlife disability prevalence and disability definitions *(Continued)*

| | | | | |
|---|---|---|---|---|
| | | Women | • 35–39 years | 3.48 %<br>(3.41, 3.55) |
| | | | • 40–44 years | 4.18 %<br>(4.10, 4.26) |
| | | | • 45–49 years | 5.32 %<br>(5.21, 5.34) |
| | | | • 50–54 years | 6.38 %<br>(6.27, 6.49) |
| | | | • 55–59 years | 8.77 %<br>(8.62, 8.92) |
| | | | • 60–64 years | 12.35 %<br>(12.15, 12.55) |
| Hairi *et al.* 2010 [59] | Alor Gajah Older People Health Survey, 2007–2008, Malaysia | 60–64 years | Level of independence in ADLs. 5-item scale included feeding, dressing, bathing, toileting and transferring. 6-item scale additionally included walking. 10-item scale additionally included grooming, bladder control, bowel control, and stair climbing. | |
| | | Women | • 10 item ADL dependence | 5.3 %<br>(2.6, 10.1) |
| | | | • 6 item ADL dependence | 4.7 %<br>(2.2, 9.4) |
| | | | • 5 item ADL dependence | 2.9 %<br>(1.1, 7.9) |

and several different questionnaire and performance-based assessment tools are in operation, thereby resulting in highly variable prevalence estimates for disability. For example, two studies reporting disability rates among mid-aged women in Finland report wildly different estimates (7.8 % vs. 25.8 %) when using different definitions of disability [39, 40].

As shown in Table 1, many United States studies use either ADLs or IADLs as a disability measure. While these measures are relevant among elderly cohorts, the focus on self-care and ability to live independently may not be adequate to capture early deficits in functioning experienced by younger populations. As evidenced in Table 1, midlife disability prevalence estimates are lowest among studies using ADL or IADL definitions of disability among the general population where the prevalence ranges from 4.1 to 6.7 % [5, 33]. Notably, pre-admission ADL and IADL disability is much higher among a midlife sample of hospitalized patients (29–36 %) [41], suggesting the importance of ADLs and IADLs as a marker of poor health status.

Instead, studies among midlife populations often focus on physical functioning assessment with the assumption that deficits in physical functioning are a predictor of incident disability. The integrated nature of disability, rooted in the interaction between an individual and their environment, cannot be fully measured based upon physical functioning because variability in physical functioning does not full capture the full spectrum of limitations described by the ICF, particularly those that are contextual in nature and particularly relevant to mid-aged cohorts. For example, limitations in physical functioning may not lead to disability given one's access to and use of adaptive strategies or resources. Further, one may

be considered disabled for reasons other than limitations in physical functioning.

When physical functioning is used as a proxy for disability, it is assessed either based upon self-report using a variety of standardized and non-standardized questionnaires or based upon objective, performance-based measures which are often mobility-based. Evidence supports that self-reported and performance-based assessments measure distinct, yet related domains of physical functioning [42–44] but little work has been done to understand the correlation between physical functioning and ICF-based disability among community-based populations. Because physical functioning is only one aspect of an individual's overall health and functioning, caution should be used when using physical functioning as a proxy for disability.

Many studies have considered self-reported limitation in (work, home, leisure, functioning) activities as a measure of disability. This paradigm is more closely aligned with the ICF framework by consideration of not only functioning but individual context. As shown in Table 1, disability prevalence using definitions based upon activity limitation are higher than those for ADL or IADL disability and increase by 40 % from early- to late-middle age in some [45, 46] but not all [47, 48] studies.

In many countries, work disability claims represent a potentially valuable resource for quantifying and studying the burden of disability among mid-life adults, as they are of working age. While such studies have contributed substantially to the literature and identified the importance of musculoskeletal functioning and mental health as major factors related to work-related disability, there are limitations in utilizing such databases for population research. First, work-related functioning and disability is often assessed in the context of one's diagnosis and physical health and do not fully capture the impact of the psychosocial domains of disability [49]. Second, in occupational databases, there is often limited individual-level information about important causes, correlates, or consequences of disability such as that which is available from epidemiologic studies. This type of data is critical to identify potential strategies to prevent disability or to alleviate the individual burden of such limitations.

To support assessment of ICF-conceptualized disability, the WHO developed the Disability Assessment Schedule (WHO-DAS). The WHO-DAS questionnaire assesses disability in 6 domains including (a) understanding and communicating, (b) getting around, (c) self-care, (d) getting along with people, (e) engaging in life activities, and (f) participation in society, in addition to a global disability score. It is recognized and promoted as a universal and standardized measure of disability, suitable for national and international comparisons of disability prevalence and determinants across populations and age groups [50, 51]. While the WHO-DAS has been used to examine disability and its correlates in several clinical populations including those with mental health conditions, migraine, Parkinson's Disease, multiple sclerosis, and traumatic brain injury, only two United States studies have examined WHO-DAS assessed disability in a general population of midlife adults. In the Michigan Study of Women's Health Across the Nation (SWAN), WHO-DAS assessed disability prevalence was 25 % overall and at least 1 in 5 women reported moderate, severe or extreme problems with the understanding and communicating, getting around, getting along with people, work-related life activities and participation in society domains [32]. Data from a sample of women aged 40–65 years recruited from Group Health, a health insurance and care delivery system in the state of Washington, found that 45 % of women reported disabilities with work and non-work (i.e., household) activities and 27 % reported mobility disability [52]. Unlike studies among elderly cohorts [53] where the prevalence of self-care associated disability is nearly 40 %, only 1 in 10 midlife women in Michigan SWAN or the Group Health cohorts reported disability in the self-care domain [32, 52]. While WHO-DAS disability prevalence estimates (based upon the summary score) are similar to those published in the literature using other definitions of disability [5, 32, 33], the wide variation in domain-specific prevalence [33, 52] demonstrate the strength of the ICF framework in understanding the scope of disability during the mid-life.

Given national differences in medical care, support systems, and acceptability of aging, it is expected that international comparisons of disability prevalence would yield global variability. Unfortunately, cross-national comparisons of disability rates are complicated by variations in assessment method and definitions. As shown in Table 1, most disability work among midlife populations from Africa has focused on mobility disability or activity limitations and so prevalence rates range from 20 to 56 % [54–56]. While disability prevalence in Asia is appreciably lower (3–13 %), definitions are more conservative, based upon doctor diagnosis [57, 58] or ADL dependence [59]. The WHO-DAS has been used to assess disability among mid-life populations in the United States [32, 52] and Spain [60]. Disability prevalence rates were higher in the United States populations as compared to the Spanish population. However, the Spanish population included both men and women whereas the United States studies were among women only.

Differences in disability definitions, assessment strategies, and data sources can make it difficult to make comparisons between different studies, including national surveys, census-based data, and international agreements. Evaluation of trends in disability must be undertaken within longitudinal or panel studies using consistent measures and definitions. When synthesizing the literature and data regarding disability prevalence, incidence, and correlates, and particularly when making comparisons between studies, one must be careful to be cognizant of the constructs used to define disability.

**Functioning and disability are dynamic processes**
Further complicating the consideration of disability among mid-life populations is that unlike elderly populations, mid-aged individuals may be more likely to experience disability due to acute, non-chronic events. Using data from NHIS of adults ≥18 years of age from 1988 to 2011, Iezzoni et al. [61] found a high proportion of non-chronic disability among respondents, ranging from 1 % for non-chronic social limitation disability to 40 % for non-chronic sensory difficulties. Similarly, data from SWAN has demonstrated that the presence of functional limitations during the mid-life is a highly dynamic process. While most SWAN women maintained their physical functioning level over a two-year period, 6–22 % of women worsened to a poorer level of functioning and 11–30 % of women actually improved their functioning [36]. Older adults also exhibit dynamic patterns of disability transitions, but unlike midlife populations, the vast majority exhibit worsening disability. In the Leiden 85-plus Study, a prospective cohort study of adults age 85 years and older, the prevalence of worsening disability after 5-years was 86 % [62], nearly 4 times greater than that among midlife women in SWAN [36]. Thus, the mid-life may be a highly malleable period during which interventions may be most efficacious because individuals may be more likely to have a propensity for improvement rather than deterioration. Consideration of the dynamic, non-chronic nature of disability status among mid-life populations is critical because most assessments

are not designed to capture transient difficulties; estimates suggest that up to 40 % of disability complaints are missed among mid-aged populations because discordance between measurement window and timing of disability [61]. Thus, in mid-aged populations, repeated assessment and data collection is critical to fully understand the burden of disability during this life stage.

### Improving disability among mid-life women

Mid-life factors including stress, low social support, decreased social activity, physical inactivity, poor physical functioning, smoking, obesity and diabetes [63–65] are known to predict old age disability. The high prevalence of disability during the mid-life period [5, 11, 32, 33], however, raises the urgent need to intervene to prevent not only future disability but also present disability. The mid-life period is a time of dynamic changes in physical functioning and mid-aged individuals have a high capacity for improvement [36], so there is an imperative need to understand correlates of mid-age disability so that we may develop appropriate and efficacious interventions. Correlates of mid-age disability include obesity [52, 66, 67], depression symptoms [32, 52, 68], economic strain [32] and chronic disease comorbidity [69] and burden [47] including knee osteoarthritis and peripheral neuropathy [32]. Further, incident disability later in life is predicted by mid-life depression [70], increased body mass index [70–72], poor physical functioning performance [68, 73], low levels of physical activity [71, 73] and smoking [72].

As chronic conditions are the leading causes of disability in the United States [5] and globally [6], efforts to prevent disease or reducing symptomatology at earlier ages is one critical strategy to prevent or forestall disability. Many of the conditions which are major correlates of disability emerge or are more bothersome during the mid-life, including osteoarthritis [74], heart trouble [75], low back pain [76] and mental and emotional health problems [77] and are further exacerbated by obesity [78–80]. Among mid-life women, arthritis and back pain have the largest contribution to disability prevalence [81]. Thus, while much work has been done to intervene on disease-specific conditions in older adults as an effort to improve functioning and reduce disability, evidence suggests that interventions starting in midlife or earlier may be most beneficial in reducing disability risk among both midlife and older adults [47].

Individuals may be most amenable to interventions during the mid-life, as evidenced by the success of ergonomic, vocational rehabilitation, and strength training work-place interventions shown to reduce back and upper limb pain-associated work disability [82–84]. However, there has been a dearth of intervention studies among mid-life adults beyond work-place interventions to reduce

sick leave or work-related disability. One potential reason for this is the belief that a prohibitively long follow-up period will be needed to observe any effects of an intervention. While recommendations for high-impact interventions for disability reductions among late-life adults have been published [85], no such statement has been issued for mid-life adults. However, given the high prevalence of disability and functional limitations among mid-life populations, this concern is mitigated by the opportunity to improve functioning and disability *during* the midlife. Given increasing trends in disability prevalence [31] and chronic conditions [2, 3] among mid-life adults, efforts to improve the health and functioning during this life stage is highly needed to appropriately address the unique health needs this population. Additionally, to fully understand how to *prevent* disability and improve health for late-life individuals, we must identify interventions that, when implemented early, have the ability for sustained benefit as one ages.

Studies among older adults, however, do provide insight to interventions that may be efficacious among mid-life populations. Multi-component exercise interventions [86] including the Lifestyle Interventions and Independence for Elders (LIFE) study [87, 88] and interventions to reduce depression symptoms [89] have showed promising results in reducing incident disability among older adults. Depressive symptoms and decreased physical activity are predictors of mid-life incident disability. This knowledge – the utility of depression and physical activity interventions among older adults and the importance of these factors for predicting mid-life disability suggest that they may be relevant areas for mid-life intervention studies. Further, a simulation study using data from the Nurses' Health Study suggest that midlife weight loss and physical activity interventions would be most efficacious in preventing chronic disease incidence, reducing risk by up to 10 percentage points [90]. The current pressing challenge, however, is to develop and implement interventions that, when begun during the mid-life, have the capacity for long-term adherence and effectiveness so as to impact long-term health, functioning and wellness trajectories.

Another challenge to intervention studies among mid-life populations is the highly dynamic nature of mid-life functioning and disability, thereby signaling a need for different frameworks and interventions to impact the onset and recovery from functional limitations and disability. In HRS among adults age 51–61 years, recovery from mobility disability over 2 years was predicted by lack of diabetes, lung disease and pain whereas onset of mobility disability was predicted by being female, less educated, obese, and having frequent pain [91]. Among women SWAN, highly dynamic patterns of functioning, characterized as both worsening and improving over time, were observed among obese women and women who had arthritis [36]. Therefore, different intervention programs and paradigms may need to be considered which target midlife factors to prevent old age disability versus those that can prompt recovery from current mid-life disability.

## Conclusion

Disability prevalence is high during the mid-life, yet domains of disability among younger populations differ substantially from those among older adults. Despite a high burden, evidence suggests that the presence of mid-life disability does not inevitably worsen. Instead, encouraging data suggests that mid-aged individuals are highly capable of recovering from non-chronic disability. This observation, combined with the known detrimental effect of poor functioning and disability on current and further health should prompt a concentrated public health effort to target interventions to improve functioning and prevent disability among mid-aged adults. Focused efforts on treatment of depression and physical activity interventions to reduce obesity and prevent mobility disability may be most efficacious during this life stage.

### Abbreviations
SIPP: Survey of Income and Program Participation; WHO: World Health Organization; ICF: International Classification of Functioning; ADL: Activities of daily living; IADL: Instrumental activities of daily living; WHO-DAS: World Health Organization Disability Assessment Schedule; SWAN: Study of Women's Health Across the Nation; NHANES: National Health and Nutrition Examination Survey; NHIS: National Health Interview Survey; HRS: Health and Retirement Survey ; BRFSS: Behavioral Risk Factor Surveillance System; .

### Competing interests
The author declares that she has no competing interests.

### Authors' contributions
CKG conceived of the manuscript, drafted and revised the manuscript, has approved the final version of the manuscript and is accountable for all aspects of work associated with this manuscript.

### Authors' information
CKG is an Assistant Research Professor whose research focuses on the impact of chronological and reproductive aging and obesity as risk factors for the development of knee osteoarthritis, functional limitations and disability.

### References
1. World Health Organization. World Health Report 2003. Geneva: World Health Organization; 2003.
2. Crimmins E, Saito Y. Change in the prevalence of diseases among older Americans: 1984–1994. Demogr Res. 2000;3:9.
3. Freedman VA, Schoeni RF, Martin LG, Cornman JC. Chronic conditions and the decline in late-life disability. Demography. 2007;44(3):459–77.
4. Paez KA, Zhao L, Hwang W. Rising out-of-pocket spending for chronic conditions: a ten-year trend. Health Aff (Millwood). 2009;28:15–25.
5. Hootman JM, Brault MW, Helmick CG, Theis KA, Armour BS. Prevalence and most common causes of disability among adults-United States, 2005. MMWR Morb Mortal Wkly Rep. 2009;58(16):421–6.
6. Vos T, Flaxman AD, Naghavi M, Lozano R, Michaud C, Ezzati M, et al. Years lived with disability (YLDs) for 1160 sequelae of 289 diseases and injuries 1990–2010: a systematic analysis for the Global Burden of Disease Study 2010. Lancet. 2012;380(9859):2163–96.
7. UN World Health Organization (WHO). World Report on Disability: Summary. 2011. WHO/NMH/VIP/11.01, available at: http://www.refworld.org/docid/50854a322.html [accessed 29 April 2015].
8. Brault MW. Americans With Disabilities: 2010. Washington (DC): U.S. Census Bureau; 2012 Jul. (Current Population Reports; 70-131).
9. Centers for Disease Control and Prevention (CDC). Trends in aging – United States and worldwide. MMWR Morb Mortal Wkly Rep. 2003;52(6):101–6.
10. United Nations, Department of Economic and Social Affairs, Population Division, 2013. World Population Ageing 2013. ST/ESA/SER.A/348, available at: http://www.un.org/en/development/desa/population/publications/pdf/ageing/WorldPopulationAgeing2013.pdf [accessed 29 April 2015].
11. Murray CJ, Vos T, Lozano R, Naghavi M, Flaxman AD, Michaud C, et al. Disability-adjusted life years (DALYs) for 291 diseases and injuries in 21 regions, 1990–2010: a systematic analysis for the Global Burden of Disease Study 2010. Lancet. 2012;380(9859):2197–223.
12. United Nations, Department of Economic and Social Affairs, Population Division, 2001. World Population Ageing 1950–2050. ST/ESA/SER.A/207, available at: http://www.un.org/esa/population/publications/worldageing19502050/ [accessed 29 April 2015].
13. Romero-Ortuno R, Fouweather T, Jagger C. Cross-national disparities in sex differences in life expectancy with and without frailty. Age Ageing. 2014;43(2):222–8.
14. Oksuzyan A, Bronnum-Hansen H, Jeune B. Gender gap in health expectancy. Eur J Ageing. 2010;7:213–8.
15. Gill TM, Gahbauer EA, Lin H, Han L, Allore HG. Comparisons between older men and women in the trajectory and burden of disability over the course of nearly 14 years. J Am Med Dir Assoc. 2013;14(4):280–6.
16. Hosseinpoor AR, Williams JS, Jann B, Kowal P, Officer A, Posarac A, et al. Social determinants of sex differences in disability among older adults: a multi-country decomposition analysis using the World Health Survey. Int J Equity Health. 2012;11:52.
17. Tseng LA, Delmonico MJ, Visser M, Boudreau RM, Goodpaster BH, Schwartz AV, et al. Body composition explains sex differential in physical performance among older adults. J Gerontol A Biol Sci Med Sci. 2014;69(1):93–100.
18. Yount KM, Hoddinott J, Stein AD. Disability and self-rated health among older women and men in rural Guatemala: the role of obesity and chronic conditions. Soc Sci Med. 2010;71:1418–27.
19. Hammond JM. Multiple jeopardy or multiple resources? The intersection of age, race, living arrangement and education level and the health of older women. J Women Aging. 1995;7(3):5–24.
20. Kuh D, Bassey EJ, Butterworth S, Hardy R, Wadsworth ME. Grip strength, postural control, and functional leg power in a representative cohort of British men and women: associations with physical activity, health status, and socioeconomic conditions. J Gerontol A Biol Sci Med Sci. 2005;60(2):224–31.
21. Bassey EJ, Mockett SP, Fentem PH. Lack of variation in muscle strength with menstrual status in healthy women aged 45–54 years: data from a national survey. Eur J Appl Physiol Occup Physiol. 1996;73(3–4):382–6.
22. Danneskiold-Samsoe B, Bartels EM, Bulow PM, Lund H, Stockmarr A, Holm CC, et al. Isokinetic and isometric muscle strength in a healthy population with special reference to age and gender. Acta Physiol (Oxf). 2009;197 Suppl 673:1–68.
23. Samson MM, Meeuwsen IB, Crowe A, Dessens JA, Duursma SA, Verhaar HJ. Relationships between physical performance measures, age, height and body weight in healthy adults. Age Ageing. 2000;29(3):235–42.
24. Phillips SK, Rook KM, Siddle NC, Bruce SA, Woledge RC. Muscle weakness in women occurs at an earlier age than in men, but strength is preserved by hormone replacement therapy. Clin Sci (Lond). 1993;84(1):95–8.
25. Greeves JP, Cable NT, Reilly T, Kingsland C. Changes in muscle strength in women following the menopause: a longitudinal assessment of the efficacy of hormone replacement therapy. Clin Sci (Lond). 1999;97:79–84.
26. Tseng LA, El Khoudary SR, Young EA, Farhat GN, Sowers M, Sutton-Tyrrell K, et al. The association of menopause status with physical function: the Study of Women's Health Across the Nation. Menopause. 2012;19(11):1186–92.
27. Kumari M, Stafford M, Marmot M. The menopausal transition was associated in a prospective study with decreased health functioning in women who report menopausal symptoms. J Clin Epidemiol. 2005;58:719–27.
28. Nagi SZ. An epidemiology of disability among adults in the United States. Milbank Mem Fund Q Health Soc. 1976;54(4):439–67.

29. Verbrugge LM, Jette AM. The disablement process. Soc Sci Med. 1994;38(1):1–14.

30. Nuru-Jeter AM, Thorpe Jr RJ, Fuller-Thomson E. Black-white differences in self-reported disability outcomes in the U.S.: early childhood to older adulthood. Public Health Rep. 2011;126(6):834–43.

31. Freedman VA, Spillman BC, Andreski PM, Cornman JC, Crimmins EM, Kramarow E, et al. Trends in late-life activity limitations in the United States: an update from five national surveys. Demography. 2013;50(2):661–71.

32. Karvonen-Gutierrez CA, Ylitalo KR. Prevalence and correlates of disability in a late middle-aged population of women. J Aging Health. 2013;25(4):701–17.

33. Martin LG, Freedman VA, Schoeni RF, Andreski PM. Trends in disability and related chronic conditions among people ages fifty to sixty-four. Health Aff (Millwood). 2010;29:725–31.

34. Seeman TE, Merkin SS, Crimmins EM, Karlamangla AS. Disability trends among older Americans: National Health and Nutrition Examination Surveys, 1988–1994 and 1999–2004. Am J Public Health. 2010;100(1):100–7.

35. Martin LG, Schoeni RF. Trends in disability and related chronic conditions among the forty-and-over population: 1997–2010. Disabil Health J. 2014;7(1 suppl):S4–S14.

36. Ylitalo KR, Karvonen-Gutierrez CA, Fitzgerald N, Zheng H, Sternfeld B, El Khoudary SR, et al. Relationship of race-ethnicity, body mass index, and economic strain with longitudinal self-report of physical functioning: the Study of Women's Health Across the Nation. Ann Epidemiol. 2013;23(7):401–8.

37. Murray ET, Hardy R, Strand BH, Cooper R, Guralnik JM, Kuh D. Gender and life course occupational social class differences in trajectories of functional limitations in midlife: findings from the 1946 British birth cohort. J Gerontol A Biol Sci Med Sci. 2011;66(12):1350–9.

38. Adams PF, Marano MA. Current estimates from the National Health Interview Survey, 1994. Vital Health Stat 10. 1995;193(Pt1):1–260.

39. Kattainen A, Reunanen A, Koskinen S, Martelin T, Knekt P, Sainio P, et al. Secular changes in disability among middle-aged and elderly Finns with and without coronary heart disease from 1978–1980 and 2000–2001. Ann Epidemiol. 2004;14(7):479–85.

40. Krishnan E, Sokka T, Hakkinen A, Hubert H, Hannonen P. Normative values for the Health Assessment Questionnaire disability index: benchmarking disability in the general population. Arthritis Rheum. 2004;50(3):953–60.

41. Brown RT, Pierluissi E, Guzman D, Kessell ER, Goldman LE, Sarkar U, et al. Functional disability in late-middle-aged and older adults admitted to a safety-net hospital. J Am Geriatr Soc. 2014;62(11):2056–63.

42. Simonsick EM, Newman AB, Nevitt MC, Kritchevsky SB, Ferrucci L, Guralnik JM, et al. Measuring higher level physical function in well-functioning older adults: expanding familiar approaches in the Health ABC study. J Gerontol A Biol Sci Med Sci. 2011;56(10):M644–649.

43. Wittink H, Rogers W, Sukiennik A, Carr DB. Physical functioning: self-report and performance measures are related but distinct. Spine. 2003;28(20):2407–13.

44. Bean JF, Olveczky DD, Kiely DK, LaRose SI, Jette AM. Performance-based versus patient-reported physical function: what are the underlying predictors? Phys Ther. 2011;91(12):1804–11.

45. Altman BM, Gulley SP. Convergence and divergence: differences in disability prevalence estimates in the United States and Canada based on four health survey instruments. Soc Sci Med. 2009;69(4):543–52.

46. Mitra S, Findley PA, Sambamoorthi U. Health care expenditures of living with a disability: total expenditures, out-of-pocket expenses, and burden, 1996 to 2004. Arch Phys Med Rehabil. 2009;90(9):1532–40.

47. Zhao G, Ford ES, Li C, Crews JE, Mokdad AH. Disability and its correlates with chronic morbidities among US adults aged 50-<65 years. Prev Med. 2009;48(2):117–21.

48. Mann J, Balte P, Clarkson J, Nitchea D, Graham CL, McDermott S. What are the specific disability and limitation types underlying responses to the BRFSS disability questions? Disability Health J. 2015;8:17–28.

49. Schellekens JM, Abma FI, Mulders HP, Brouwer S. Measuring clients' perception of functional limitations using the Perceived Functioning & Health questionnaire. J Occup Rehabil. 2010;20(4):512–25.

50. Garin O, Ayuso-Mateos JL, Almansa J, Nieto M, Chatterji S, Vilagut G, et al. Validation of the World Health Organization Disability Assessment Schedule, WHODAS-2 in patients with chronic diseases. Health Qual Life Outcomes. 2010;8:51.

51. Ustun TB, Chatterji S, Kostanjsek N, Rehm J, Kennedy C, Epping-Jordan J, et al. WHO/NIH joint project: developing the world health organization

disability assessment schedule 2.0. Bull World Health Organ. 2010;88(11):815–23.

52. Arterburn D, Westbook EO, Ludman EJ, Operskalski B, Linde JA, Rohde P, et al. Relationship between obesity, depression and disability in middle-aged women. Obes Res Clin Pract. 2012;6(3):e197–206.

53. de Pedro-Cuesta J, Alberquilla A, Virues-Ortega J, Carmona M, Alcalde-Cabero E, Bosca G, et al. ICF disability measured by WHO-DAS II in three community diagnostic groups in Madrid, Spain. Gac Sanit. 2011;25 Suppl 2:21–8.

54. Miszkurka M, Zunzunegui MV, Langlois EV, Freeman EE, Kouanda S, Haddad S. Gender differences in mobility disability during young, middle and older age in West African adults. Glob Public Health. 2012;7(5):495–508.

55. Payne CF, Mkandawire J, Kohler HP. Disability transitions and health expectancies among adults 45 years and older in Malawi: a cohort-based model. PLoS Med. 2013;10(5):e1001435.

56. Wandera SO, Notzi J, Kwagala B. Prevalence and correlates of disability among older Ugandans: evidence from the Uganda National Household Survey. Glob Health Action. 2014;7:25686.

57. Zheng X, Chen G, Song X, Liu J, Yan L, Du W, et al. Twenty-year trends in the prevalence of disability in China. Bull World Health Organ. 2011;89(11):788–97.

58. Peng X, Song S, Sullivan S, Qiu J, Wang W. Ageing, the urban–rural gap and disability trends: 19 years of experience in China – 1987 to 2006. PLoS One. 2010;5(8):e12129.

59. Hairi NN, Bulgiba A, Cumming RG, Naganathan V, Mudla I. Prevalence and correlates of physical disability and functional limitation among community dwelling older people in rural Malaysia, a middle income country. BMC Public Health. 2010;10:492.

60. Almazan-Isla J, Comin-Comin M, Damian J, Alcalde-Cabero E, Ruiz C, Franco E, et al. Analysis of disability using WHODAS 2.0 among middle-aged and elderly in Cinco Villas, Spain. Disabil Health J. 2014;7(1):78–87.

61. Iezzoni LI, Kurtz SG, Rao SR. Trends in US adult chronic disability rates over time. Disabil Health J. 2014;7(4):402–12.

62. van Houwelingen AH, Cameron ID, Gussekloo J, Putter H, Kurrle S, de Craen AJ, et al. Disability transitions in the oldest old in the general population; The Leiden 85-plus study. Age (Dordr). 2014;26(1):483–93.

63. Kulmala J, von Bonsdorff MB, Stenholm S, Tormakangas T, von Bonsdorff ME, Nygard CH, et al. Perceived stress symptoms in midlife predict disability in old age: a 28-year prospective cohort study. J Gerontol A Biol Sci Med Sci. 2013;68(8):984–91.

64. Agahi N, Lennartsson C, Kareholt I, Shaw BA. Trajectories of social activities from middle age to old age and late-life disability: a 36-year follow-up. Age Ageing. 2013;42(6):790–3.

65. Deshpande N, Metter EJ, Guralnik J, Bandinelli S, Ferrucci L. Predicting 3-year incident mobility disability in middle-aged and older adults using physical performance tests. Arch Phys Med Rehabil 2013;94(5):994–997.

66. Imai K, Gregg EW, Chen YJ, Zhang P, de Rekeneire N, Williamson DF. The association of BMI with functional status and self-rated health in US adults. Obesity. 2008;16:40240–8.

67. Nosek MA, Robinson-Whelen S, Hughes RB, Petersen NJ, Taylor HB, Bryne MM, et al. Overweight and obesity in women with physical disabilities: Associations with demographic disability characteristics and secondary conditions. Disabil Health J. 2008;1:89–98.

68. Wolinsky FD, Miller TR, Malmstrom TK, Miller JP, Schootman M, Andresen EM, et al. Four-year lower extremity disability trajectories among African American men and women. J Gerontol A Biol Sci Med Sci. 2007;62:525–30.

69. Khoury AJ, Hall A, Andresen E, Zhang J, Ward R, Jarjoura C. The association between chronic disease and physical disability among female Medicaid beneficiaries 18–64 years of age. Disabil Health J. 2013;6(2):141–8.

70. Dunlop DD, Manheim LM, Song J, Lyons JS, Chang RW. Incidence of disability among preretirement adults: the impact of depression. Am J Public Health. 2005;95(11):2003–8.

71. Clarke P, Latham K. Life course health and socioeconomic profiles of Americans aging with disability. Disabil Health J. 2014;7(1 Suppl):S15–22.

72. Wong E, Stevenson C, Backholer K, Woodward M, Shaw JE, Peeters A. Predicting the risk of physical disability in old age using modifiable mid-life risk factors. J Epidemiol Community Health. 2015;69(1):70–6.

73. den Ouden ME, Schuurmans MJ, Brand JS, Arts IE, Mueller-Schotte S, van der Schouw YT. Physical functioning is related to both an impaired physical ability and ADL disability: a ten year follow-up study in middle-aged and older persons. Maturitas. 2013;74(1):89–94.

74. Oliveria SA, Felson DT, Reed JI, Cirillo PA, Walker AM. Incidence of symptomatic hand, hip, and knee osteoarthritis among patients in a health maintenance organization. Arthritis Rheum. 1995;38:1134–41.

75. Matthews KA, Crawford SL, Chae CU, Everson-Rose SA, Sowers MF, Sternfeld B, et al. Are changes in cardiovascular disease risk factors in midlife women due to chronological aging or to the menopausal transition? J Am Coll Cardiol. 2009;54(25):2366–73.

76. Andersson GB. Epidemiological features of chronic low-back pain. Lancet. 1999;354:581–5.

77. Takayanagi Y, Spira AP, Roth KB, Gallo JJ, Eaton WW, Mojtabai R. Accuracy of reports of lifetime mental and physical disorders: results from the Baltimore Epidemiological Catchment Area study. JAMA Psychiatry. 2014;71(3):273–80.

78. Koonce RC, Bravman JT. Obesity and osteoarthritis: more than just wear and tear. J Am Acad Orthop Surg. 2013;21(3):161–9.

79. Okifuji A, Hare BD. The association between chronic pain and obesity. J Pain Res. 2015;8:399–408.

80. Luppino FS, de Wit LM, Bouvy PF, Stijnen T, Cuijpers P, Penninx BW, et al. Overweight, obesity and depression: a systematic review and meta-analysis of longitudinal studies. Arch Gen Psychiatry. 2010;67(3):220–9.

81. Klijs B, Nusselder WJ, Looman CW, Mackenback JP. Contribution of chronic disease to the burden of disability. PLoS One. 2011;6(9):e25325.

82. Sundstrup E, Jakobsen MD, Andersen CH, Jay K, Persson R, Aagaard P, et al. Effect of two contrasting interventions on upper limb chronic pain and disability: a randomized controlled trial. Pain Physician. 2014;17(2):145–54.

83. Linton SJ, Boersma K, Traczyk M, Shaw W, Nicholas M. Early workplace communication and problem solving to prevent back disability: results of a randomized controlled trial among high-risk workers and their supervisors. J Occup Rehabil. 2015. [Epub ahead of print].

84. Del Pozo-Cruz B, Adsuar JC, Parraca J, Del Pozo-Cruz J, Moreno A, Gusi N. A web-based intervention to improve and prevent low back pain among office workers: a randomized controlled trial. J Orthop Sports Phys Ther. 2012;42(10):831–41.

85. Freedman VA, Hodgson N, Lynn J, Spillman B, Waidmann T, Wilkinson A, Wold DA. US Department of Health and Human Services Assistant Secretary for Planning and Evaluation Office of Disability, Aging and Long-Term Care Policy. A framework for identifying high-impact interventions to promote reductions in late-life disability. 2006. Available at http://aspe.hhs.gov/daltcp/reports/2006/prodecl.htm, [accessed 29 April 2015].

86. Daniels R, van Rossum E, de Witte L, Kempen GI, van den Heuvel W. Interventions to prevent disability in frail community-dwelling elderly: a systematic review. BMC Health Serv Res. 2008;8:278.

87. Cesari M, Vellas B, Hsu FC, Newman AB, Doss H, King AC, et al. A physical activity intervention to treat the frailty syndrome in older persons – results from the LIFE-P study. J Gerontol A Biol Sci Med Sci. 2015;70(20):216–22.

88. Pahor M, Guralnik JM, Ambrosius WT, Blair S, Bonds DE, Church TS, et al. Effect of structured physical activity on prevention of major mobility disability in older adults: the LIFE study randomized clinical trial. JAMA. 2014;311(23):2387–96.

89. Gitlin LN, Szanton SL, Huang J, Roth DL. Factors mediating the effects of a depression intervention on functional disability in older African Americans. J Am Geriatr Soc. 2014;62(12):2280–7.

90. Danaei G, Pan A, Hu FB, Hernan MA. Hypothetical midlife interventions in women and risk of type 2 diabetes. Epidemiology. 2013;24(1):122–8.

91. Clark DO, Stump TE, Wolinsky FD. Predictors of onset and recovery from mobility difficulty among adults age 51–61 years. Am J Epidemiol. 1998;148(1):63–71.

# 3

# Rheumatic autoimmune diseases in women and midlife health

Wendy Marder[1,2], Évelyne Vinet[3,4] and Emily C. Somers[1,2,5*]

## Abstract

Autoimmune diseases such as systemic lupus erythematosus (SLE), rheumatoid arthritis (RA), and systemic sclerosis (scleroderma) preferentially affect women, and are characterized by systemic inflammation leading to target organ dysfunction. The public health burden of autoimmune diseases, which collectively represent a leading cause of morbidity and mortality among women throughout adulthood, is substantial. While some features of these diseases have been observed to improve over the menopausal transition, such as disease flare rate in SLE and skin softening and thinning in scleroderma, others, such as swollen and tender joints and radiographically confirmed damage in RA may worsen. The general trends, however, are not consistent or conclusive for all disease-related manifestations. Of great importance is the recognition that comorbid diseases, including osteoporosis and accelerated cardiovascular disease, contribute excess morbidity and mortality that becomes increasingly apparent as women with autoimmune diseases undergo the menopausal transition.

**Keywords:** Autoimmune diseases, Rheumatic diseases, Systemic lupus erythematosus, Rheumatoid arthritis, Scleroderma

## Background

Autoimmune diseases are characterized by systemic inflammation, in which a dysregulated immune system causes damage or dysfunction to target organs. Rheumatic autoimmune diseases include conditions such as systemic lupus erythematosus (SLE), rheumatoid arthritis (RA) and systemic sclerosis (scleroderma), in which the connective tissues (cartilage, joint synovium, skin) are most frequently targeted. Collectively, the autoimmune diseases are estimated to afflict over 7 % of the general population [1]; RA is among the most common autoimmune diseases, with RA prevalence of greater than 1 % of the adult female population in the United States [2]. While rheumatic autoimmune diseases can occur across the lifespan, the typical presentation occurs in mid- or late- adulthood [3]. These diseases are considerably more common in women than in men, with approximately 90 % of prevalent cases being female for SLE and scleroderma, and approximately 75 % for RA [3]. Effective targeted therapies for RA have rapidly expanded over the last decade, leading to improved outcomes, but treatment options for SLE and scleroderma remain largely based on traditional immunosuppressive and anti-inflammatory agents which are associated with a range of toxicities [4]. Major comorbidities for the rheumatic autoimmune diseases include premature cardiovascular disease and osteoporosis, due both to underlying disease and chronic exposure to glucocorticoids [5–7]. Data from the last 15 years have demonstrated that when autoimmune diseases are considered as a group, they rank among the 10 leading causes of death among women under age 75 years [8, 9].

While varying effects of estrogen and other sex hormones have been proposed related to the predisposition and development of autoimmune diseases and their comorbidities, the roles of genetics, environmental factors, and their interactions undoubtedly play significant roles [10]. This review will discuss the epidemiology and clinical features of three systemic rheumatic autoimmune diseases—SLE, RA and scleroderma—in relation to women in midlife.

* Correspondence: emsomers@umich.edu
[1]Division of Rheumatology, Department of Internal Medicine, University of Michigan, Ann Arbor, MI, USA
[2]Department of Obstetrics & Gynecology, University of Michigan, Ann Arbor, MI, USA
Full list of author information is available at the end of the article

## Review

This review is aimed at providing an overview of key topics related to women's midlife health that are thought to have distinct features and implications for women with autoimmune diseases compared to the general population. While not intended to serve as an exhaustive review of the literature, the authors screened and reviewed studies predominantly from the last two decades related to epidemiologic patterns and clinical features of SLE, RA and scleroderma in relation to midlife, with emphasis on large, population-based studies when available, in order to synthesize recurrent themes.

### Epidemiologic overview

It is well-recognized that the majority of autoimmune diseases disproportionately afflict females. This is true for the rheumatic autoimmune diseases, with few exceptions, such as granulomatosis with polyangiitis (formerly termed Wegener's granulomatosis) and vasculitis, which have sex ratios closer to 1:1 [3]. However, for the female-predominant diseases, the magnitude of female preponderance tends to wane in older age groups. In terms of lifestage of greatest risk, a long-held perception has been that SLE and other rheumatic disease are most likely to occur in women during their reproductive years. Recent epidemiologic data have provided the basis for a more nuanced view related to sex-specific patterns of disease, with SLE perhaps serving as the clearest example. A study of SLE incidence during the 1990s in the United Kingdom including 1638 incident cases revealed that among females in this population of predominantly European ancestry, risk of SLE rose steadily with age among females until 50–54 years of age, and thereafter steadily declined; in males, incidence increased steadily until 70–74 years of age before declining [11]. This data-driven observation of peak incidence in females occurring around the time of menopause was a novel finding, and contrasted with the premise of SLE as a "disease of women of childbearing age." More recently, lupus registries from sociodemographically diverse populations in the United States have provided evidence for disparities in the risk of disease in different population subsets [12]. Data from the Michigan Lupus Epidemiology & Surveillance (MILES) Program [13] demonstrate a clear peak in incidence among black females during the 25–29 year age range; the magnitude and young age of peak incidence in this group are striking in comparison to other groups (Fig. 1). White females in the Michigan population experienced highest incidence between the ages of 30 and 34, but their peak was much less distinct and tapered slowly throughout the midlife years. With the younger risk of developing disease among black females, the highest prevalence occurred in midlife, at 40–44 years of age. MILES Registry data has also documented a

higher SLE incidence and younger age of diagnosis in the Arab/Chaldean American population compared to non-Arab/Chaldean American whites, with prevalence among the Arab/Chaldean American population peaking in the 30–39 year age group [14].

Another registry in the United States, focused on the American Indian/Alaska Native population, found high rates of lupus, with incidence among American Indian/Alaska Native females similar to that of black females, and prevalence approximately 1.5 times higher [15]. Peak incidence in the American Indian/Alaska Native population (for females and males combined) occurred in the 40–49 year age span [15]. Together, contemporary SLE epidemiology data underscore varying patterns of risk in different population subsets, but clearly a high burden of disease among women in midlife.

### Primary ovarian insufficiency among women with rheumatic autoimmune diseases

When considering the subject of menopausal timing and its effects among populations of women with rheumatic autoimmune diseases, the possibility of exposure to gonadotoxic therapies used to treat severe manifestations of these conditions must be considered [16]. Potent first line immunosuppressive therapy for target-organ threatening manifestations of autoimmune diseases (e.g., lupus nephritis, systemic vasculitis, scleroderma) has historically been the combination of high dose corticosteroids and a gonadotoxic alkylating agent including cyclophosphamide, chlorambucil and even nitrogen mustard. Many women who received and continue to receive cyclophosphamide for rheumatic diseases, as well as for hematologic and solid organ malignancies, experience irreversible gonadal toxicity as a result of this therapy, leading to primary ovarian insufficiency [17–20]. Primary ovarian insufficiency, also known as premature ovarian failure, is defined as menopause before the age of 40 years [21]. Unlike with natural menopause, which occurs on average around age 50 years, 50 % of women with primary ovarian insufficiency still have variations in ovarian function and 5–10 % conceive following this diagnosis [22, 23]. There is lack of evidence that assisted reproductive technologies have efficacy in this population [23].

A major focus over the past two decades has been the development of alternate therapeutic regimens that minimize cyclophosphamide exposure in this patient population, as well as the use of adjuvant therapy such as with gonadotropin-releasing hormone analogues (e.g., leuprolide acetate), to preserve ovarian function during cyclophosphamide therapy [24]. Practice has evolved in recent years towards increased utilization of less toxic immunosuppressive therapies such as rituximab and mycophenolate mofetil in vasculitis and lupus nephritis

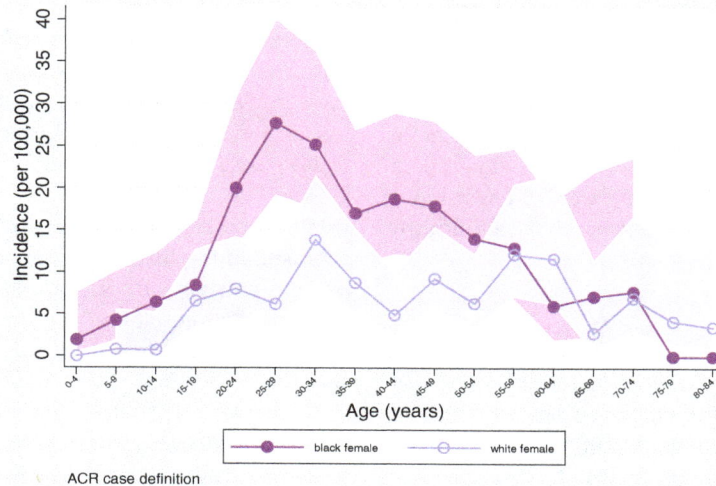

**Fig. 1** SLE incidence data from the Michigan Lupus Epidemiology & Surveillance (MILES) Program Registry [13]. SLE was defined according to the American College of Rheumatology (ACR) classification criteria for SLE [69, 70]

respectively, as well as the adoption of lower-dose cyclophosphamide regimens (e.g., "Euro-Lupus" [25, 26]) for treating many cases of lupus nephritis. In addition to the increase in widespread off-label use of gonadotropin-releasing hormone analogues during cyclophosphamide therapy, these changes in standard of care therapy are allowing for rheumatic disease patients to achieve natural menopause at a rate that may soon mirror that of the general public.

## Systemic lupus erythematosus

SLE is a chronic, systemic inflammatory disease with a waxing and waning course, that can affect multiple organs, with the kidneys, joints, and skin most commonly involved. Symptoms can range from mild, including photosensitive rashes, mucosal ulcerations, and pleurisy, to severe and even life threatening, with rapidly progressive glomerular nephritis, central nervous system inflammation or hemolytic anemia. Lupus is classically considered an autoantibody-mediated disease, with evidence of immune complex deposition seen in renal and dermal biopsies of patients with active disease. Lupus patients also have heightened risk of cardiovascular disease that is not explained by traditional Framingham risk factors [27, 28], due at least in part to disease associated endothelial dysfunction that contributes to the accelerated atherosclerotic disease that also characterizes SLE [29–31]. Long-term studies of lupus outcomes have therefore included several means of quantifying disease. For example, the Systemic Lupus Erythematosus Disease Activity Index (SLEDAI) [32] is a widely used tool that measures recent

disease activity, incorporating clinical history, physical exam and laboratory findings. The "SLICC/ACR" Damage Index [33] is used in lupus patients to quantify cumulative damage in 12 different target organs over time regardless of etiology; notably, it captures disease burden induced by cardiovascular disease, osteoporosis due to prolonged corticosteroid use and chronic inflammation, and the additive sequelae of premature menopause due to gonadotoxic therapy.

As stated previously, SLE incidence for women of predominantly European ancestry has been observed to rise steadily with age until the 50s, and decline thereafter. Multiple population based studies support the observation that the clinical course and disease manifestations of SLE are different if the disease onset occurs after natural menopause. Some studies have described a milder course associated with later disease onset, with general observations of less renal and mucocutaneous involvement, but higher rates of interstitial lung disease, neurologic complications and sicca symptoms [34–38]. Other studies have noted no difference in the clinical course of SLE between these two populations [39, 40]. However, data from a longitudinal and multiethnic cohort of 73 women with late-onset SLE (onset at age ≥ 50 years) and 144 matched women with earlier onset SLE found late-onset SLE to be independently associated with both damage (measured by the "SLICC/ACR" Damage Index [33]; OR 23.3, 95 % CI 4.0–141.6) and mortality (OR 10.7, 95 % CI 3.1–37.6) [37]. Thus, while in general it seems that most studies support a more mild course of lupus activity in later onset disease, the accrual of lupus damage as reflected in part by comorbid disease is probably greater in this group [41].

Varying degrees of improvement in lupus disease activity have been observed after women go through hormone withdrawal, whether due to natural menopause, hysterectomy or primary ovarian insufficiency after cyclophosphamide [41–44]. Although heterogeneous and somewhat difficult to compare given differences in age of the study populations and duration of follow-up, in general the research supports a trend toward fewer lupus disease flares after hormone withdrawal, but significantly more damage accrual.

### Rheumatoid arthritis

RA is a systemic disease that can lead to erosive, destructive joint damage, as well as "extra-articular" disease involving not just the joints, but target organ tissues of the body including the lungs, blood vessels, eyes and nervous system. This is particularly true for those people who are "seropositive" for the characteristic autoantibodies of rheumatoid factor and anti-cyclic citrullinated peptide antibodies. As mentioned above, RA is also associated with excess mortality compared with the general population, which is predominantly due to accelerated atherosclerotic cardiovascular disease [45–47]. As is true with antinuclear antibody positive diseases, RA preferentially affects women, in ratios around 4:1 [48], and has a peak incidence in females following menopause (age 55–64 years), a full two decades prior to age of peak incidence in men (75–84 years) [48]. Interestingly, the female-to-male incidence ratio after age 60 years is approximately 1:1, potentially implicating changes in sex hormones in the development of RA [49]. A disease with waxing and waning activity, RA is clearly influenced by sex hormones throughout adult life: multiple population-based studies have found that women with RA have a lower mean age at menopause compared to controls [50–52] and a pattern of RA symptom improvement or even remission during pregnancy is well recognized [50].

What is less well understood, however, is the role of gonadal hormones in both the risk for developing the disease, as well as the timing and severity of its manifestations. Observational studies that have assessed menopause by patient self-report, with variable lengths of recall, do not uniformly specify surgical or non-surgical menopause among their study populations, and have produced conflicting results. For example, a prospective cohort study of 31,336 women in Iowa, aged 55 to 69 years at cohort baseline and followed for 11 years, revealed 158 incident cases of RA, with age at last pregnancy and age at menopause each significantly inversely associated with RA [53]. In this study, no effect was found related to onset of menarche, oral contraceptive use or hysterectomy/oophorectomy, though those women who underwent later menopause (after age 51 years) were

at decreased risk of developing RA compared to those who underwent menopause at or below age 45. However, a recent study, in which a group of 534 patients in a Canadian inception cohort of RA patients were divided into an "early menopause" (mean age 38.5 years) and "usual menopause" group (mean age 51.7 years), the age of RA disease onset was found to be similar between the groups [54]. Furthermore, the early menopause patients were more likely to be rheumatoid factor positive, a characteristic of the disease that is known to impart increased risk of erosive joint disease as well as extra-articular, systemic manifestations (e.g., vasculitis, interstitial lung disease). This study did include persons who underwent surgical menopause. In contrast, a subsequent study of 134 women with RA and earlier menopause (age <45 years) revealed that these women had more mild-moderate disease, and more rheumatoid factor negative disease, than women who underwent later menopause [52]; it is unclear if women who underwent surgical menopause were excluded from the earlier menopause group. It is therefore difficult to interpret these results other than to restate the observation that, like other autoimmune diseases, the role of sex hormones is significant but complex, and clearly not fully elucidated. However, general observations about the impact of menopause in this patient population are not in dispute. The heightened risk of accelerated cardiovascular disease [55], excessive bone density loss due to long-term corticosteroid therapy, and the possibility of primary ovarian insufficiency due to previous exposure to gonadotoxic therapies, in the context of ongoing underlying systemic inflammatory diseases, all confound the care and management of these patients as they age, and should prompt vigilance on the part of caregivers to address any modifiable risk factors associated with these conditions.

RA disease activity is typically measured using the 28-joint count disease activity scale (DAS-28) [56], an assessment of progression of bone X-ray changes, and patient-reported health assessment questionnaires. The largest study to address the effect of menopausal transition on RA was conducted in a cohort of early RA patients using these measures. Post-menopausal women in this cohort (n = 109) were found to have more significant joint damage on X-ray, in addition to higher scores on the DAS-28 and health assessment scores both at baseline and at 6-year follow-up, when compared to pre-menopausal women (n = 64) and age-matched men (n = 85) [51]. The menopausal state in this study was thought to be a primary factor underlying the differences observed between these groups of RA patients.

### Systemic sclerosis (or scleroderma)

Scleroderma is an inflammatory disease that causes vasculopathy and fibrosis and scarring in multiple target organs, including the vasculature, lungs, gastrointestinal tract and skin. Skin thickening is a defining feature of scleroderma, which is characterized by excessive production of extracellular matrix proteins (e.g., collagen, laminin, fibronectin) by skin fibroblasts [57]. The peak incidence of scleroderma is in the fifth and sixth decades, and scleroderma predominantly affects women (with a female-to-male ratios ranging from 3:1 to 14:1) [58].

In the general population, menopause is characterized by a low estrogenic state and is associated with skin thinning due to decreased extracellular matrix protein deposition by fibroblasts [59]. Although thinning of the dermis often accompanies aging, most studies suggest that collagen loss is more closely related to postmenopausal status than chronologic age, reflecting hormonal changes [60]. Investigators have observed a mean decline in dermal collagen of approximately 1–2 % per year after menopause [61]. Estrogen supplementation in postmenopausal women has been reported to improve skin thickness by increasing skin collagen content [62].

Although scleroderma most commonly occurs near the end of the reproductive period and predominantly affects women, there has been only one study investigating the impact of menopause on skin thickening in women with scleroderma [58]. Investigators, using previously collected data from 1070 women with scleroderma enrolled within the Canadian Scleroderma Research Group (CSRG) cohort, found that postmenopausal status in women with diffuse scleroderma was associated with a substantially lower mean modified Rodnan Skin Score, a validated measure of skin thickening, compared to premenopausal status (effect estimate of −2.62 units, 95 % CI −4.44, −0.80) [58]. This effect was independent of age, follow-up time, and disease duration. However, postmenopausal status had a smaller effect on skin thickening in women with limited scleroderma compared to women with diffuse scleroderma (effect estimate of −0.58 units, 95 % CI −1.50, 0.34).

The findings from this study are supported by previous experimental evidence showing that estrogen increases extracellular matrix protein production in skin fibroblast cultures of scleroderma patients [62]. In addition, an estrogen-receptor inhibitor (i.e., tamoxifen) induced a significant decrease of these extracellular matrix proteins in cultures of scleroderma skin fibroblasts [62]. Moreover, it is well-established that estrogen stimulates normal skin fibroblasts to produce transforming growth factor-beta 1, as well as monocytes and macrophages to produce platelet-derived growth factor, which are both key profibrotic cytokines in scleroderma skin disease [57, 63]. As scleroderma skin fibroblasts show increased expression of transforming growth factor-beta 1 receptor and platelet-derived growth factor receptor, the study

investigators postulated that estrogen might play a role in scleroderma pathogenesis through its stimulatory effect on these two cytokines [58].

Furthermore, early menopause in women with scleroderma may contribute adverse lowering of bone mineral density in affected women, though the competing effects of underlying systemic inflammation and long term treatment with corticosteroids make it difficult to assess the relative impact of early menopause. Several studies have shown a potentially reduced bone mineral density in women with scleroderma compared to control women. A recent systematic literature review summarized data about the prevalence of low bone mineral density and its risk factors in scleroderma [64]. The search resulted in ten studies, which reported a lower bone mineral density in patients with scleroderma compared to matched controls, while two studies reported no difference. Potential risk factors for low bone mineral density in women with scleroderma included early age at menopause, as well as traditional risks factors such as family history of osteoporosis, age, low vitamin D levels, in addition to disease-related factors such as diffuse disease subtype, presence of internal organ involvement, and calcinosis. However, early menopause was inconsistently assessed across included studies, which makes it difficult to draw firm conclusions about the significance and size of its effect on bone mineral density in scleroderma women [64].

As mentioned previously, vasculopathy is an important disease-related manifestation in scleroderma. Since estrogen has well-established beneficial effects on the vascular system, the low estrogenic state associated with menopause has been suggested to aggravate vascular manifestations in scleroderma women [65]. In a retrospective cohort study of 189 scleroderma women with neither pulmonary arterial hypertension nor interstitial lung disease at baseline, investigators assessed the effect of postmenopausal status on the risk of isolated pulmonary arterial hypertension. During a mean follow-up of 15.9 years [standard deviation (SD) 11.3], 63 (33 %) women developed isolated pulmonary arterial hypertension. Postmenopausal status was significantly associated with more than a 5-fold increase in the risk of isolated pulmonary arterial hypertension, accounting for disease and human leukocyte antigen (HLA) subtypes [66]. Furthermore, another retrospective cohort study from the same group evaluated the effect of hormone replacement therapy on the risk of isolated pulmonary arterial hypertension in females with scleroderma [67]. Sixty-one postmenopausal women with limited scleroderma and without evidence of isolated pulmonary arterial hypertension or interstitial lung disease at cohort entry were studied. Among these, 23 were treated with hormone replacement therapy for a mean of 6.7 years (SD 3.7), of whom none developed isolated pulmonary arterial hypertension during follow-up. However, among the 41 women unexposed to hormone replacement therapy, 8 (20 %) developed isolated pulmonary arterial hypertension over a similar period of follow-up. This difference was not accounted for by age, autoantibody profile, lung diffusing capacity at menopause onset, or calcium channel blocker use. The investigators concluded that hormone replacement therapy might prevent the onset of isolated pulmonary arterial hypertension in patients with limited scleroderma.

Observational studies have also reported a higher prevalence of atherosclerotic cardiovascular disease in scleroderma patients in comparison to healthy individuals, with its presence being associated with poorer prognosis [68]. The mechanisms leading to increased atherosclerosis in scleroderma are not completely understood, but some have proposed endothelial dysfunction due to inflammation and vasculopathy, which might potentially interact with traditional risk factors, including age and menopause, as important contributing factors [68].

Although the menopause-related decline in estrogen appears to have a beneficial effect on skin thickening in scleroderma, it might have an adverse effect on the pulmonary arterial vasculature as well as atherosclerotic cardiovascular disease in affected women. Observational studies of menopause in women with scleroderma highlight the pleiotropic role that estrogen might play in scleroderma pathophysiology and prompt further research to better understand its complexity.

## Conclusions

It is difficult to disentangle the true impact of reproductive aging on the natural history of rheumatic autoimmune diseases. However, what seems clear is that the effects of major comorbidities associated with aging, which are likely accelerated in rheumatic autoimmune diseases, are magnified as these women approach midlife and beyond. This is due in part to the compounding effects of the underlying diseases and their treatments, such as long-term corticosteroid use and gonadotoxic immunosuppression, in addition to recognized vascular endothelial dysfunction that exists across the spectrum of these diseases. The public health burden of autoimmune diseases, which collectively represent a leading cause of morbidity and mortality among women throughout adulthood, is substantial. Their impact on women's health becomes even more complex through menopause. With greater numbers of these patients achieving longer lives due to therapeutic advances, ascertaining the true impact of menopause on rheumatic autoimmune disease should be considered a priority for women's health.

## Competing interests
The authors declare that they have no competing interests.

## Authors' contributions
All authors participated in the design and drafting of this review, and approved the final manuscript.

## Acknowledgements
This work was funded in part by the following: K12HD001438 from the National Institutes of Health (NIH)/Office of Research on Women's Health; K01ES019909 from NIH/National Institute of Environmental Health Sciences; and 5U01-DP3250 from the Centers for Disease Control and Prevention (CDC). Its contents are solely the responsibility of the authors and do not necessarily represent the official views of the NIH, CDC, or Department of Health and Human Services.

## Author details
[1]Division of Rheumatology, Department of Internal Medicine, University of Michigan, Ann Arbor, MI, USA. [2]Department of Obstetrics & Gynecology, University of Michigan, Ann Arbor, MI, USA. [3]Division of Rheumatology, McGill University Health Centre, Montreal, Canada. [4]Division of Clinical Epidemiology, McGill University Health Centre, Montreal, Canada. [5]Department of Environmental Health Sciences, University of Michigan, 2800 Plymouth Rd, NCRC B14-G236, Ann Arbor, MI 48109-2800, USA.

## References
1. Cooper GS, Bynum MLK, Somers EC. Recent insights in the epidemiology of autoimmune diseases: improved prevalence estimates and understanding of clustering of diseases. J Autoimmun. 2009;33:197–207.
2. Gabriel SE. The epidemiology of rheumatoid arthritis. Rheum Dis Clin North Am. 2001;27:269–81.
3. Cooper GS, Stroehla BC. The epidemiology of autoimmune diseases. Autoimmun Rev. 2003;2:119–25.
4. Marder W, McCune WJ. Advances in immunosuppressive drug therapy for use in autoimmune disease and systemic vasculitis. Semin Respir Crit Care Med. 2004;25(5):581–94.
5. Wasko MCM. Comorbid conditions in patients with rheumatic diseases: an update. Curr Opin Rheumatol. 2004;16:109–13.
6. Pineau CA, Urowitz MB, Fortin PJ, Ibanez D, Gladman DD. Osteoporosis in systemic lupus erythematosus: factors associated with referral for bone mineral density studies, prevalence of osteoporosis and factors associated with reduced bone density. Lupus. 2004;13:436–41.
7. Manzi S, Meilahn EN, Rairie JE, Conte CG, Medsger TA, Jansen-McWilliams L, et al. Age-specific incidence rates of myocardial infarction and angina in women with systemic lupus erythematosus: comparison with the Framingham Study. Am J Epidemiol. 1997;145:408–15.
8. Walsh SJ, Rau LM. Autoimmune diseases: a leading cause of death among young and middle-aged women in the United States. Am J Public Health. 2000;90:1463–6.
9. Thomas SL, Griffiths C, Smeeth L, Rooney C, Hall AJ. Burden of mortality associated with autoimmune diseases among females in the United Kingdom. Am J Public Health. 2010;100:2279–87.
10. Somers EC, Richardson BC. Environmental exposures, epigenetic changes and the risk of lupus. Lupus. 2014;23:568–76.
11. Somers EC, Thomas SL, Smeeth L, Schooen WM, Hall AJ. Incidence of systemic lupus erythematosus in the United Kingdom, 1990–1999. Arthritis Rheum. 2007;57:612–8.
12. Lim SS, Drenkard C, McCune WJ, Helmick CG, Gordon C, Deguire P, et al. Population-based lupus registries: advancing our epidemiologic understanding. Arthritis Rheum. 2009;61:1462–6.
13. Somers EC, Marder W, Cagnoli P, Lewis EE, DeGuire P, Gordon C, et al. Population-based incidence and prevalence of systemic lupus erythematosus: the Michigan lupus epidemiology and surveillance program. Arthritis Rheumatol. 2014;66:369–78.
14. Housey M, DeGuire P, Lyon-Callo S, Wang L, Marder W, McCune WJ, et al. Incidence and prevalence of systemic lupus erythematosus among Arab and Chaldean Americans in Southeastern Michigan: the Michigan Lupus Epidemiology and Surveillance Program. Am J Public Health. 2015;105(5):e74–9.

15. Ferucci ED, Johnston JM, Gaddy JR, Sumner L, Posever JO, Choromanski TL, et al. Prevalence and incidence of systemic lupus erythematosus in a population-based registry of american Indian and alaska native people, 2007–2009. Arthritis Rheumatol (Hoboken, NJ). 2014;66:2494–502.

16. Marder W, Fisseha S, Ganser MA, Somers EC. Ovarian damage during chemotherapy in autoimmune diseases: broad health implications beyond fertility. Clin Med insights Reprod Heal. 2012;2012:9–18.

17. Boumpas DT, Austin HA, Vaughan EM, Yarboro CH, Klippel JH, Balow JE. Risk for sustained amenorrhea in patients with systemic lupus erythematosus receiving intermittent pulse cyclophosphamide therapy. Ann Intern Med. 1993;119:366–9.

18. Blumenfeld Z, Shapiro D, Shteinberg M, Avivi I, Nahir M. Preservation of fertility and ovarian function and minimizing gonadotoxicity in young women with systemic lupus erythematosus treated by chemotherapy. Lupus. 2000;9(6):401–5.

19. Koyama H, Wada T, Nishizawa Y, Iwanaga T, Aoki Y. Cyclophosphamide-induced ovarian failure and its therapeutic significance in patients with breast cancer. Cancer. 1977;39:1403–9.

20. Hoffman GS, Kerr GS, Leavitt RY, Hallahan CW, Lebovics RS, Travis WD, et al. Wegener granulomatosis: an analysis of 158 patients. Ann Intern Med. 1992;116(6):488–98.

21. Nelson LM. Clinical practice. Primary ovarian insufficiency. N Engl J Med. 2009;360:606–14.

22. Rebar RW, Connolly HV. Clinical features of young women with hypergonadotropic amenorrhea. Fertil Steril. 1990;53:804–10.

23. Van Kasteren YM, Schoemaker J. Premature ovarian failure: a systematic review on therapeutic interventions to restore ovarian function and achieve pregnancy. Hum Reprod Update. 1999;5(5):483–92.

24. Somers EC, Marder W, Christman GM, Ognenovski V, McCune WJ. Use of a gonadotropin-releasing hormone analog for protection against premature ovarian failure during cyclophosphamide therapy in women with severe lupus. Arthritis Rheum. 2005;52:2761–7.

25. Houssiau FA, Vasconcelos C, D'Cruz D, Sebastiani GD, De Ramon Garrido E, Danieli MG, et al. Immunosuppressive therapy in lupus nephritis: the Euro-Lupus Nephritis Trial, a randomized trial of low-dose versus high-dose intravenous cyclophosphamide. Arthritis Rheum. 2002;46:2121–31.

26. Wofsy D, Diamond B, Houssiau FA. Commentary: crossing the Atlantic: the Euro-Lupus Nephritis Regimen in North America. Arthritis Rheumatol. 2015;67:1144–6.

27. Ward MM. Premature morbidity from cardiovascular and cerebrovascular diseases in women with systemic lupus erythematosus. Arthritis Rheum. 1999;42:338–46.

28. Esdaile JM, Abrahamowicz M, Grodzicky T, Li Y, Panaritis C, Du Berger R, et al. Traditional Framingham risk factors fail to fully account for accelerated atherosclerosis in systemic lupus erythematosus. Arthritis Rheum. 2001;44:2331–7.

29. Denny MF, Thacker S, Mehta H, Somers EC, Dodick T, Barrat FJ, et al. Interferon-α promotes abnormal vasculogenesis in lupus: a potential pathway for premature atherosclerosis. Blood. 2007;110:2907–15.

30. Somers EC, Marder W, Kaplan MJ, Brook RD, McCune WJ. Plasminogen activator inhibitor-1 is associated with impaired endothelial function in women with systemic lupus erythematosus. Ann N Y Acad Sci. 2005;1051:271–80.

31. Somers EC, Zhao W, Lewis EE, Wang L, Wing JJ, Sundaram B, et al. Type I interferons are associated with subclinical markers of cardiovascular disease in a cohort of systemic lupus erythematosus patients. PLoS One. 2012;7:e37000.

32. Bombardier C, Gladman DD, Urowitz MB, Caron D, Chang CH. Derivation of the SLEDAI. A disease activity index for lupus patients. The Committee on Prognosis Studies in SLE. Arthritis Rheum. 1992;35:630–40.

33. Gladman DD, Goldsmith CH, Urowitz MB, Bacon P, Fortin P, Ginzler E, et al. The Systemic Lupus International Collaborating Clinics/American College of Rheumatology (SLICC/ACR) Damage Index for systemic lupus erythematosus international comparison. J Rheumatol. 2000;27:373–6.

34. Font J, Pallarés L, Cervera R, López-Soto A, Navarro M, Bosch X, et al. Systemic lupus erythematosus in the elderly: clinical and immunological characteristics. Ann Rheum Dis. 1991;50:702–5.

35. Ho CT, Mok CC, Lau CS, Wong RW. Late onset systemic lupus erythematosus in southern Chinese. Ann Rheum Dis. 1998;57:437–40.

36. Wojdyla D, Jacobelli S, Massardo L, Chaco R, Alvarellos A, Saurit V, et al. Late-onset systemic lupus erythematosus in Latin Americans : a distinct subgroup ? 2014. p. 1–8.

37. Bertoli AM, Alarcón GS, Calvo-Alén J, Fernández M, Vilá LM, Reveille JD. Systemic lupus erythematosus in a multiethnic US cohort. XXXIII. Clinical [corrected] features, course, and outcome in patients with late-onset disease. Arthritis Rheum. 2006;54:1580–7.

38. Formiga F, Moga I, Pac M, Mitjavila F, Rivera A, Pujol R. Mild presentation of systemic lupus erythematosus in elderly patients assessed by SLEDAI. SLE Disease Activity Index. Lupus. 1999;8:462–5.

39. Padovan M, Govoni M, Castellino G, Rizzo N, Fotinidi M, Trotta F. Late onset systemic lupus erythematosus: no substantial differences using different cut-off ages. Rheumatol Int. 2007;27:735–41.

40. Sayarlioglu M, Cefle A, Kamali S, Gul A, Inanc M, Ocal L, et al. Characteristics of patients with late onset systemic lupus erythematosus in Turkey. Int J Clin Pract. 2005;59:183–7.

41. Urowitz MB, Ibañez D, Jerome D, Gladman DD. The effect of menopause on disease activity in systemic lupus erythematosus. J Rheumatol. 2006;33:2192–8.

42. Mok CC, Lau CS, Ho CTK, Wong RWS. Do ̄ ares of systemic lupus erythematosus decline after menopause ? 1999. p. 357–62.

43. Sánchez-Guerrero J. Disease activity during the premenopausal and postmenopausal periods in women with systemic lupus erythematosus. Am J Med. 2001;111:464–8.

44. Mok CC, Wong RW, Lau CS. Ovarian failure and flares of systemic lupus erythematosus. Arthritis Rheum. 1999;42:1274–80.

45. Goodson N, Symmons D. Rheumatoid arthritis in women: still associated with an increased mortality. Ann Rheum Dis. 2002;61:955–6.

46. Goodson NJ, Wiles NJ, Lunt M, Barrett EM, Silman AJ, Symmons DPM. Mortality in early inflammatory polyarthritis: cardiovascular mortality is increased in seropositive patients. Arthritis Rheum. 2002;46:2010–9.

47. Solomon DH, Karlson EW, Rimm EB, Cannuscio CC, Mandl LA, Manson JE, et al. Cardiovascular morbidity and mortality in women diagnosed with rheumatoid arthritis. Circulation. 2003;107:1303–7.

48. Doran MF, Pond GR, Crowson CS, O'Fallon WM, Gabriel SE. Trends in incidence and mortality in rheumatoid arthritis in Rochester, Minnesota, over a forty-year period. Arthritis Rheum. 2002;46:625–31.

49. Goemaere S, Ackerman C, Goethals K, De Keyser F, Van Der Straeten C, Verbruggen G, et al. Onset of symptoms of rheumatoid arthritis in relation to age, sex and menopausal transition. J Rheumatol. 1990;17:1620–2.

50. De Man Y, Dolhain RJEM, van de Geijn FE, Willemsen SP, Hazes JMW. Disease activity of rheumatoid arthritis during pregnancy: results from a nationwide prospective study. Arthritis Rheum. 2008;59:1241–8.

51. Kuiper S, Van Gestel AM, Swinkels HL, De Boo TM, Da Silva JAP, Van Riel PLCM. Influence of sex, age, and menopausal state on the course of early rheumatoid arthritis. J Rheumatol. 2001;28:1809–16.

52. Pikwer M, Nilsson J-A, Bergstrom U, Jacobsson LT, Turesson C. Early menopause and severity of rheumatoid arthritis in women over 45 years of age. Arthritis Res Ther. 2012;14:R190.

53. Merlino LA, Cerhan JR, Criswell LA, Mikuls TR, Saag KG. Estrogen and other female reproductive risk factors are not strongly associated with the development of rheumatoid arthritis in elderly women. Semin Arthritis Rheum. 2003;33:72–82.

54. Wong LE, Huang W-T, Pope JE, Haraoui B, Boire G, Thorne JC, et al. Effect of age at menopause on disease presentation in early rheumatoid arthritis: results from the Canadian Early Arthritis Cohort. Arthritis Care Res (Hoboken). 2015;67(5):616–23.

55. Bertone-Johnson ER, Manson JE. Early menopause and subsequent cardiovascular disease. Menopause. 2015;22:1–3.

56. Prevoo MLL, Van'T Hof MA, Kuper HH, Van Leeuwen MA, Van De Putte LBA, Van Riel PLCM. Modified disease activity scores that include twenty-eight-joint counts: development and validation in a prospective longitudinal study of patients with rheumatoid arthritis. Arthritis Rheum. 1995;38:44–8.

57. Gabrielli A, Avvedimento EV, Krieg T. Scleroderma. N Engl J Med. 2009;360:1989–2003.

58. Vinet E, Bernatsky S, Hudson M, Pineau C, Baron M. Effect of menopause on the modified Rodnan skin score in systemic sclerosis. Arthritis Res Ther. 2014;16:R130.

59. Soldano S, Montagna P, Brizzolara R, Sulli A, Parodi A, Seriolo B, et al. Effects of estrogens on extracellular matrix synthesis in cultures of human normal and scleroderma skin fibroblasts. Ann N Y Acad Sci. 2010;1193:25–9.

60. Hall G, Phillips TJ. Estrogen and skin: the effects of estrogen, menopause, and hormone replacement therapy on the skin. J Am Acad Dermatol. 2005;53:555–68. quiz 569–72.

61. Brincat M, Kabalan S, Studd JW, Moniz CF, de Trafford J, Montgomery J. A study of the decrease of skin collagen content, skin thickness, and bone mass in the postmenopausal woman. Obstet Gynecol. 1987;70:840–5.

62. Maheux R, Naud F, Rioux M, Grenier R, Lemay A, Guy J, et al. A randomized, double-blind, placebo-controlled study on the effect of conjugated estrogens on skin thickness. Am J Obstet Gynecol. 1994;170(2):642–9.

63. Kanda N, Watanabe S. Regulatory roles of sex hormones in cutaneous biology and immunology. J Dermatol Sci. 2005;38(1):1–7.

64. Omair MA, Pagnoux C, McDonald-Blumer H, Johnson SR. Low bone density in systemic sclerosis. A systematic review. J Rheumatol. 2013;40:1881–90.

65. Sammaritano LR. Menopause in patients with autoimmune diseases. Autoimmun Rev. 2012;11:A430–6.

66. Scorza R, Caronni M, Bazzi S, Nador F, Beretta L, Antonioli R, et al. Post-menopause is the main risk factor for developing isolated pulmonary hypertension in systemic sclerosis. Ann N Y Acad Sci. 2002;966:238–46.

67. Beretta L, Caronni M, Origgi L, Ponti A, Santaniello A, Scorza R. Hormone replacement therapy may prevent the development of isolated pulmonary hypertension in patients with systemic sclerosis and limited cutaneous involvement. Scand J Rheumatol. 2006;35:468–71.

68. Cannarile F, Valentini V, Mirabelli G, Alunno A, Terenzi R, Luccioli F, et al. Cardiovascular disease in systemic sclerosis. Ann Transl Med. 2015;3:1–11.

69. Tan EM, Cohen AS, Fries JF, Masi AT, McShane DJ, Rothfield NF, et al. The 1982 revised criteria for the classification of systemic lupus erythematosus. Arthritis Rheum. 1982;25:1271–7.

70. Hochberg MC. Updating the American College of Rheumatology revised criteria for the classification of systemic lupus erythematosus. Arthritis Rheum. 1997;40:1725.

# 4

# Chronic vulvar pain in a cohort of post-menopausal women: Atrophy or Vulvodynia?

Susanna D. Mitro[1], Siobán D. Harlow[1*], John F. Randolph[2] and Barbara D. Reed[2]

## Abstract

**Background:** Although postmenopausal vulvar pain is frequently attributed to vaginal atrophy, such symptoms may be due to vulvodynia, a chronic vulvar pain condition. Given the limited research on vulvodynia in postmenopausal women, the objective of this study was to provide preliminary population-based data on the associations of vaginal symptoms, serum hormone levels and hormone use with chronic vulvar pain in a multiethnic sample of post-menopausal women.

**Methods:** We used data from 371 participants at the Michigan site of the Study of Women's Health Across the Nation (SWAN) who participated in the 13th follow-up visit. Women completed a validated screening instrument for vulvodynia and provided information on additional vaginal symptoms as well as demographic characteristics, and hormone use by questionnaire. Blood samples were obtained to assess hormone levels. We compared women who screened positive for vulvodynia and women with past or short-duration vulvar pain to women without vulvar pain, using Chi-squared and Fisher's Exact tests. Relative odds ratios and 95 % confidence intervals were calculated using multinomial logistic regression models adjusting for age, body mass index, and race/ethnicity.

**Results:** Current chronic vulvar pain consistent with vulvodynia was reported by 4.0 % of women, while 13.7 % reported past but not current chronic vulvar pain or short-duration vulvar pain symptoms. One quarter of women who reported current chronic vulvar pain did not report vaginal dryness. Women with current chronic and with past/short duration vulvar pain symptoms were more likely to have used hormones during the preceding year than women without vulvar pain symptoms (13.3 %, 17.6 %, 2.0 %, respectively; *p* < .01). Increased relative odds of current vulvar pain symptoms were associated with each log unit decrease in serum dehydroepiandrosterone-sulfate, estradiol and testosterone levels at the previous year's visit.

**Conclusion:** Some women who experience chronic vulvar pain symptoms do not report vaginal dryness, and others report continued or first onset of pain while using hormones. Vulvodynia should be considered in the differential diagnosis of postmenopausal women presenting with vulvar pain symptoms.

## Background

Although vulvar pain symptoms can occur at any time over the life span, it is not uncommon for symptoms to begin for the first time after menopause [1–3]. In fact, the prevalence of chronic vulvar pain in mid-life women has been estimated to be 8.9-38 % percent, making chronic vulvar pain a major health concern for women in this age group [4, 5]. However, despite recognition of the burden of chronic vulvar pain symptoms in the mid-life, research on vulvodynia, a chronic pain condition characterized by pain in the vulva, has mainly focused on premenopausal women [1, 2].

Until recently, research on postmenopausal vulvar pain symptoms has largely focused on vaginal dryness and vulvar atrophy, secondary to estrogen deprivation. However, evidence indicates that postmenopausal vulvar pain may occur for other reasons as well [6–9]. Additionally, women with atrophy do not all experience pain [7], episodes of postmenopausal vulvar pain are not all successfully treated using estrogen therapy [8, 9], and in a

* Correspondence: harlow@umich.edu
[1]Department of Epidemiology, School of Public Health, 1415 Washington Heights, Ann Arbor, MI 48109, USA
Full list of author information is available at the end of the article

recent study serum estradiol, estrone, and progesterone levels of postmenopausal women were not tightly correlated with vulvar pain [3]. These findings suggest that some vulvar pain reported by postmenopausal women may be a condition other than atrophy, such as vulvodynia, and present independent of estrogen-or atrophy-related changes.

This paper evaluates chronic vulvar pain reported by African American and white women participating in the Michigan site of the longitudinal, multiethnic Study of Women's Health Across the Nation (SWAN). Although the sample size is limited, prospective measurements of age at final menstrual period, symptoms of vaginal dryness, and hormone therapy (HT) use, as well as serum hormone levels obtained prior to the assessment of current pain status, provide preliminary data on the estimated prevalence of chronic vulvar pain, consistent with vulvodynia in post-menopausal women and its association with hormones, HT use and vaginal dryness in this population-based sample of postmenopausal women.

## Methods

This study used data from the Michigan site of SWAN, a multiethnic prospective cohort study addressing health-related changes in the midlife and menopausal transition. The cohort has been described in detail previously [10]. Briefly, in 1996, each SWAN clinic site enrolled white women and one targeted minority population. The Michigan SWAN population, established using a community census, was composed of women aged 42–52 years at baseline, who were not using exogenous hormones at the time of enrollment, had an intact uterus and at least one ovary and had had a menstrual period in the three months before enrollment, were not pregnant or lactating, and self-identified as either white or African American. At baseline and each follow-up visit a blood sample was collected, height and weight measures were taken while demographic characteristics, medication use, and symptoms of vaginal dryness were ascertained by questionnaire. Over the next 17 years women participated in follow-up visits approximately annually. At the 13th follow-up visit in 2012, the Michigan site added several screening instruments for chronic pain conditions including a validated screening instrument for vulvodynia [11].

At baseline, the Michigan SWAN cohort was composed of 543 women, 60 % of whom were African American by design. In 2012, 32 (5.9 %) women had died and 411 (80.4 % of the non-deceased cohort) were still active, 380 (92.5 %) of whom participated in follow-up Visit 13. Nine women who did not answer any questions pertaining to vulvar pain were excluded, leaving 371 womeN (61.7 % African American) eligible for this analysis. For analyses including endogenous serum hormone levels, we evaluated hormone levels at Visit 12, to ensure hormone levels preceded the report of vulvar pain status at Visit 13. These analyses include 319 women as we excluded the 37 women who did not have blood drawn and the 15 women who reported HT use at Visit 12.

### Ethics and consent

This study was approved by Health Sciences and Behavioral Sciences Institutional Review Board of the University of MichigaN (HUM00083308). Women provided informed consent at baseline and each follow-up interview.

In Visit 13, Michigan participants completed a validated screening questionnaire for vulvodynia [11] that obtained information on symptoms of vulvar pain or discomfort, including date of pain onset, duration of pain, and whether pain continues. We interpret a positive screen in this postmenopausal population to be consistent with vulvodynia but acknowledge that this screening tool may not adequately differentiate vulvodynia from atrophy in this postmenopausal cohort. Therefore we use the term "chronic vulvar pain" in lieu of vulvodynia when presenting the results.

Based on responses to the vulvodynia questionnaire, each participant was categorized into one of three groups: women with current chronic (lasting 3 months or longer) vulvar pain, women who reported ever having chronic vulvar pain in the past or reported having short-duration (less than 3 months duration) vulvar pain symptoms, and women reporting no current or past vulvar pain symptoms. Current chronic vulvar pain was defined by a history of vulvar pain or discomfort at the opening to the vagina that had lasted for at least three months and had been experienced in the preceding three months. The past chronic vulvar pain/short-duration vulvar pain symptom group included women who had a history of vulvar pain lasting for at least three months but who had not experienced pain in the preceding three months and women with current vulvar pain lasting for less than three months. This group represents a heterogeneous symptomatic group who, based on prior work [12], are more likely than the non-symptomatic group to develop vulvodynia, and hence we categorize them separately from the no pain group.

Age was modeled as a continuous variable. Race/ethnicity was self-reported as either white or African American. Measured height and weight were used to calculate body mass index (BMI) (weight in kilograms (kg) divided by height in meters (m) squared). BMI was further categorized as normal weight, overweight, or obese (<25, 25-<30, and >= 30 kg/m$^2$). Socioeconomic status was assessed by self-reported difficulty paying for basics (very hard versus somewhat or not hard) and education at baseline (high school or less versus at least some college). Marital status was categorized as either married or not married.

In addition to questions about vulvar pain, we asked about other specific vulvovaginal symptoms at Visit 13 including self-reported number of days in the past 2 weeks of vaginal dryness, soreness, and irritation categorized into three duration levels (0 days, 1–5 days, or >6 days). In addition, we created variables to reflect whether women ever reported vaginal dryness before, and after, the final menstrual period (FMP) or hysterectomy (yes/no) based on responses at each follow-up visit. Although women were not eligible to enroll in SWAN ff they were using HT, women who began using HT after enrollment remained in the study. Two HT variables were considered: current HT use (yes/no), and ever used HT during the study (yes/no).

At each visit, a fasting blood sample was collected, refrigerated for 1–2 h after collection, and then centrifuged. Serum hormone levels of estradiol (E2), dehydro-epiandrosterone-sulfate (DHEA-S), follicle stimulating hormone (FSH), sex hormone-binding globuliN (SHBG), and testosterone (T) were determined.

All assays were performed on the ACS-180 automated analyzer (Bayer Diagnostics Corporation, Tarrytown, NY) at the CLASS laboratory at the University of Michigan, utilizing a double-antibody chemiluminescent immunoassay with a solid phase anti-IgG immunoglobulin conjugated to paramagnetic particles, anti-ligand antibody, and competitive ligand labeled with dimethylacridinium ester (DMAE). The FSH assay is a modification of a manual assay kit (Bayer Diagnostics) utilizing two monoclonal antibodies directed to different regions on the beta subunit, with a lower limit of detection (LLD) of 1.05 mIU/mL. Inter-and intra-assay coefficients of variation were 12.0 % and 6.0 %, respectively. The E2 assay modifies the rabbit anti-E2-6 ACS-180 immunoassay to increase sensitivity, with a LLD of 1.0 pg/mL and inter- and intra-assay coefficients of variation averaging 10.6 % and 6.4 %, respectively. The T assay modifies the rabbit polyclonal anti-T ACS-180 immunoassay, with a LLD of 2.19 ng/dL and inter-and intra-assay coefficients of variation of 10.5 % and 8.5 %, respectively. The DHEA-S and SHBG assays were developed using rabbit anti-DHEA-S and anti-SHBG antibodies, with LLDs of 1.52 mcg/dL and 1.95 nM, respectively. For DHEA-S, the inter- and intra-assay coefficient of variation were 11.3 % and 8.0 %, respectively. For SHBG, the inter- and intra-assay coefficient of variation were 9.9 % and 6.1 %, respectively. Duplicate E2 assays were conducted, with results reported as the arithmetic mean for each subject, with a CV of 3-12 %. All other assays were single determinations. Hormone levels below the lower limit of detection were assigned a random number between 0 and the lower limit of detection.

The prevalence of vulvar symptoms overall and stratified by demographic characteristics were calculated and compared using Chi-squared and Fisher's Exact tests as appropriate. Hormone levels were log-transformed for regression analyses. The median values of the log-transformed E2, DHEA-S, SHBG, FSH, and T at Visit 12 were compared overall and across symptoms groups using Kruskal-Wallis tests. Relative odds ratios (OR) and 95 % confidence intervals (CI) comparing the current chronic vulvar pain and past/short-duration vulvar pain groups to the no vulvar pain group were calculated using multinomial logistic regression models appropriate for outcomes with more than two categories [13]. These models compare odds for reporting current chronic vulvar pain symptoms in relation to the no pain category and odds for reporting past/short-term vulvar pain symptoms in relation to the no pain category. In addition to an unadjusted model, models adjusted for race, BMI, and age were also assessed. Analyses were performed using SAS 9.3 (Cary, NC).

## Results

At follow-up Visit 13, participants ranged in age from 56 to 68 years (median 61.3 years). Of the 371 women eligible for this analysis, 15 women (4.0 %; 95 % CI: 2.5 %, 6.6 %) reported current chronic vulvar pain, 51 (13.7 %; 95 % CI: 10.6 %, 17.6 %) reported past chronic or short-duration vulvar pain, and 305 (82.2 %; 95 % CI: 78.0 %, 85.8 %) reported no vulvar pain. Of the 15 women reporting current chronic vulvar pain, one did not provide an age of symptom onset, four experienced symptom onset before age 45, two experienced onset between age 46 and 55, and the remaining 8 experienced onset between ages 56 and 64 years. Five of the 15 women reported first onset since their previous follow-up visit, representing an incidence of 1.3 %.

Median age, marital status, and proportion sexually active in the previous 6 months did not differ by chronic vulvar pain status (Table 1). However, women with current chronic vulvar pain were more likely to be white, less likely to be obese, and more likely to have completed at least some college compared to women in the other vulvar pain groups (Table 1).

Although few women reported current HT use, both the current chronic and past/short-duration vulvar pain groups were more likely than women with no vulvar pain symptoms to report having used HT during the preceding year (Table 1). Women with past/short-duration vulvar pain were more likely to have ever used HT and more likely to have had a hysterectomy than women in the other two groups (Table 1). Two of the 15 women with current symptoms (13.3 %) began HT after pain onset but did not report remission while 3 of the 32 women with current or past chronic vulvar pain

**Table 1** Demographic and clinical characteristics of women in the MI SWAN population, by self-reported vulvar pain

| Variable | Total N (%) | Current Chronic Vulvar Pain n (%) | Past/Short-term Vulvar Pain n (%) | No Vulvar Pain n (%) | p-value[6] |
|---|---|---|---|---|---|
| Race | | | | | < .01 |
| White | 142 (38.3 %) | 10 (66.7 %) | 27 (52.9 %) | 105 (34.4 %) | |
| African American | 229 (61.7 %) | 5 (33.3 %) | 24 (47.1 %) | 200 (65.5 %) | |
| Education at Baseline[1] | | | | | .05 |
| High School or less | 108 (30.1 %) | 2 (15.4 %) | 9 (18.0 %) | 97 (32.8 %) | |
| At least some college | 251 (69.9 %) | 11 (84.6 %) | 41 (82.0 %) | 199 (67.2 %) | |
| Marital Status[2] | | | | | .65 |
| Married | 188 (55.8 %) | 10 (66.7 %) | 27 (57.5 %) | 151 (54.9 %) | |
| Not Married | 149 (44.2 %) | 5 (33.3 %) | 20 (42.5 %) | 124 (45.1 %) | |
| Sexually Active in Last 6 Months [3] | | | | | .40 |
| Yes | 120 (39.7 %) | 7 (58.3 %) | 18 (40.0 %) | 95 (38.8 %) | |
| No | 182 (60.3 %) | 5 (41.7 %) | 27 (60.0 %) | 150 (61.2 %) | |
| BMI[4] | | | | | .02 |
| <25 kg/m$^2$ | 47 (14.2 %) | 3 (21.4 %) | 12 (26.7 %) | 32 (11.7 %) | |
| 25 - <30 kg/m$^2$ | 81 (24.4 %) | 6 (42.9 %) | 9 (20.0 %) | 66 (24.2 %) | |
| > = 30 kg/m$^2$ | 204 (61.4 %) | 5 (35.7 %) | 24 (53.3 %) | 175 (64.1 %) | |
| Currently Use HT | | | | | < .01 |
| Yes | 17 (4.6 %) | 2 (13.3 %) | 9 (17.6 %) | 6 (2.0 %) | |
| No | 354 (95.4 %) | 13 (86.7 %) | 42 (82.4 %) | 299 (98.0 %) | |
| Ever Used HT | | | | | < .01 |
| Yes | 137 (36.9 %) | 7 (46.7 %) | 30 (58.8 %) | 100 (32.8 %) | |
| No | 234 (63.1 %) | 8 (53.3 %) | 21 (41.2 %) | 205 (67.2 %) | |
| History of Hysterectomy | | | | | .21 |
| Yes | 63 (17.0 %) | 2 (13.3 %) | 13 (25.5 %) | 48 (15.7 %) | |
| No | 308 (83.0 %) | 13 (86.7 %) | 38 (74.5 %) | 257 (84.3 %) | |
| *Urogenital Symptoms in previous 2 weeks* | | | | | |
| Dryness | | | | | < .01 |
| 0 days | 272 (73.3 %) | 4 (26.7 %) | 33 (64.7 %) | 235 (77.1 %) | |
| 1-5 days | 53 (14.3 %) | 3 (20.0 %) | 9 (17.6 %) | 41 (13.4 %) | |
| 6-14 days | 46 (12.4 %) | 8 (53.3 %) | 9 (17.6 %) | 29 (9.5 %) | |
| Soreness[2] | | | | | < .01 |
| 0 days | 318 (94.4 %) | 10 (66.7 %) | 44 (93.6 %) | 264 (96.0 %) | |
| 1-5 days | 15 (4.4 %) | 3 (20.0 %) | 3 (6.4 %) | 9 (3.3 %) | |
| 6-14 days | 4 (1.2 %) | 2 (13.3 %) | 0 (0.0 %) | 2 (0.7 %) | |
| Irritation[2] | | | | | < .01 |
| 0 days | 280 (83.1 %) | 8 (53.3 %) | 35 (74.5 %) | 237 (86.2 %) | |
| 1-5 days | 43 (12.8 %) | 3 (20.0 %) | 10 (21.3 %) | 30 (10.9 %) | |
| 6-14 days | 14 (4.2 %) | 4 (26.7 %) | 2 (4.3 %) | 8 (2.9 %) | |
| *History of Reported Dryness* | | | | | |
| Dry Before FMP/Hysterectomy[5] | | | | | .46 |
| Yes | 126 (46.7 %) | 7 (63.6 %) | 16 (50.0 %) | 103 (45.4 %) | |
| No | 144 (53.3 %) | 4 (36.4 %) | 16 (50.0 %) | 124 (54.6 %) | |

**Table 1** Demographic and clinical characteristics of women in the MI SWAN population, by self-reported vulvar pain *(Continued)*

| Dry After FMP/Hysterectomy[5] | | | | .01 |
|---|---|---|---|---|
| Yes | 232 (62.5 %) | 10 (90.9 %) | 23 (71.9 %) | 124 (54.6 %) |
| No | 139 (37.5 %) | 1 (9.1 %) | 9 (28.1 %) | 103 (34.3 %) |

Missing observations: [1]12, [2] 34, [3]69, [4]39 , [5]101.
[6]All p-values calculated using Chi-squared tests except BMI, Difficulty Paying for Basics, Currently Use HT, Vaginal Dryness, Vaginal Soreness, and Vaginal Irritation, which were calculated using Fisher's Exact test

symptoms (9.4 %) reported first onset of vulvar pain while taking HT.

Prevalences of self-reported dryness, soreness, and/or irritation were lowest in the no vulvar pain symptoms group and highest in the current chronic vulvar pain group (Table 1). However, although over half of women with current vulvar pain indicated they had "dryness" for over 6 days in the past 2 weeks, approximately a quarter (26.7 %) of women with current vulvar pain did not report vaginal dryness. Similarly, although reporting of "soreness" or "irritation" was most frequent in women with current chronic vulvar pain, over half of the women with current chronic vulvar pain did not report soreness or irritation.

In the multinomial logistic regression models adjusted for race, odds of having current chronic vulvar pain symptoms were significantly elevated in white women, current HT users, and individuals reporting dryness, soreness, or irritation for 6 or more days in the preceding 2 weeks (Table 2). Odds of past/short-duration vulvar pain symptoms were significantly elevated in white women, current and past HT users, women who had had a hysterectomy, and individuals reporting vaginal irritation 1–5 days in the previous 2 weeks. Adjusting the logistic models for age or BMI did not substantially alter results (data not shown).

At Visit 12, median serum hormone levels of E2 and DHEA-S tended to be lower ($p = 0.06$) in women who subsequently reported current chronic vulvar pain symptoms at Visit 13 compared to those who reported no vulvar symptoms (Table 3). The unadjusted relative odds of current chronic vulvar pain symptoms versus no vulvar symptoms at Visit 13 were elevated with each log unit decrease in Visit 12 E2, DHEA-S, and T levels (Table 4). After adjustment for age, race and BMI, the odds remained elevated only for DHEA-S and T. FSH and SHBG levels were not associated with chronic vulvar pain. In an exploratory analysis we evaluated longitudinal endocrine patterns prior to pain onset in the five women reporting new onset chronic pain symptoms at visit 13. From Visit 10 to Visit 12, three of the five experienced a sharp drop in E2 levels (defined < =15 % of the Visit 10 level at Visit 12) as did only 12 of 256 women without symptoms.

## Discussion

Postmenopausal women are as likely as younger women to report chronic vulvar pain consistent with vulvodynia

[4, 14, 15]. This study is one of the first population-based studies to examine the association between symptoms of vaginal dryness, serum hormone levels, hormone use and chronic vulvar pain symptoms in postmenopausal women. We found that women with current chronic vulvar pain symptoms often experienced pain onset prior to menopause. Women with current chronic pain were more likely than women without such pain symptoms to be using HT, and some reported the onset of vulvar pain symptoms while already taking HT. Despite the possibility of inadequate hormonal treatment in some cases, vulvar pain unresponsive to HT further supports the presence of a chronic pain condition such as vulvodynia that is likely to require alternative, non-hormonal, treatment modalities. Notably, more than a quarter of women who reported current chronic vulvar pain did not report vaginal dryness, a common complaint associated with vaginal atrophy. Lower average DHEA-S, and T levels prior to ascertainment of vulvar pain symptoms were associated with elevated odds of subsequently reporting chronic vulvar pain, further supporting that for some, hormonal levels may contribute to symptoms experienced. These results provide additional evidence that chronic vulvar pain in postmenopausal women has a heterogeneous etiology and, in many women, may not be explained by estrogen deficiency-related atrophy alone [6, 14, 15].

In this sample of postmenopausal women, the prevalence and incidence of chronic vulvar pain was somewhat lower than that observed in other studies. One previous study reported prevalences in women age 40–65 years of 13.9 % and 8.9 % among women who had and had not used HT, respectively [4, 5], and an incidence of approximately 3.3 per 100 person-years in women age 50 and older [16]. A second paper reported a prevalence of vulvovaginal symptoms suggestive of atrophy in 38 % of women aged 45–65 [5]. The low prevalence of chronic vulvar pain reported in this study reflects the large proportion of African Americans who have been shown to be less likely than white women to report chronic vulvar pain. Vulvodynia is more prevalent in white women than African American women in most [2, 4, 16], although not all studies [17]. The low prevalence reported here also reflects the older average age of the study population, as previous reports have indicated that vulvodynia prevalence and incidence decline with

**Table 2** Relative odds ratios (OR) and 95 % confidence intervals (CI) for selected variables, adjusted for race

| Variable | Current Chronic Vulvar Pain vs none | | Past/Short-term Vulvar Pain vs none | |
|---|---|---|---|---|
| | OR (95 % CI) | P | OR (95 % CI) | P |
| Categorical BMI | | | | |
| <25 kg/m$^2$ | REF | – | REF | – |
| 25-<30 kg/m$^2$ | 0.96 (0.22, 4.13) | 0.34 | 0.36 (0.14, 0.95) | .21 |
| > = 30 kg/m$^2$ | 0.30 (0.07, 1.35) | 0.12 | 0.36 (0.16, 0.81) | .01 |
| Currently Use HT | | | | |
| Yes | 7.12 (1.27, 39.94) | 0.03 | 10.24 (3.42, 30.68) | < .01 |
| No | REF | – | REF | – |
| Ever Use HT | | | | |
| Yes | 1.79 (0.63, 5.13) | 0.28 | 2.93 (1.59, 5.40) | < .01 |
| No | REF | – | REF | – |
| Sexually Active in Last 6 months. | | | | |
| Yes | 2.17 (0.66, 7.11) | 0.20 | 1.04 (0.54, 2.01) | .90 |
| No | REF | – | REF | – |
| Hysterectomy | | | | |
| Yes | 0.91 (0.20, 4.23) | 0.91 | 1.95 (0.96, 3.97) | .07 |
| No | REF | – | REF | – |
| Vaginal Dryness | | | | |
| 0 days | REF | – | REF | – |
| 1-5 days | 5.47 (1.14, 26.12) | 0.03 | 1.79 (0.78, 4.07) | .17 |
| 6-14 days | 16.34 (4.53, 58.85) | <0.01 | 2.22 (0.96, 5.16) | .06 |
| Vaginal Soreness | | | | |
| 0 days | REF | – | REF | – |
| 1-5 days | 14.43 (2.95, 70.56) | <0.01 | 2.46 (0.63, 9.68) | .20 |
| 6-14 days | 28.28 (2.99, 267.5) | <0.01 | (Insufficient data) | .99 |
| Vaginal Irritation | | | | |
| 0 days | REF | – | REF | – |
| 1-5 days | 3.30 (0.81, 13.42) | 0.09 | 2.40 (1.07, 5.41) | < .01 |
| 6-14 days | 12.60 (3.00, 52.86) | 0.03 | 1.53 (0.31, 7.65) | .60 |

**Table 3** Serum hormone levels (median and interquartile range (IQR)) at Visit 12 for all women not using hormonal therapy, by self-reported vulvar pain symptoms at Visit 13

| Variable | Total | Current Chronic Vulvar Pain | Past/Short-term Vulvar Pain | No Vulvar Pain | |
|---|---|---|---|---|---|
| | Median (IQR) | Median (IQR) | Median (IQR) | Median (IQR) | p-value |
| Age (yr) | 61.3 (59.4-63.7) | 59.3 (58.6-60.4) | 61.4 (60.0-63.7) | 61.3 (59.4-63.7) | .23 |
| *Hormones (log transformed)* | | | | | |
| | N = 319 | n = 12 | n = 38 | n = 264 | |
| E2 (average, pg/mL) | 19.8 (12.0-27.2) | 15.2 (3.7-24.4) | 23.2 (18.8-26.9) | 19.4 (12.0-27.3) | 0.06 |
| DHEA-S (ug/dL) | 63.7 (36.8-88.6) | 28.5 (8.0-73.1) | 62.0 (49.3-83.2) | 65.0 (37.7-90.1) | 0.06 |
| FSH (mIU/mL) | 52.2 (36.8-70.7) | 55.4 (38.7-64.6) | 52.7 (31.5-79.6) | 51.5 (36.9-70.6) | 0.92 |
| SHBG (nM) | 48.8 (35.7-68.7) | 56.4 (31.8-94.1) | 53.1 (34.8-68.5) | 48.8 (35.8-67.8) | 0.83 |
| T (ng/dL) | 49.8 (38.5-61.8) | 45.2 (22.5-54.9) | 54.7 (41.7-65.4) | 49.8 (38.7-61.6) | 0.22 |

**Table 4** Relative odds ratios (OR) and 95 % confidence intervals (CI) for having chronic vulvar pain by log-transformed serum hormone levels at Visit 12 among women not using hormones

| Hormone (log) | Unadjusted Model | | Adjusted Model* | |
|---|---|---|---|---|
| | Current Chronic Vulvar Pain vs none | Past/Short-term Chronic Pain vs none | Current Chronic Vulvar Pain vs none | Past/Short-term Vulvar Pain vs none |
| | OR (95 % CI) | OR (95 % CI) | OR (95 % CI) | OR (95 % CI) |
| *Visit 12 (N = 319)* | | | | |
| E2 (average, pg/mL) | 0.49 (0.28, 0.86)** | 1.37 (0.86, 2.19) | 0.58 (0.32, 1.04) | 1.52 (0.92, 2.50) |
| DHEA-S (ug/dL) | 0.46 (0.29, 0.75)*** | 1.09 (0.69, 1.73) | 0.45 (0.28, 0.72)*** | 1.07 (0.66, 1.74) |
| FSH (mIU/mL) | 1.13 (0.39, 3.28) | 1.11 (0.60, 2.05) | 0.76 (0.28, 2.10) | 1.15 (0.56, 2.39) |
| SHBG (nM) | 1.45 (0.49, 4.31) | 0.99 (0.52, 1.89) | 1.00 (0.29, 3.47) | 0.99 (0.47, 2.11) |
| T (ng/dL) | 0.13 (0.04, 0.48)*** | 1.38 (0.55, 3.47) | 0.14 (0.04, 0.56)*** | 1.39 (0.53, 3.68) |

* adjusted for age, categorical BMI, and race
** $p = .01$; *** $p < .01$

age, especially if those not having sexual intercourse are included in the analysis [4, 16].

Previous research has suggested that a drop in estrogen may be associated with onset of chronic vulvar pain that will not necessarily be reversed by subsequent estrogen supplementation [8]. We observed that lower levels of E2, DHEA-S, and T were associated with increased odds of reporting current chronic vulvar pain, although only DHEA-S and T remained significant after adjustment. When we evaluated longitudinal endocrine patterns prior to pain onset only in the five women reporting new onset chronic pain symptoms at visit 13, three of the five had experienced a prior sharp drop in E2 levels compared to just five percent of women with no symptoms. Although consistent with the theory that a variable hormonal environment may contribute to chronic vulvar pain, we observed only a small number of new onset cases. Further study of the relationship between longitudinal endocrine patterns and risk for chronic vulvar pain is warranted.

Lower DHEA-S levels at visit 12 were associated with higher odds of reporting current chronic vulvar pain symptoms, a finding that should be explored in future studies. An association between low DHEAS and sexual dysfunctio*N* (as measured by the Female Sexual Function Index) [18] and a weak association of serum androgens and sexual well-being in women with premature ovarian failure have been reported [19]. However, a mechanism to explain a direct relationship between DHEAS and vulvar symptoms is unclear. The topical application of DHEA to the vagina in women with severe atrophy has been reported to improve all domains of sexual function, including pain with sexual activity, in controlled clinical trials [20–22], potentially due to local conversion to androgens and estrogens. Future studies are needed to confirm and further assess these findings.

This study adds to the literature indicating that post-menopausal vulvar pain may be caused by factors other than vulvovaginal atrophy [6–9, 14, 15]. Hormone use did not always prevent symptom onset and was not associated with symptom remission in all women. However, as the vulvodynia screening instrument was administered at only Visit 13, timing of vulvar pain onset was ascertained by retrospective report. Also, information on details of HT such as dose, route of administration, indication and duration of use was limited or unavailable; thus, we are not able to assess adequacy of treatment for presumed estrogen deficiency. However, those with vulvar pain symptoms secondary to atrophy who had been adequately treated with estrogen would not be included in the chronic vulvar pain group–hence only those with persistent symptoms despite hormone therapy, and those with persistent symptoms who have not taken HT, were included in the chronic vulvar pain group.

This analysis was constrained by the limited sample size, particularly the small number of women with current vulvar pain symptoms meeting our screening criteria. As a categorization of chronic pain requires a minimum duration of three months and categorization as a past case depends on participant recall, it is possible that some participants forgot to report past episodes, thus attenuating the findings. Nonetheless, a unique strength of this study is the availability of longitudinal data on HT use, serum hormone levels, and self-reports of vaginal dryness in postmenopausal women within a defined timeframe after the final menstrual period permitting a more detailed, though preliminary, look at the relationship between vaginal symptoms, hormone levels and vulvar pain in a population-based, multi-ethnic sample of midlife women. Future studies might consider evaluation of additional pain symptoms such as dyspareunia in relation to reporting of chronic vulvar pain.

## Conclusion

This preliminary but rich longitudinal population-based study adds to the growing literature suggesting that vulvar atrophy may not be the sole cause of postmenopausal vulvar pain. Postmenopausal women may be experiencing new onset, exacerbated and/or long-term chronic vulvar pain consistent with a diagnosis of vulvodynia. Health care providers should consider and evaluate for vulvodynia when treating postmenopausal women with chronic vulvar pain, especially those women who fail to respond to HT. The best tool for distinguishing if chronic vulvar pain consistent with both atrophy and vulvodynia will respond to HT is to give a trial of HT, followed by alternative vulvodynia treatments in those not responding. Future research should focus on the diagnosis and treatment of women who do not respond to this intervention.

### Abbreviations
BMI, body mass index; DHEA-S, dehydroepiandrosterone-sulfate; E2, estradiol; FSH, follicle stimulating hormone; HT, hormone therapy; Kg, kilograms; M, meters; SHBG, steroid hormone binding globulin; SWAN, Study of Women's Health Across the Nation; T, testosterone

### Acknowledgements
Clinical Centers: *University of Michigan, Ann Arbor—Siobán Harlow, PI 2011 –present, MaryFran Sowers, PI 1994–2011; Massachusetts General Hospital, Boston, MA—Joel Finkelstein, PI 1999–present; Robert Neer, PI 1994–1999; Rush University, Rush University Medical Center, Chicago, IL—Howard Kravitz, PI 2009 –present; Lynda Powell, PI 1994–2009; University of California, Davis/Kaiser –Ellen Gold, PI; University of California, Los Angeles—Gail Greendale, PI; Albert Einstein College of Medicine, Bronx, NY—Carol Derby, PI 2011–present, Rachel Wildman, PI 2010–2011; Nanette Santoro, PI 2004–2010; University of Medicine and Dentistry–New Jersey Medical School, Newark—Gerson Weiss, PI 1994–2004; and the University of Pittsburgh, Pittsburgh, PA—Karen Matthews, PI.* NIH Program Office: *National Institute on Aging, Bethesda, MD—Winifred Rossi 2012-present; Sherry Sherman 1994–2012; Marcia Ory 1994–2001; National Institute of Nursing Research, Bethesda, MD—Program Officers.* Central Laboratory: *University of Michigan, Ann Arbor—Daniel McConnell* (Central Ligand Assay Satellite Services). Coordinating Center: *University of Pittsburgh, Pittsburgh, PA –Maria Mori Brooks, PI 2012-present; Kim Sutton-Tyrrell, PI 2001–2012; New England Research Institutes, Watertown, MA-Sonja McKinlay, PI 1995–2001.* Steering Committee: Susan Johnson, Current Chair, Chris Gallagher, Former Chair. We thank the study staff at each site and all the women who participated in SWAN.
The Study of Women's Health Across the NatioN (SWAN) has grant support from the National Institutes of Health (NIH), DHHS, through the National Institute on Aging (NIA), the National Institute of Nursing Research (NINR) and the NIH Office of Research on Women's Health (ORWH) (Grants U01NR004061; U01AG012505, U01AG012535, U01AG012531, U01AG012539, U01AG012546, U01AG012553, U01AG012554, U01AG012495). The content of this article is solely the responsibility of the authors and does not necessarily represent the official views of the NIA, NINR, ORWH or the NIH. SDH gratefully acknowledges use of the services and facilities of the Population Studies Center at the University of Michigan, funded by NICHD Center Grant R24 HD041028.

### Authors' contributions
SM contributed to the literature review, conducted the data analysis and had primary responsibility for drafting the manuscript. SDH, JFR, and BDR made substantial contributions to conception, design, and acquisition and interpretation of the data. SDH oversaw the data analysis, contributed to the drafting and critical revisions of the manuscript. BDR and JFR contributed to the critical revision of the manuscript for important intellectual content. All authors have read and approved the final manuscript.

### Competing interests
The authors have no competing interests.

### Author details
[1]Department of Epidemiology, School of Public Health, 1415 Washington Heights, Ann Arbor, MI 48109, USA. [2]School of Medicine, University of Michigan Ann Arbor, Ann Arbor, MI, USA.

### References
1. Harlow BL, Stewart EG. A population-based assessment of chronic unexplained vulvar pain: have we underestimated the prevalence of vulvodynia? JAMWA. 2003;58:82–8.
2. Harlow BL, Wise LA, Stewart EG. Prevalence and predictors of chronic lower genital tract discomfort. Am J Obstet Gynecol. 2001;185(3):545–50.
3. Kao A, Binik YM, Amsel R, Funaro D, Leroux N, Khalife S. Biopsychosocial predictors of postmenopausal dyspareunia: the role of steroid hormones, vulvovaginal atrophy, cognitive-emotional factors, and dyadic adjustment. J Sex Med. 2012;9:2066–76.
4. Reed BD, Harlow SD, Sen A, Legocki LJ, Edwards RM, Arato N, et al. Prevalence and demographic characteristics of vulvodynia in a population-based sample. Am J Obstet Gynecol. 2012;206:170.e1–9.
5. Kingsberg SA, Wysocki S, Magnus L, Krychman ML. Vulvar and vaginal atrophy in postemenopausal women: findings from the REVIVE (REAl women's VIews of treatment options for menopausal Vaginal changEs) survey. J Sex Med. 2013;10:1790–9.
6. Kao A, Binik K, Amsel R, Funaro D, Leroux N, Khalife S. Challenging atrophied perspectives on postmenopausal dyspareunia: a systematic description and synthesis of clinical pain characteristics. J Sex Marital Ther. 2012;38:128–50.
7. Goetsch MF. Unprovoked vestibular burning in late estrogen-deprived menopause: a case series. J Low Genit Tract Di. 2012;16(4):442–6.
8. Leclair CM, Goetsch MF, Li H, Morgan TK. Histopathologic characteristics of menopausal vestibulodynia. Obstet Gynecol. 2013;122:787–93.
9. McKay M. Dysesthetic ("essential") vulvodynia: treatment with amitriptyline. J Reprod Med. 1993;38(1):9–13.
10. Sowers MF, Crawford S, Sternfeld B, Morganstein D, Gold E, Greendale G, Evans D, Neer R, Matthews KA, Sherman S, Lo A, Weiss G, Kelsey J. SWAN: A multi-center, multi-ethnic, community-based cohort study of women and the menopause transition. In: Lobo RA, Kelsey J, Marcus R, editors. Menopause. New York: Academic; 2000. p. 175–88.
11. Reed BD, Haefner HK, Harlow SD, Gorenflo DW, Sen A. Reliability and validity of self-reported symptoms for predicting vulvodynia. Obstet Gynecol. 2006;108:906–13.
12. Reed BD, Haefner HK, Sen A, Gorenflo DW. Vulvodynia incidence and remission rates among adult women: a 2-year follow-up study. Obstet Gynecol. 2008;112:231–7.
13. Agresti A. Categorical Data Analysis. 3rd ed. New York, NY: John Wiley & Sons; 2012.
14. Phillips N, Bachmann G. Vulvodynia: An often overlooked cause of dyspareunia in the menopausal population. Menopausal Medicine. 2010; 18(S1):S3–5.
15. Phillips NA, Brown C, Foster D, Bachour C, Rawlinson L, Wan J, Bachman G. Presenting symptoms among premenopausal and postmenopausal women with vulvodynia: a case series. Menopause. 2015;22:1296–300.
16. Reed BD, Legocki LJ, Plegue MA, Sen A, Haefner HK, Harlow SD. Factors associated with vulvodynia incidence. Obstet Gynecol. 2014;123:225–31.
17. Bachmann G, Rosen R, Arnold L, Burd I, Rhoads GG, Leiblum SR, et al. Chronic vulvar and other gynecologic pain: prevalence and characteristics in a self-reported survey. J Reprod Med. 2006;51:3–9.
18. Gracia CR, Freeman EW, Sammel MD, Lin H, Mogul M. Hormones and sexuality during transition to menopause. Obstet Gynecol. 2007;109: 831–40.
19. van der Stege JG, Groen H, Van Zadelhoff SJ, Lambalk CB, Braat DD, Van Kasteren YM, et al. Decreased androgen concentrations and diminished general and sexual well-being in women with premature ovarian failure. Menopause. 2008;15:23–31.
20. Labrie F, Archer D, Bouchard C, Fortier M, Cusan L, Gomez JL, Girard G, Baron M, Ayotte N, Moreau M, Dubé R, Côté I, Labrie C, Lavoie L, Berger L, Gilbert L, Martel C, Balser J. Effect of intravaginal dehydroepiandrosterone (Prasterone) on libido and sexual dysfunction in postmenopausal women. Menopause. 2009;16:923–31.

21.  Labri F, Archer DF, Bouchard C, Fortier M, Cusan L, Gomez JL, Girard G,
     Baron M, Ayotte N, Moreau M, Dubé R, Côté I, Labrie C, Lavoie L, Berger L,
     Gilbert L, Martel C, Balser J. Intravaginal dehydroepiandrosterone
     (prasterone), a highly efficient treatment of dyspareunia. Climacteric. 2011;
     14(2):282–8.
22.  Archer D, Larie F, Bouchard C, Portman DJ, Koltun W, Cusan L, Labrie C,
     Cote I, Lavoie L, Martel C, Balser J and the VVA Prasterone Group.
     Treatment of pain at sexual activity (dyspareunia) with intravaginal
     dehydroepiandrosterone (prasterone). Menopause 2015; 22, DOI:
     10.1097/gme.0000000000000428.

# The Seattle Midlife Women's Health Study: a longitudinal prospective study of women during the menopausal transition and early postmenopause

Nancy Fugate Woods[1*] and Ellen Sullivan Mitchell[2]

## Abstract

**Background:** The need for longitudinal, population-based studies to illuminate women's experiences of symptoms during the menopausal transition motivated the development of the Seattle Midlife Women's Health Study.

**Methods:** Longitudinal, population-based study of symptoms women experienced between the Late Reproductive stage of reproductive aging and the early postmenopause. Data collection began in 1990 with 508 women ages 35–55 and continued to 2013. Entry criteria included age, at least one period in past 12 months, uterus intact and at least 1 ovary. Women were studied up to 5 years postmenopause. Data collection included yearly health questionnaires, health diaries, urinary hormonal assays, menstrual calendars and buccal cell smears.

**Results:** Contributions of the study included development of a method for staging the menopausal transition; development of bleeding criteria to differentiate bleeding episodes from intermenstrual bleeding from menstrual calendars; identification of hormonal changes associated with menopausal transition stages; assessment of the effects of menopausal transition factors, aging, stress-related factors, health factors, social factors on symptoms, particularly hot flashes, depressed mood, pain, cognitive, sexual desire, and sleep disruption symptoms, and urinary incontinence symptoms; identification of naturally occurring clusters of symptoms women experienced during the menopausal transition and early postmenopause; and assessment of gene polymorphisms associated with events such as onset of the early and late menopausal transition stages and symptoms.

**Conclusions:** Over the course of the longitudinal Seattle Midlife Women's Health Study, investigators contributed to understanding of symptoms women experience during the menopausal transition and early postmenopause as well as methods of staging reproductive aging.

**Keywords:** Menopausal transition, Staging reproductive aging, Menopause, Midlife cohort, Symptoms, Endocrine changes

## Background

During the 1970s and 1980s attention to women's health research increased in the US, culminating in several important milestones, among them establishment of the Office of Women's Health Research in the National Institutes of Health in 1991 and development of the first US Women's Health Research Agenda [1]. In 1993 the National Institutes of Health/National Institute on Aging, National Institute of Child Health and Development, and collaborating organizations convened a workshop on Menopause to provide focus for future research about midlife women and menopause. This work was preceded by the landmark longitudinal study of the menopausal transition (MT): the Massachusetts Women's Health Study begun in 1982 [2], a longitudinal study developed to expand knowledge about the experiences of a community-based population of women as they traversed the MT. This focus on a community-based population was in

* Correspondence: nfwoods@uw.edu
[1]Department of Biobehavioral Nursing, University of Washington, Seattle, WA 98195, USA
Full list of author information is available at the end of the article

contrast to earlier studies of clinical populations. Another early effort by Matthews and colleagues recruited women from the state of Pennsylvania (The Healthy Women Study) to determine the natural history of the MT, and behavioral and biological changes that occurred during the MT and postmenopause (PM) and their effects on cardiovascular disease risk [3].

The Seattle Midlife Women's Health Study (SMWHS) was built on the foundational studies of the 1980s, including our longitudinal studies of perimenstrual symptoms that focused on women after they had reached age 40 years [4–6]. The SMWHS originated as one component of a Center for Women's Health Research (CWHR) at the University of Washington School of Nursing in 1989. Funded by the National Institute of Nursing Research, the CWHR was created by an interdisciplinary cadre of investigators to support research development in women's health [7].

## Overview of the SMWHS
The initial phase of SMWHS from September 1989 to July 1996, as part of the CWHR, was designed to test a model relating MT status, stress exposure, socialization for midlife, personal and social factors modulating midlife experiences, reproductive health history, and health behaviors to health status and health-seeking behavior in midlife women between the ages of 35 and 55. A model including menopausal changes, socialization for midlife, health status, stressful life context, and vasomotor symptoms guided analysis of depressed mood symptoms, an outcome of interest [8]. The model was generalized to other symptoms, for example, by testing outcomes including hot flashes, sleep, cognitive, mood, and pain symptoms, to name a few. (The Aims for Phase 1 are included in Table 1)

Based on results of the initial study, additional funding was obtained for the SMWHS from July 1996 to February 2001. This second funding phase focused on the MT and its relationship to symptoms, altered ovarian function, perceived stress and stress arousal, as well as symptom management. A major addition to the measures for this study included hormonal assays (urinary estrone, FSH, testosterone, cortisol and catecholamines). (Aims for Phase 2 are included in Table 1).

A third funding phase spanned 2002 through 2006. Phase 3 of SMWHS continued to focus on symptoms as the primary endpoints. In addition to linking the symptoms to endocrine patterns, the effect of gene polymorphisms in estrogen synthesis, metabolism and receptor genes was added to the aims. (Detailed aims for Phase 3 are given in Table 1).

A fourth and final phase of data collection, after the end of major funding, continued from 2007 to 2013. The focus of this phase was to complete the data collection for the study. Women who had not yet reached 5 years PM, were not taking any estrogen and had an intact uterus were entered into this final phase. Aims for this phase were a combination of the aims for the three prior phases of funding. The model guiding the longitudinal analysis of symptom data across all 4 phases is depicted in Fig. 1.

Two small grants supported the fourth phase of the study. The first was "Menopausal Transition Symptom Clusters: Genetic, Endocrine, and Social Correlates" that focused on the secondary analyses of symptom data, particularly on multiple co-occurring symptoms called symptom clusters that women experienced during the MT and early PM. Symptom data were analyzed to identify clusters of symptoms women experienced and to relate them to stress, health behaviors, health status, endocrine patterns, and gene polymorphisms. (Aims for this study are in Table 1). A second small grant during the fourth phase of the study, Urinary Incontinence during the Menopausal Transition and Early Postmenopause, was awarded by Pfizer, Inc, Medical Division, that supported the secondary analysis of urinary incontinence data over time. (Aims for this study are in Table 1).

In addition, research support was provided by intramural funds to develop a scannable health diary form, for a pilot study of gene polymorphisms related to symptoms, and to complete collection of data from women as they experienced the early PM (Research Intramural Funding Program, University of Washington School of Nursing).

## Methods
### Design
A prospective, repeated measures design was used to study a population-based sample of women who were about to begin or had begun the transition to menopause at the time of entry into the study. Data were collected throughout the study at intervals described below for a total of 23 years. The study was divided into 4 phases based on the aims associated with each funding period. Each phase expanded the aims of the previous phase.

### Sample
From early 1990 to early 1992, 508 women were enrolled. This original population-based sample from the Seattle area was obtained by telephone screening of all households in over 20 census tracts selected for mixed ethnicity and mixed income. There were 13,120 households enumerated. Of the 11,222 households able to be contacted (85.5 % of those enumerated), 1,428 women between the ages of 35 and 55 were screened (12.7 % of those contacted) and 820 were eligible (57.4 % of those screened). In addition to age, a woman was eligible if

**Table 1** Aims for the Seattle Midlife Women's Health Study by Phase

**Phase 1: 1990–1996**

The aim of Phase I was to test a model relating menopausal status, stress exposure, socialization for midlife, personal and social factors modulating midlife experiences, reproductive health history, and health behaviors to health status and health-seeking behavior in midlife women between the ages of 35 and 55.

**Phase 2: 1996–2001**

**Aim 1.** Describe the **progression through stages of the perimenopuse** (pre transition, early transition, middle transition, late transition, and postmenopause as determined from annual health updates and daily menstrual calendars) for women over a nine year period with respect to:

a) **Symptoms**, including vasomotor, dysphoric mood, insomnia, somatic, and discomfort symptoms, recorded in a daily health diary for three days monthly (coinciding with hormone assays);

b) **Altered ovarian function** (estrone, testosterone (T), and FSH), measured in first morning urine samples at monthly intervals;

c) **perceived stress** (stressful life events, income inadequacy) measured annually and perceived stress measured 3 days each month in the health diary;

d) **stress arousal** (urinary levels of cortisol and catecholamines) measured in the first morning urine samples at monthly intervals; and

e) **symptom management**, including use of health services and hormone replacement therapy assessed annually in a health update questionnaire and interview.

**Aim 2.** Test the following **hypotheses regarding symptoms** during the three stages of the transition to menopause (early to middle to late):

a) women who experience more severe **vasomotor symptoms** during the transition to menopause will have: higher levels of perceived stress, lower levels of estrone, and higher levels of catecholamines and cortisol;

b) women who experience more severe **dysphoric mood symptoms** during the transition to menopause will have: higher levels of perceived stress, higher levels of cortisol, and norepinepherine, and a lower estrogen:androgen ratio;

c) women who experience more sever **insomnia symptoms** during the transition to menopause will have: higher levels of perceived stress, lower levels of estrone, and higher levels of catecholamines.

**Aim 3.** Test the relationship within individual women among HPO axis hormones (estrone, FSH, testosterone), indicators of physiologic stress arousal (cortisol and catecholamines), daily stress ratings, and symptoms (especially vasomotor, dysphoric mood, and insomnia), measured monthly over a nine year period, using auto-correlation and cross-correlation techniques.

**Aim 4.** To estimate the stability of symptom patterns women have recorded in daily health diaries each year with symptom patterns women experience during the menopausal transition (over the period of 1991 to 1995, 1996–2000 and 2001–2005).

**Phase 3: 2002–2006**

**Aim 1.** Describe and compare women in the menopausal transition (early, middle and late transition), in the early postmenopause, and those who use HRT, on indicators of pituitary-ovarian hormone changes, perceived stress, physiologic stress arousal, vasomotor, dysphoric mood, somatic, discomfort and insomnia symptoms.

*Aim 1 Hypotheses:*

Hypothesis 1: Women in late transition will have higher levels of urinary FSH, cortisol and norepinepherine, higher perceived stress and higher vasomotor symptom severity than women in early or middle transition.

Hypothesis 2: Women in the postmenopause will have lower levels of urinary estrone and testosterone, lower perceived stress and higher levels of FSH and vasomotor symptoms than women in the three menopausal transition stages.

Hypothesis 3: There will be no group differences among women in the three menopausal transition stages for urinary estrone,

**Table 1** Aims for the Seattle Midlife Women's Health Study by Phase (*Continued*)

testosterone and epinephrine, depressed mood or the 5 symptom clusters except for vasomotor symptoms.

Hypothesis 4: Women on HRT will have higher estrone levels and lower perceived stress, urinary cortisol, and vasomotor symptoms than women who are not on HRT, those in the menopausal transition or those who are postmenopausal.

**Aim 2.** Compare women in the menopausal transition and early postmenopause with different *estrogen metabolism and catabolism gene polymorphisms* with respect to estradiol and estrone levels, age of onset of middle and late menopausal transition stage and menopause, and heaviness of menstrual blood flow.

**Aim 3.** Compare women in the menopausal transition and early postmenopause with different *estrogen receptor gene polymorphisms* with respect to estradiol and estrone levels, age of onset of middle and late menopausal transition stage and menopause, and heaviness of menstrual blood flow.

**Phase 4: 2007–2013**

Continuation of aims from Phases 1 –3.

Additional aims for the Symptom Cluster Study that was part of Phase 4.

1. Identify symptom clusters (SC) SMWHS participants experienced during the late reproductive, early menopausal transition stages and early postmenopause using latent class analysis to complement the preliminary analyses of the late stage SCs;

2. Determine the consistency of SCs with the clusters identified for the late menopausal transition stage across the late reproductive stage, early menopausal transition stage and early postmenopause;

3. Test models hypothesizing the relationship between SC groups and profiles of:

a) gene polymorphisms in the estrogen synthesis pathways (CYP 19 and 17 HSD) and genes polymorphisms in neuroendocrine pathways (5HTTLPR, NPY, BDNF);

b) hypothalamic-pituitary-ovarian (HPO) biomarkers (E, T, FSH), and hypothalamic-pituitary-adrenal (HPA – cortisol) and autonomic nervous system (ANS- epinephrine, norepinephrine) biomarkers;

c) reproductive aging stages (late reproductive, early and late menopausal transition, and early postmenopause);

d) socio-behavioral risk factors (e.g. high stress, role burden, low income adequacy, employment, education, social support);

e) symptom vulnerability factors (e.g. history of sexual abuse, low mastery, self-consciousness, low self esteem); and outcomes of well-being and interference with work and relationships;

4. Based on a systematic review of controlled clinical trials for managing hot flashes, identify treatment effects on co-occuring symptoms and reported adverse treatment effects, including sleep disturbances, mood, pain and cognitive symptoms;

5. Synthesize results of the empirical analyses (aims 1–3) and systematic review (aim 4) to develop novel symptom cluster management protocols to be tested in a future feasibility study.

Additional aims for Urinary Incontinence Study that was part of Phase 4.

1. Determine the influence of age and menopausal transition factors on the experience of urinary incontinence (stress, urge and any incontinence) among midlife women;

2. Assess the influence of lifespan health factors and life context (personal and social resources and stress) on urinary incontinence; and

3. Determine the relationship between urinary incontinence and well-being, symptoms (fatigue, disrupted sleep, anxiety and depressed mood) and interference with daily living (work and relationships).

she had an intact uterus and at least one ovary, had at least one menstrual period within the past 12 months, was not pregnant or lactating, and could read and understand English. Of the 820 women eligible, 620 agreed to participate (75.6 % of those eligible) and 508 actually began the study and provided initial cross-

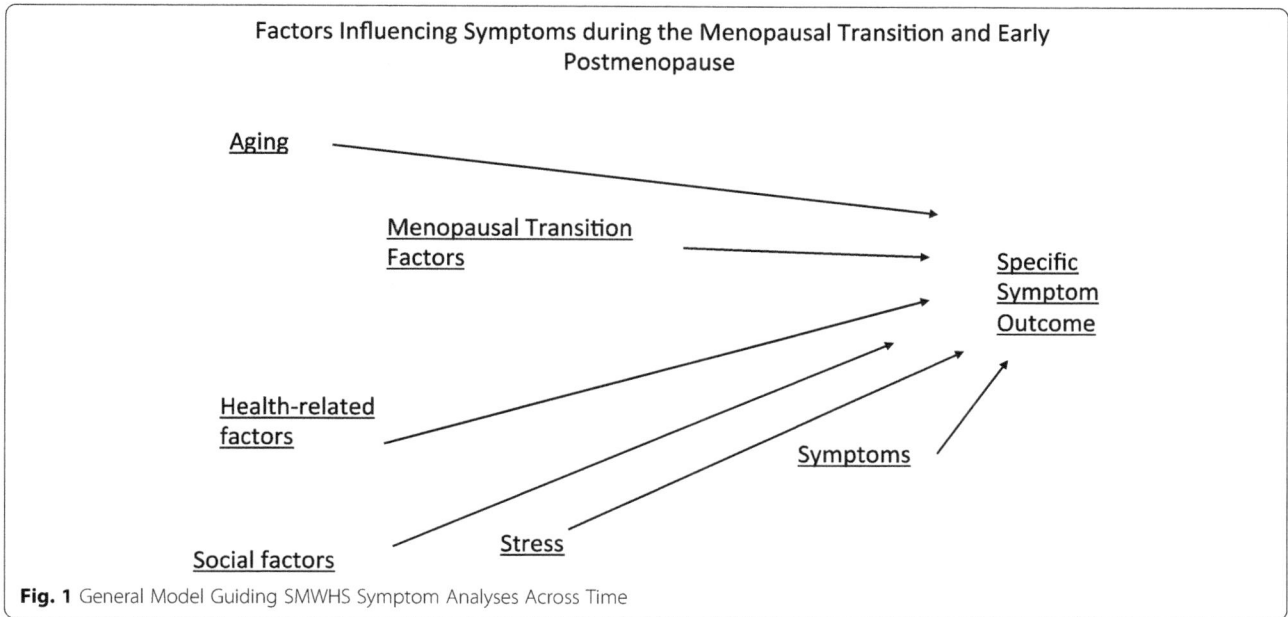

**Fig. 1** General Model Guiding SMWHS Symptom Analyses Across Time

sectional data (81.9 % of those who initially agreed to participate) (See Table 2). 390 of the 508 women entered the longitudinal component of the study (76.8 % of the cross-sectional sample) by agreeing to provide data over time. A description of the characteristics of the women who agreed to participate in the longitudinal component ($N = 390$) and those who only completed the initial cross sectional component ($N = 118$) is shown in Table 3. Those who entered the longitudinal component compared to those who did not enter were more likely to be partnered, not a parent and not Black. There were no significant differences for education, employment, age, BMI, income and stress level.

For entry into the second major funding phase of the study (mid-1996), women still enrolled at the end of the previous phase of this longitudinal project, plus those who had dropped out of phase 1 but had contributed at least two years of data, were contacted by phone about participating in this second phase. A total of 300 women were contacted in mid-1996 and screened for continuing eligibility (5 years or less PM or, if taking hormones, age less than 60 years old, uterus intact and at least one ovary intact). Of

those 300 women screened, 243 were eligible and agreed to enroll in phase 2 (62 % of the 390 who began the longitudinal component). In addition, between 2000 and 2002, 174 women provided a buccal cell smear for genotyping. See Fig. 2 for retention across the entire project.

For entry into the third major funding phase of the study (2001–2006) all eligible women (5 years or less PM or, if taking hormones, age less than 60, uterus intact and at least one ovary) who were still participating ($N = 160$) were contacted and screened (66 % of those who entered phase 2). Of these 160 women, 144 (90 %) agreed to continue for a third phase. At the end of phase three 67 women were still eligible and participating.

Research funds from the UW School of Nursing Research Intramural Funding Program were obtained in 2007 to continue data collection from those still eligible for the study. Of these 67 women, 64 were eligible and agreed to continue participation in the fourth and final phase until no longer eligible. This part of the study continued until February 2013 when all data collection was completed. Of the original 508 women who entered the study, by the end of the study in 2013, 173 had dropped due to personal reasons (34 %), 162 were lost to contact (32 %) and 173 became ineligible sometime during the study (34 %).

**Retention efforts**
Numerous efforts were taken to retain the eligible sample throughout the study. These include the following:

- yearly birthday card with a personal note
- yearly thank you checks through the first two funding periods

**Table 2** Smwhs sample identification and screening

| Sampling Identification | N and (% of total enumerated) |
| --- | --- |
| Households enumerated | 13,120 (100 %) |
| Households contacted by phone | 11,222 (86 %) |
| Women in households 35–55 years of age screened | 1,428 (11 %) |
| Women eligible after screening | 820 (6 %) |
| Women who agreed to participate | 620 (5 %) |
| Women who actually began study | 508 (4 %) |

**Table 3** Baseline Sample Characteristics for women who participated in the Longitudinal Component Compared with women who participated only in the Cross Sectional Component (1990–1991)

| Characteristic | Women in Longitudinal Component (n = 390) Mean (SD) | Women in Cross Sectional Component (n = 118) Mean (SD) | p value* |
|---|---|---|---|
| Age (years) | 41.5 (4.3) | 41.4 (4.4) | 0.43 |
| Years of education | 15.7 (2.8) | 15.3 (3.2) | 0.15 |
| Family gross income ($) | 37360 (15,800) | 35,500 (17,460) | 0.27 |
| Number live births | 1.97 (1.4) | 1.57 (1.4) | .006 |
| Perceived stress | 2.2 (0.55) | 2.3 (0.55) | 0.31 |
| Characteristic | N (Percent) | N (Percent) | p value** |
| Currently employed | | | |
| Yes | 336 (86.1) | 102 (86.4) | 0.94 |
| No | 54 (13.8) | 16 (13.6) | |
| Race/ethnicity | | | |
| African American | 32 (8.2) | 26 (22.0) | .001 |
| Asian /Pacific Islander | 34 (8.7) | 9 (7.6) | |
| Caucasian | 311 (79.7) | 80 (67.8) | |
| Other (Hispanic, Mixed) | 13 (3.3) | 3 (2.5) | |
| Marital Status | | | |
| Married/partnered | 277 (71.0) | 71 (60.2) | 0.03 |
| Never partnered/ divorced/widowed | 113 (29.0) | 47 (39.8) | |
| Never married/partnered | 21 (7.2) | 14 (6.5) | |

*Independent t-test
**Chi-square test

- personal and consistent contact by the research staff
  - reminder postcards about data collection
  - in-person pick-up of urine and diaries at a community site or at home
  - reminder phone calls about pick-up of data
- flexibility regarding schedules; negotiating alternatives
- periodic sharing of findings with women
- yearly newsletter, The Midlife Times
- two Health Fairs at community sites
- a web site
- a certification of appreciation after 10 years of participation
- easy access to research staff via phone and email

**Data collection**

In the first phase of the study all measures were pencil and paper measures. This included measures of symptom severity, stress, personal and social resources, socialization for midlife and aging, reproductive health experiences including menstrual cycle changes, social environmental demands, and personal health practices. These measures were obtained in an annual daily health diary across two to three menstrual cycles, an annual health questionnaire and a menstrual calendar.

In the second phase of the study measures of pituitary-ovarian and pituitary-adrenal function were added. These additional measures were obtained by collecting monthly first AM urine specimens on day 6 of the menstrual cycle, if the woman was still cycling. Women were instructed not to eat, drink, smoke, take medications or exercise before each urine collection. The health diary was collected on 3 consecutive days (days 5, 6 and 7) to coordinate with the time of the urine collection (day 6). For those with very erratic bleeding and those no longer having periods a consistent 3 days of the month was used for data collection. This procedure was used from late 1996 through 2000.

The data collection time for the diary and urine specimens was modified from 2001 through 2005. The timing was changed from monthly to quarterly for both the diary and urine collections. During all phases of the study the yearly health questionnaire and menstrual calendars were continued (See Table 4 for sample size for each measure by year).

In addition, buccal cell smears were obtained from 174 of these women between 2000 and 2002. Urine collections stopped at the end of 2005. From 2006 to the end of the study quarterly health diaries, yearly health questionnaires and menstrual calendars, if still bleeding, were obtained.

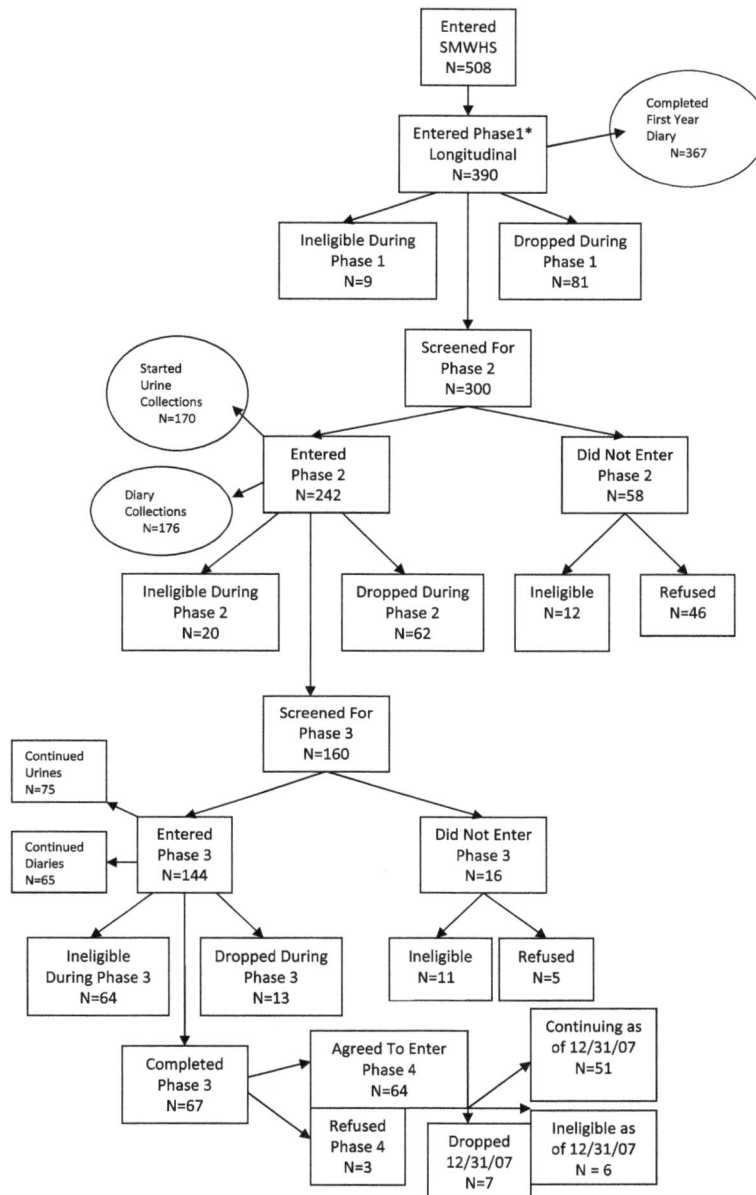

**Fig. 2** Retention Flow Chart. *Funding phases

## Data handling

Except for the interview at the start of the study, all data in phase 1 and phase 4 were collected by mail (yearly questionnaire, diaries, menstrual calendars). In phases 2 and 3 the diaries and urine samples were collected in person while the annual questionnaire and menstrual calendar were collected by mail. For the urine samples, after the first morning urine was collected by the participant it was immediately frozen in a home freezer at 0°. These specimens were either brought frozen to a community site by the participant at a prearranged time or were picked up by a research associate within 56 days

(8 weeks) of collection. Each specimen was kept frozen during transport and then taken to the University of Washington School of Nursing Biobehavioral Lab and placed in a –70° centigrade freezer. The specimens were then assayed by the laboratory staff. (See Additional file 1: Assay Descriptions and Laboratory Assay Procedure). A maximum of 56 days for home freezing was determined by the laboratory staff using various intervals and testing for sample degradation. The diaries were picked up in a similar manner as the urine during phases 2 and 3. If urine was not collected, the diaries were mailed to the study personnel.

**Table 4** Frequencies for data sources (1990–2013)

|  | Questionnaire N | Diary N | Assay N (# specimens) |
|---|---|---|---|
| 1990–1992 | 508 | 367 | NA |
| 1993 | 347 | 259 | NA |
| 1994 | 309 | 261 | NA |
| 1995 | 250 | 141 | NA |
| 1996 | 192 | 146 | NA |
| 1997 | 233 | 176 | 170 (1783) |
| 1998 | 205 | 162 | 167 (1820) |
| 1999 | 212 | 149 | 157 (1478) |
| 2000 | 190 | 103 | 106 (1036) |
| 2001 | 175 | 79 | 85 (340) |
| 2002 | 157 | 65 | 74 (279) |
| 2003 | 140 | 59 | 59 (236) |
| 2004 | 110 | 46 | 54 (208) |
| 2005 | 95 | 44 | 49 (179) |
| 2006 | 84 | 30 | NA |
| 2007 | 57 | 20 | NA |
| 2008 | 47 | 18 | NA |
| 2009 | 37 | 15 | NA |
| 2010 | 31 | 10 | NA |
| 2011 | 20 | 10 | NA |
| 2012 | 17 | 5 | NA |
| 2013 | 12 | 5 | NA |

## Measures

A blank **menstrual calendar** was mailed at the end of each calendar year for completion during the following year. Any occurrence of bleeding (B) or spotting (S) was recorded. Beginning in 1996, the amount of B on a scale of 1 (light flow) to 4 (very heavy/flooding) was recorded with each occurrence. Spotting was any bloody vaginal discharge that did not require any protection [9]. (See Additional file 1 for sample calendar). The menstrual calendars were returned at the start of the following year and reviewed for completeness.

Definitions of bleeding events used for the study, called standard bleeding events, were modifications of those recommended by WHO [9] [Gray, RH. WHO Meeting on the Analysis of Bleeding Patterns, Feb 28, 1978, unpublished]. A standard bleeding episode was defined as ≥2 days of B or a mix of ≥2 B and S days but not all S days with ≤2 bleed free days. A standard bleeding interval was any series of ≥4 consecutive bleed-free days bounded by bleeding episodes. A bleeding segment was a bleeding episode and the subsequent bleeding interval.

The WHO standard definitions did not differentiate bleeding episodes from intermenstrual bleeding (IMB)

or non-menses bleeding such as S or B days between consecutive bleeding episodes and within a bleeding interval. A limitation of the WHO standard definition of a bleeding episode (≥1 days B or S) was the creation of many very short bleeding segments. Short bleeding segments can overstate the incidence of irregularity, bias downward the age of onset of each MT stage and bias upward the duration of MT stages. To address this problem of short bleeding segments additional criteria were developed by the study staff and Sybil Crawford, PhD, to determine if a bleeding event with 1 B day or 1 or more S days only was an episode or IMB and whether 3 bleed free days between B or S days represented a bleeding interval or was part of the episode. The criteria were applied using the woman as the unit of analysis as recommended by Treloar [10] (See Additional file 1 for Nonstandard Bleeding Criteria). The basic premise behind these additional criteria was that the typical bleeding pattern of some women can reflect a slight variation from the standard definitions and that IMB or non-menses bleeding is a phenomenon that needs to be accounted for as part of a woman's bleeding pattern.

A reduction in the number of short bleeding segments was the result of this procedure. In the SMWHS sample. The majority of instances of 1 S day or ≥2 S days together occurred between episodes, in the bleeding interval (unpublished data).

After all the bleeding criteria were applied to the calendar data each calendar was assigned a subgroup for staging using staging criteria developed by the study personnel [11] and modified based on the findings of the ReSTAGE Collaboration [12] (See Additional file 1 for Staging Criteria).

A **health questionnaire** was mailed at the end of each year. This questionnaire obtained data about changes in health, the menstrual cycle, current health practices, medication use, stress, social support, mental health, symptoms and well-being. (See Additional file 1 for a summary of measures included in the annual health questionnaires).

A **health diary** was kept by a subset of the original 508 women. Initially this diary was kept daily for two to three menstrual cycles. It was completed once a year for three years (at the start of the study, 12 months later, and 24 months from the start). The data from this early diary was hand entered into the computer. In 1994 the diary was converted to a scannable format and for 1995 and 1996 was kept daily for two weeks once a year (around the time of the yearly health questionnaire). Beginning in late 1996 to the end of 2000 this scannable diary was kept for 3 days every menstrual cycle on days 5, 6, and 7, if there were identifiable menstrual periods, to correspond with the urine collection on day 6. Otherwise it was kept monthly on the same 3 days every month. Starting in 2001 the diary was completed once a quarter for the same 3 consecutive days instead of monthly. The diary included items such as symptoms commonly experienced by midlife women, medication use, stress levels and health practices (smoking, drinking alcohol, caffeine use, exercise, sleep). (See Additional file 1 for sample pages of the diary).

**Urine specimens** were obtained from a subset of women one time per menstrual cycle on day 6 or once a month if there were no identifiable periods. These urine collections began in late 1996 and continued until the end of 2005. This was a first morning specimen and was assayed for estrone glucuronide, FSH, total testosterone, cortisol, epinephrine and norepinephrine. (See Additional file 1 for assay descriptions).

A **buccal cell smear** was obtained for genetic analysis from 174 women sometime between 2000 and 2002. (See Additional file 1 for buccal cell smear collection procedure and Additional file 1 for genotyping sequencing).

## Analytic strategies

A variety of analytic strategies was used over the course of the study. Examples include discriminant function analysis [9], confirmatory factor analysis and LISREL [8–14], content analysis with cross tabulations [15–17], ANOVA and regression analysis [18], cluster analysis [19], t-tests [20], time series analysis [21], general estimating equation [22] and numerous papers since 2006 using multilevel modeling (MLM) [23–35]. The analytic method called multi-level modeling (MLM) was used for most of the longitudinal analyses once most of the data were collected and processed (from 2006 on). For all MLM analyses age was used as the measure of time. This method was specifically adapted for the SMWHS data by a statistician (Don Percival, PhD) and was developed using an R program to account for specific characteristics of the data such as an unbalanced design, serial correlation, and missing data [30]. (See Additional file 1 for a detailed description of the MLM procedure).

## Results

Selected results are presented to illustrate the contributions of each phase of the SMWHS. A complete list of publications from the Seattle Midlife Women's Health Study is appended to the References section.

### Phase 1

Data collected during phase I of the study were used to amplify our understanding of women's views of midlife and menopause, as well as to evaluate models of women's health and health-seeking behavior during midlife. In response to open-ended questions, women described midlife as a time of many transitions: getting older and changing bodies, outlooks and relationships.

Personal achievements and employment were central to the lives of midlife women in this study [16]. Women viewed menopause as a period of transition. When women were asked about their anticipation of menopause they indicated it was a time of uncertainty that elicited mixed feelings [17]. Women also revealed their meanings of menopause as the cessation of periods, experiencing the end of fertility and reproductive capacity, hormonal changes, new or different life stage, changing emotions, changing bodies, symptoms, and part of the aging process. Few referred to menopause as a time of risk for disease or of need for health care.

A model of depressed mood symptoms was developed, evaluating 3 pathways to depressed mood, comparing the influence of the MT, stressful life context, and health status pathways in a multiethnic sample ($N = 337$). The stressful life context pathway was most influential in accounting for depressed mood. Health status had a direct effect on depressed mood and an indirect effect through perceived stress. The menopausal changes pathway had little explanatory power. At the time this model was tested, the majority of participants were in the Late Reproductive stage or the Early MT stage. Nonetheless, these results suggested the need for clinicians to look beyond menopausal status to the broader context of midlife women's lives [8].

The primary endpoint throughout the study was type and severity of symptoms women experienced and reported during the MT and early PM. When the symptoms women experienced during midlife were first examined, measured during the premenses week, several groups were identified, including: dysphoric mood, vasomotor, somatic, neuromuscular,and insomnia symptoms. Notably the stability of vasomotor and somatic symptoms was lowest over the three year period studied, but dysphoric mood, neuromuscular, and insomnia symptoms were relatively stable, suggesting their chronic experience in this cohort [13]. The variability of the vasomotor and somatic symptoms over the three year period led to a focus on the role of the MT and related hormonal changes during subsequent phases of the study.

During phase 1 women's health-seeking behavior was also investigated and was then tracked during subsequent phases. After publication of Women's Health Initiative findings in 2002 linking hormone therapy (HT) with increased risk of breast cancer, stroke, heart attacks and other health problems, the percent of women taking hormones during the MT decreased from 49 % in 1999 to 35 % in 2003 [23].

### Phases 2, 3, and 4
#### Development of a staging system

Phase 2 of the study focused on the development of a staging system for the MT that eventually informed and was integrated with the Staging Reproductive Aging Workshop (STRAW) efforts [36], and later validated by the multi-country work of the Re-STAGE Collaboration [11, 37–39]. Mitchell led development of the MT staging system from detailed observation and analysis of menstrual calendar data over a seven year period (1990–1997) [11]. Development of the staging system for the MT provided a useful framework to organize subsequent analyses and demonstrate the influence of the MT stages on endocrine patterns, symptoms, and other aspects of the MT.

An important measurement issue related to staging reproductive aging was whether retrospective and prospective reporting of menstrual irregularity by women would influence staging efforts. Agreement between women's reporting on a menstrual calendar and questionnaires with retrospective reports was weak, thus we incorporated only prospective reporting on menstrual calendars in the SMWHS staging approach [40].

The original and modified stages and criteria for staging used by SMWHS were as follows:

**Pretransition stage** when cycles were regular with no change in length of periods, amount of flow or cycle length from the previous year. This stage was later called Late Reproductive stage to correspond to STRAW recommendations.

**Early stage** when cycles were still regular but there was a change in length of periods, amount of flow or cycle length from the previous year. This stage was later called Late Reproductive stage to correspond to STRAW recommendations.

**Middle stage** when cycles became irregular, i.e., start of consecutive cycles were 7 or more days apart. This stage was later called Early stage to correspond to STRAW recommendations.

**Late stage** when periods were skipped, i.e., twice the modal cycle length between consecutive cycles. The criteria for this stage were later changed to 60 or more days of amenorrhea between the start of consecutive periods to correspond to the findings from the ReSTAGE Collaboration [39].

The original focus of staging in the SMWHS was on the menopausal transition. When the Staging Reproductive Aging Workshop (STRAW) investigators proposed use of stages of reproductive aging across the lifespan, we adopted the STRAW staging approach derived from consensus of investigators who participated in the STRAW workship in 2001. Our initial staging system had included an early, middle, and late stage of the menopausal transition. Because the STRAW investigators believed that the menopausal transition did not begin until cycle intervals became irregular, we adapted our staging to fit their recommendations. We no longer used our old definition of early menopausal transition, which included regular cycles with more subtle changes in the length of the period and cycle length, and instead adopted the STRAW definition of early stage. We also changed our pretransition stage to use the nomenclature of STRAW: late reproductive stage.

**Age of onset** of MT stages and the final menstrual period (FMP), and **duration** of the Early and Late MT stages were identified. On average, women ($N = 121$) entered Early stage at age 46.4 (SD = 3.4) and stayed in the stage ($N = 82$) for an average of 2.8 years (SD = 1.5). On average, women ($N = 130$) entered Late stage at age 49.4 (SD = 2.7) and stayed in this stage ($N = 84$) for an average of 2.5 years (SD = 1.3). The average age ($N = 114$) for the FMP (start of PM) for this cohort was 52.1 (SD = 2.9) years [37].

To identify an onset of each MT stage it was necessary to have bleeding data about the prior stage for the previous 12 months so the time of change could be identified. For example, using the staging criteria, if a woman was in Early stage for one year and the next year met the criteria for Late stage, the onset of Late stage could be identified. However, if she was in Late stage for one year but the prior 12 months of calendar data were not available, her onset of Late stage would be unknown. This same situation also would apply to onset of Early stage. Content analysis of women's descriptions of irregularity and skipping of periods revealed that using simple questions about these was not adequate to apply the staging criteria. Instead, it was important to use the menstrual calendars to collect actual bleeding data [40].

*Hormonal changes across the menopausal transition*
An inspection of changes in urinary **FSH** (follicle-stimulating hormone) levels across the MT showed a rise as women progressed from Early MT to Late MT stage and to early PM and urinary **estrone** levels rose slightly from the Early to the Late MT stage and then dropped substantially the final year before and the first year after the FMP. **Urinary testosterone** levels remained flat across all MT stages and early PM. When these 3 hormones were analyzed for an association with MT stage across time, early PM had a significant negative effect on estrone and both Late MT stage and early PM had a significant positive effect on FSH. Testosterone was not affected by stage (unpublished data). (See Figs. 3 a,b,c)

When these same hormone levels were graphed based on number of **years before and after FMP** (from 8 years before to 5 years after FMP) FSH began to rise at 3 years before FMP and steadily increased to 3 years after FMP

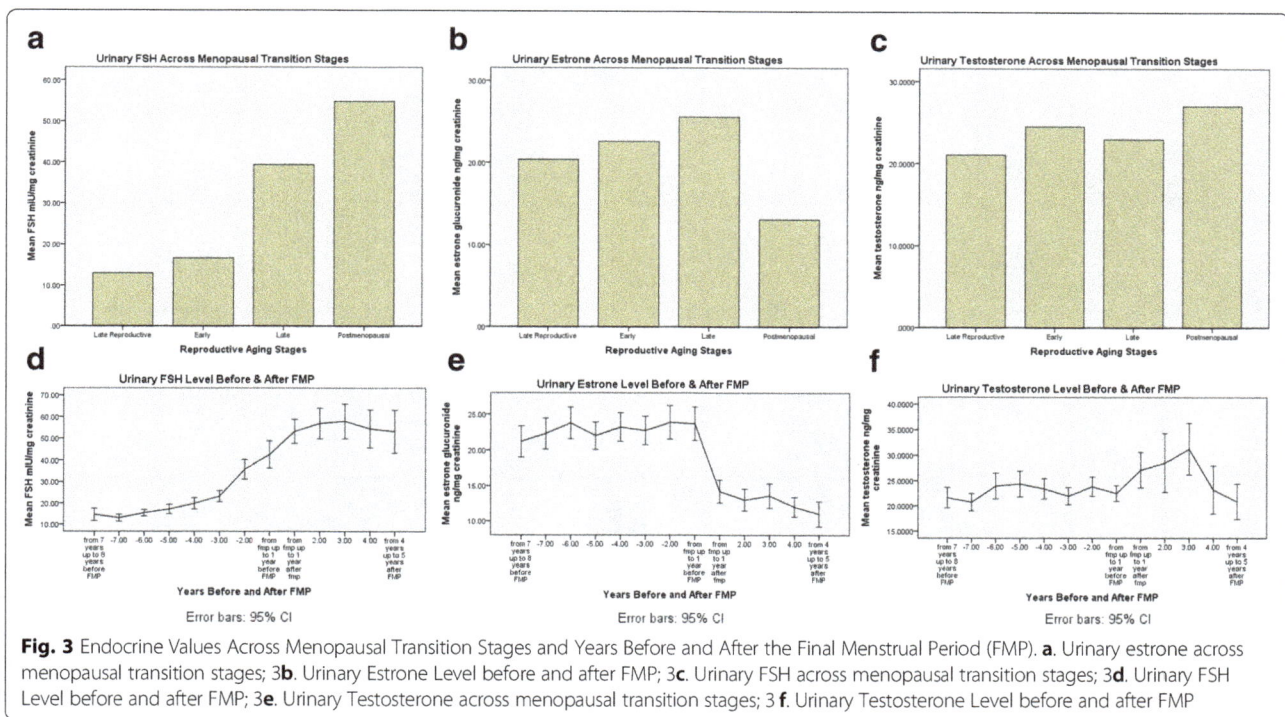

**Fig. 3** Endocrine Values Across Menopausal Transition Stages and Years Before and After the Final Menstrual Period (FMP). **a**. Urinary estrone across menopausal transition stages; 3**b**. Urinary Estrone Level before and after FMP; 3**c**. Urinary FSH across menopausal transition stages; 3**d**. Urinary FSH Level before and after FMP; 3**e**. Urinary Testosterone across menopausal transition stages; 3 **f**. Urinary Testosterone Level before and after FMP

when it leveled off to at least 5 years FMP. Estrone showed a drop in level within 1 year before FMP and then slowly continued to decline to at least 5 years after FMP. Testosterone began to rise within 1 year before FMP, peaked at 3 year after FMP and declined steadily to at least 5 years after FMP (See Figs. 3 d,e,f).

Because of the important relationship of stress during midlife to symptoms, urinary **cortisol** was studied. The findings showed an increase in cortisol in the 7 to 12 months after onset of Late stage compared to the 7 to 12 months before onset of Late stage [20]. Also, women with increased cortisol levels during the Late stage had more severe hot flashes than those without a cortisol increase during the same stage [20]. In another study of cortisol using multilevel modeling there was a significant positive relationship between urinary epinephrine, norepinephrine, estrone, FSH, testosterone and hot flashes with cortisol levels in a univariate model. Health-related and social factors and symptoms other than hot flashes did not show a significant effect on cortisol levels. When the significant variables were combined in a multivariate model only estrone and FSH had a significant effect on cortisol [25].

An inspection of changes in urinary cortisol revealed a rise in the late MT stage, as seen in earlier analyses (See Fig. 4a) [15] and inspection revealed a gradual increase from 7 years before to 5 years after FMP (Fig. 4b). An inspection of urinary epinephrine and norepinephrine levels across MT stages showed a minimal change in epinephrine across stages and a slight rise in norepinephrine from

Early MT stage to early PM (Fig. 4 c and d). When a multilevel analysis of these catecholamines across MT stage was done no significant effect of stage was found on epinephrine or on norepinephrine (unpublished data). In contrast, when number of years before and after FMP were examined, epinephrine showed no definitive pattern while norepinephrine slowly rose from 8 years before FMP to 5 years after FMP (Fig. 4 e and f).

### Well-being and the menopausal transition

General well-being as measured by the 4 item subscale of the General Well-Being Scale [41] was positively associated with satisfaction with social support and a sense of mastery [27]. A decrease in well-being was associated with negative life events. Being in Late Stage of MT was associated with a decrease in well-being only in the univariate analysis.

### Symptom patterns across the menopausal transition

Because the primary end points throughout the SMWHS were symptoms, of interest was identifying effects of MT stages on various types of symptoms. In addition, we used a general model (See Fig. 1) to guide analyses of women's symptom experiences over time that included the following concepts and examples of indicators for each: menopausal transition factors, aging, health-related factors, stress-related factors, and other co-occurring symptoms. In the following paragraphs, findings related to each of the symptom groups studied are summarized.

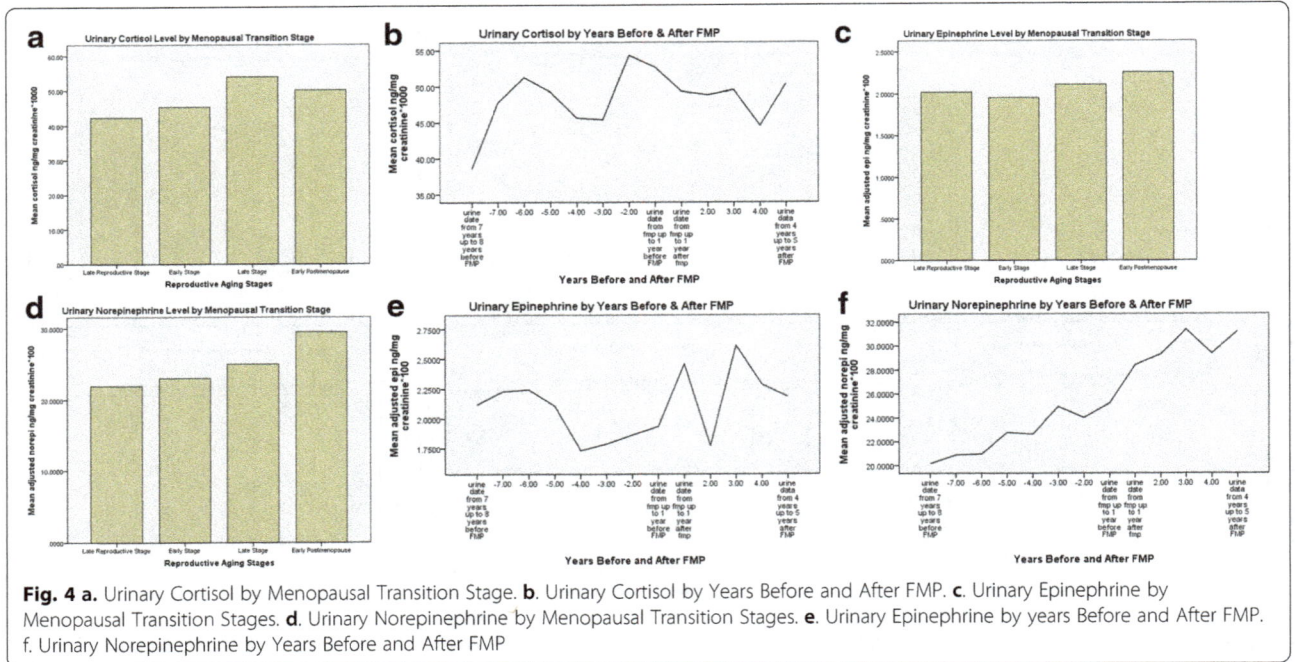

**Fig. 4 a.** Urinary Cortisol by Menopausal Transition Stage. **b**. Urinary Cortisol by Years Before and After FMP. **c**. Urinary Epinephrine by Menopausal Transition Stages. **d**. Urinary Norepinephrine by Menopausal Transition Stages. **e**. Urinary Epinephrine by years Before and After FMP. f. Urinary Norepinephrine by Years Before and After FMP

### Hot flashes

An analysis of women using and not using hormone therapy (HT) revealed that increases in hot flash severity were associated with late transition stage, early postmenopause, use of HT, duration of early transition stage, age of entry into early PM and level of FSH. Age of entry into early transition and estrone levels were associated with decreased hot flash severity. Not associated with hot flash severity were being in early transition stage, age of entry into or duration of late transition stage and all of the psychosocial (anxiety, stress, depressed mood) and lifestyle variables (BMI, activity level, sleep, alcohol use). Use of HT ameliorated but did not eliminate severe hot flashes [23].

Hot flash severity persisted through the MT stages, peaking in the Late MT stage and diminishing only after the second year PM. Hot flash severity was associated with being older, being in the Late MT stage or early PM, beginning the Late MT stage at a younger age and reporting greater anxiety. In a model including only endocrine factors, hot flash severity was significantly associated with higher FSH and lower estrone levels [34].

### Sleep symptoms

Severity of **nighttime awakening** was significantly associated with age, Late MT stage and early PM, higher FSH, lower E1G, more severe hot flashes, depressed mood, anxiety, joint pain, backache, and perceived stress, history of sexual abuse, poorer perceived health, and less alcohol use [30]. Severity of **problems going to sleep** was associated with hot flashes, depressed mood,

anxiety, joint pain, backache, perceived stress, history of sexual abuse, poorer perceived health, less alcohol use, and lower cortisol, but not with MT stages or hormone levels. Severity of **early morning awakening** was significantly associated with age, hot flashes, depressed mood anxiety, joint pain, backache, perceived stress, history of sexual abuse, poorer perceived health, but not MT stages, estrone, or FSH.

### Depressed mood

Most women experienced the MT without a high level of depressed mood. A small group of women experienced worsening of their mood. Another small group experienced improvement in their mood [19]. Women with consistently depressed mood were more likely to have hot flashes, stress, history of premenstrual syndrome and postpartum blues than women with occasional depressed mood or those without depressed mood [19, 42].

Depressed mood symptoms (measured by CES-D scores) were associated with being in the Late MT stage, severity of hot flashes, life stress, family history of depression, history of postpartum blues, sexual abuse history, body mass index, and use of antidepressants. Hormonal levels and age of entry into and duration of Late MT stage were unrelated [24]. In another multivariate analysis, when covariates were examined individually, a decrease in depressed mood as a single symptom was associated with early PM, higher estrone, more exercise and being partnered. An increase in depressed mood was associated with perceived stress, a history of sexual abuse and more severe sleep disruption symptoms (problem getting to sleep, awakening at night, early morning awakening). FSH level, BMI, alcohol use, number of live births and hot flash severity were not associated with depressed mood. In a model with multiple covariates that individually had a significant effect, awakening at night no longer significantly increased depressed mood. Also, estrone level and early PM were no longer associated with a decrease in depressed mood [Mitchell, ES and Woods, NF Depressed Mood during the Menopausal Transition, Reproductive Aging and Life: Observations from the Seattle Midlife Women's Health Study. Unpublished].

## Cognitive symptoms

Women in the Late Reproductive and Early MT stages and those who used hormones reported more problems with memory measured by the Memory Functioning Questionnaire than women in Late stage [18]. About 72 % of women reported problems remembering names at least some of the time. About 50 % had a problem remembering where they put things, recent phone numbers, things others told them (or they told others), keeping up correspondence and forgetting what they were doing. However, none of these events was considered a serious problem [18]. Many types of problems with memory were related to lower ratings of health and depressed mood. Problems with current memory and remembering past events were associated with higher levels of reported stress, which women attributed to the burden of meeting multiple role demands [18].

**Memory changes** most noted by women (mean age 47 years) who responded to open-ended questions about their memory were difficulty remembering words or numbers, i.e., verbal memory. These changes were attributed to increased role burden and stress, getting older, physical health, menstrual cycle changes/hormones, inadequate concentration, and emotional factors [15].

As individual covariates and in a multivariate model, age, anxiety, depressed mood, night-time awakening, perceived stress, perceived health, and employment were each significantly related to **difficulty concentrating**. Hot flashes, amount of exercise and history of sexual abuse had a significant effect as individual covariates but not in the final multivariate model. The best predictors of **forgetfulness** when analyzed as individual covariates and in the multivariate model were age, hot flashes, anxiety, depressed mood, perceived stress, perceived health and history of sexual abuse [32].

## Pain symptoms

Pain symptoms rose slightly with age. A significant increase in **back pain** was reported during the Early and Late MT stages and early PM, but urinary E1G, FSH and testosterone levels were unrelated. Of the stress-related factors, perceived stress and lower overnight urinary

cortisol levels were associated with more severe back pain; history of sexual abuse and catecholamines did not have a significant effect. Women most troubled by symptoms of hot flashes, depressed mood, anxiety, night-time awakening, and difficulty concentrating reported significantly greater back pain. Of the health-related factors, having worse perceived health, exercising more, using analgesics, and having a higher body mass index were associated with more back pain, but alcohol use and smoking did not have significant effects. Of the social factors, only having more years of formal education was associated with less back pain; parenting, having a partner, and employment did not have significant. Factors associated with joint pain included age but not menopausal transition-related factors. Symptoms of hot flashes, night-time awakening, depressed mood, and difficulty concentrating were each significantly associated with **joint pain**. Poorer perceived health, more exercise, higher body mass index, and greater analgesic use were all associated positively with joint pain. History of sexual abuse was the only stress-related factor significantly related to joint pain severity [29].

## Sexual desire symptoms

Women's concerns about decreasing sexual desire during midlife prompted analysis of factors influencing sexual desire as recorded in the symptom diaries. Women reported a significant reduction in sexual desire during the Late MT stage and early PM. Those with higher urinary E1G and T reported significantly higher levels of sexual desire whereas those with higher FSH levels reported significantly lower sexual desire. Women using hormone therapy also reported higher sexual desire. Those reporting higher perceived stress reported lower sexual desire, but having a history of sexual abuse did not have a significant effect. Those most troubled by symptoms of hot flashes, fatigue, depressed mood, anxiety, difficulty getting to sleep, early morning awakening, and awakening during the night also reported significantly lower sexual desire, but there was no effect of vaginal dryness. Women with better perceived health and those reporting more exercise and more alcohol intake also reported greater sexual desire. Having a partner was associated with lower sexual desire [26].

## Urinary incontinence symptoms

**Stress urinary incontinence** (SUI) was associated significantly with individual predictors of worse perceived health, history of ≥3 live births, being in the Early MT stage, having less formal education and being white. **Urge incontinence** (UUI) was associated significantly with individual predictors of increasing age, worse perceived health, BMI ≥30, history of ≥3 live births, and lower FSH levels. Both SUI and UUI were significantly associated with lower self-esteem and with age included in the models as a measure of time. UI effects on mood symptoms, attitudes toward aging and menopause, perceived health and consequences for daily life were not significant [22, 33].

### Interference of symptoms with work and relationships

Women reported the effects of their symptoms on work and relationships in the symptom diary. Analyses of the extent to which symptoms interfered with daily living revealed that **interference with work** was significantly associated with perceived health, stress, hot flashes, depressed mood, anxiety, difficulty getting to sleep, awakening during the night, early morning awakening, backache, joint pain, forgetfulness and difficulty concentrating. **Interference with relationships** was significantly associated with age and individual covariates perceived health, estrone, perceived stress, depressed mood, anxiety, sleep symptoms, backache, joint pain, forgetfulness and difficulty concentrating [31].

### Genetic influences and the menopausal transition

Polymorphisms in the estrogen synthesizing, metabolizing, and receptor genes were genotyped and associated with both symptoms and the timing of the events of the MT. Women with the CYP19 11r polymorphism reported more severe and frequent hot flashes during the Early and Late MT stages and early PM and higher E1G levels during Early and Late stages. [43]. In addition, polymorphisms in the 17 beta HSD gene (rs 5942 and rs 2389) were related to a symptom cluster incuding high severity hot flashes and moderate levels of 5 other symptom groups (sleep, mood, cognitive, pain symptoms). Moreover the rs2389 heterozygous allele had a significant positive effect on estrone and rs2830 homozygous mutant allele had a significant negative effect on FSH. The rs5942 17 HSD had no effect on either estrone or FSH (unpublished data).

Women with two CYP19 7r alleles had menarche earlier (11.5 y) than those with one CYP19 7r allele (13.1 y). Women with two CYP19 11r alleles were 2 years older at onset of Late stage than those with one CYP19 11r allele (50.7 y vs 48.6 y). Those with two CYP19 7r(−3) alleles were 2 years older at FMP than those without this allele (53.9 y vs 51.3 y). Women with the homozygous wild-type allele for HSDB1 (rs2830) were younger at FMP by 2 years than those with the heterozygous allele (50.8 y vs 52.9 y). Women with the heterozygous allele for CYP1B1*2 had a later age at menarche compared with women with the homozygous wild type (13 y vs 12.5 y). [44].

### Stress and symptoms during the menopausal transition

Although some would contend that the MT is inherently stressful, factors that influenced the level of perceived stress among SMWHS participants were inadequate income to meet needs, lower levels of perceived health

status, role burden and current employment [28]. Of interest was that perceived stress was related to each of the symptoms studied: hot flashes, depressed mood, lower sexual desire, difficulty getting to sleep, night-time awakening, early morning awakening, forgetfulness, difficulty concentrating, but not urinary incontinence symptoms. Perceived stress was not related to MT stage nor to the endocrine assays measured, including E1G, FSH, cortisol, and the catecholamines.

### Symptom clusters associated with the menopausal transition

Analyses of each of the symptoms studied indicated they were commonly associated with other symptoms, e.g. hot flashes with sleep problems, depressed mood, pain and cognitive symptoms. The realization that women experienced multiple, co-occurring symptoms (defined as symptom clusters) during the MT and early PM led to further study [45]. Three symptom clusters composed of hot flashes and five groups of symptoms that had been identified in prior factor analysis (depressed mood symptoms, sleep disruption symptoms, tension symptoms, cognitive symptoms, and pain symptoms) among this community-based cohort [46]. Cluster I was composed of low severity hot flashes with low severity sleep disruption symptoms, depressed mood symptoms, tension symptoms, cognitive symptoms and pain symptoms (75 %); Cluster II was high severity hot flashes with a moderate level of the 5 symptom clusters (12 %); and Cluster III was low severity hot flashes with moderate severity levels of the 5 symptom clusters (13 %). When each of the 3 clusters were compared with each other for estrone, FSH, testosterone, epinephrine and norepinephrine significant group differences were between Cluster I (low hot flash/low symptom clusters) and Cluster III (high hot flash/moderate symptom clusters), and between Cluster I and Cluster II (low hot flash/moderate symptom clusters). Cluster III had lower estrone, higher FSH, lower epinephrine and higher norepinephrine than Cluster I and Cluster II had lower epinephrine levels than Cluster I. Cortisol and testosterone had no significant group differences among the 3 clusters [47].

When perceived stress levels were compared among the 3 clusters, Clusters II and III had significantly higher levels than Cluster I (unpublished data). Finally, polymorphisms in estrogen synthesis, metabolism, and receptor genes were tested. Only the 17HSD polymorphisms (rs 5942 and rs 2389) significantly differentiated Cluster III from Cluster I. None of the polymorphisms differentiated Cluster II from I or Cluster II from III.

## Conclusions and Discussion

Contributions of the SMWHS included:

- Development of a system for staging reproductive aging with emphasis on the period from the Late

Reproductive stage through the early PM and establishment of the validity of the staging system with the ReSTAGE Collaboration and contributions to the Staging Reproductive Aging Workshop and STRAW + 10 [48];

- Incorporation of the staging system into the study of endocrine changes during the MT stages and early PM, including demonstration of changes in estrone, FSH, testosterone, cortisol, epinephrine and norepinephrine by MT stages and PM;
- Integration of the staging system into models of symptoms including hot flashes, sleep disturbances, depressed mood, pain, cognitive symptoms, incontinence, and sexual desire;
- Confirmation of effects of the MT stages and early PM on the following symptoms: hot flashes, awakening during the night, back pain, and sexual desire, but not on depressed mood, cognitive symptoms, incontinence, or joint pain;
- Identification of functional effects of symptoms on interference with work and relationships, in particular, effects of depressed mood and difficulty concentrating on work and depressed mood, anxiety, difficulty concentrating, and awakening during the night on relationships;
- Demonstration of effects of gene polymorphisms CYP 19 11r, 17 beta HSD (rs 2389 and 5942) in estrogen synthesizing genes on hot flashes as well as CYP 19 7r, CYP 19 7r(−3), 17 beta HSD (rs 2830) and estrogen metabolizing gene CYP 1B1*2 on events related to menarche and the MT; and
- Identification of naturally occurring symptom clusters and their relationship to endocrine levels (estrone, FSH), perceived stress, epinephrine, norepinephrine levels, and 17 beta HSD genotypes.

Results of this study can be generalized to women experiencing the natural menopausal transition and early postmenopause and who were not using hormone therapy. Limitations of the SMWHS included a predominantly White and well-educated sample, despite efforts to include Asian American and African American women. Another limitation was the smaller sample size relative to larger studies, such as the Study of Women and Health Across the Nation (SWAN) The limitation of sample size was compensated in part by the more frequent occasions of measurement, with some measures obtained several times per year. In addition, SMWHS was a longitudinal population-based study that enabled analysis of patterns observed in symptoms over time, up to 23 years for some participants. Efforts to recruit and retain a multi-ethnic sample were effective initially, but with waning retention during the latter years of the study. In addition, the development and application of

specific criteria for staging the MT and analyzing data to examine effects of MT stages supported our ability to distinguish between endocrine factors, stress, and symptoms that were influenced by MT stages versus those who were not [44].

Issues for further study suggested by SMWHS included the importance of studying clusters of symptoms vs single symptoms and the need for interventions targeting multiple symptoms. We have begun examination of non-pharmacologic therapies that may be effective for clusters of symptoms vs individual symptoms [49–52]. In the interim, this research is being incorporated in the clinical education of women's health care providers [53].

## Abbreviations

BMI: Body mass index; CYP: Cytochrome P450; E1G: Estrone; FMP: Final menstrual period; FSH: Follicle-stimulating hormone; HSD: Hydroxy steroid dehydrogenase; HT: Hormone therapy; MLM: Multi-level modeling; MT: Menopausal transition; PM: Postmenopause; SMWHS: Seattle Midlife Women's Health Study; STRAW: Staging Reproductive Aging Workshop; SUI: Stress urinary incontinence

## Acknowledgements

We acknowledge the contribution of the participants who provided data for the Seattle Midlife Women's Health Study, some for over 20 years. Only the authors of this paper contributed to this manuscript.

## Funding

- National Institute for Nursing Research, NIH, R01- NR 04141 need title
- National Institute for Nursing Research, NIH, P50-NR-02323, P30-NR04001 Center for Women's Health Research.
- National Institute of Environmental Health Sciences P30-07033 Center for Ecogenetics and Environmental Health.
- National Institute for Nursing Research R21-NR012218 Symptom Clusters during the Menopausal Transition and Early Postmenopause.
- Pfizer, Inc., Medical Division Research Grant (Pfizer, Inc, Medical Division. #WS1752232. Urinary Incontinence during the Menopausal Transition and Early Postmenopause.
- Research Intramural Funding Program, University of Washington School of Nursing.

## Authors' contributions

Nancy Fugate Woods and Ellen Sullivan Mitchell both contributed to writing the manuscript. Both authors read and approved the final manuscript.

## Authors' information

NFW and ESM: Study Design and Principal Investigator of the Seattle Midlife Women's Health Study. Over the course of the entire study NFW and ESM rotated roles as principal investigator.

## Competing interests

The authors declare they have no competing interests.

## Author details

[1]Department of Biobehavioral Nursing, University of Washington, Seattle, WA 98195, USA. [2]Department of Family and Child Nursing, University of Washington, Seattle, WA98195USA.

## References

1. U. S. Public Health Services. Opportunities for Research on Women's Health. Bethesda: National Institutes of Health; 1992.
2. McKinlay S, Brambilla D, Posner J. The normal menopause transition. Maturitas. 1992;14(2):103–15.
3. Matthews K, Wing R, Kuller L, et al. Influences of natural menopause on psychological characteristics and symptoms of middle-aged healthy women. J Consult Clin Psychol. 1990;58:345–51.
4. Woods N, Lentz M, Mitchell ES, Heitkemper M, Shaver J. PMS after 40: Persistence of a stress-related symptom pattern. Res Nurs Health. 1997;20:329–40.
5. Woods NF, Lentz MJ, Mitchell ES, Shaver J, Heitkemper M. Luteal phase ovarian steroids, stress arousal, premenses perceived stress and premenstrual symptoms. Res Nurs Health. 1998;21:129–42.
6. Woods N, Lentz M, Mitchell E, Heitkemper M, Shaver J, Henker R. Perceived stress, physiologic stress arousal, and premenstrual symptoms: Group diffferences and intra-individual patterns. Res Nurs Health. 1998;21:511–23.
7. Woods NF, Shaver JF. The evolutionary spiral of a specialized center for women's health research. Image. 1992;24:229–34.
8. Woods NF, Mitchell ES. Patterns of depressed mood in midlife women: Observations from the Seattle Midlife Women's Health Study. Res Nurs Health. 1996;19:111–23.
9. Belsey EM, Farley TMM. The analysis of menstrual bleeding patterns: A review. Applied Stochastic Models Data Analysis. 1987;3:125–50.
10. Treloar AE. Variation of the human menstrual cycle through reproductive life. Int J Fertil. 1967;12:77–126.
11. Mitchell ES, Woods NF, Mariella A. Three stages of the menopausal transition: Toward a more precise definition. Menopause. 2000;7:334–49.
12. Harlow SD, Crawford S, Dennerstein L, Burger HG, Mitchell ES, Sowers MF for the ReSTAGE Collaboration. Recommendations from a multi-study evaluation of proposed criteria for Staging Reproductive Aging. Climacteric. 2007;10:112–9.
13. Mitchell ES, Woods NF. Symptom experiences of midlife women: Observations from the Seattle Midlife Women's Health Study. Maturitas. 1996;25:1–10.
14. Woods NF, Mitchell ES. Pathways to depressed mood for midlife women: Observations from the Seattle Midlife Women's Health Study. Res Nurs Health. 1997;20:119–29.
15. Mitchell ES, Woods NF. Midlife women's attributions about perceived memory changes: Observations from the Seattle Midlife Women's Health Study. J Womens Health Gend Based Med. 2001;10:351–62.
16. Woods NF, Mitchell ES. Women's images of midlife: Observations from the Seattle Midlife Women's Health Study". Health Care Women Int. 1997;18:439–53.
17. Woods NF, Mitchell ES. Anticipating menopause: Observations from the Seattle Midlife Women's Health Study. Menopause. 1999;6:167–73.
18. Woods NF, Mitchell ES, Adams C. Memory functioning among midlife women: Observations from the Seattle Midlife Women's Health Study. Menopause. 2000;7:257–65.
19. Woods NF, Mariella AM, Mitchell ES. Patterns of depressed mood across the menopausal transition: Approaches to studying patterns in longitudinal data. Acta Obstet Gynecol Scand. 2002;81:623–32.
20. Woods NF, Carr MC, Tao EY, Taylor HJ, Mitchell ES. Increased urinary cortisol levels during the menopausal transition. Menopause. 2006;13(2):212–1.
21. Woods NF, Smith-DiJulio K, Percival DB, Tao EY, Taylor HJ, Mitchell ES. Symptoms during the menopausal transition and early postmenopause and their relation to endocrine levels over time: Observations from the Seattle Midlife Women's Health Study. J Women's Health. 2007;16:667–77.
22. Mitchell ES, Woods NF. Correlates of Urinary Incontinence during the Menopausal Transition and Early Postmenopause: Observations from the Seattle Midlife Women's Health Study. Climacteric. 2013;16:653–62.
23. Smith-diJulio K, Percival DB, Woods NF, Tao EY, Mitchell ES. Hot flash severity in hormone therapy users/nonusers across the menopausal transition. Maturitas. 2007;58:191 200.
24. Woods NF, Smith-diJulio K, Percival DB, Tao EY, Mariella A, Mitchell ES. Depressed mood during the menopausal transition and early postmenopause: Observations from the Seattle Midlife Women's Health Study. Menopause. 2008;15:223–32.
25. Woods NF, Smith-DiJulio K, Percival DB, Mitchell ES. Cortisol Levels during the Menopausal Transition and Early Postmenopause: Observations from the Seattle Midlife Women's Health Study. Menopause. 2009;16:708–18.
26. Woods NF, Mitchell ES, Smith-DiJulio K. Sexual desire during the menopausal transition and early postmenopause Observations from the Seattle Midlife Women's Health Study. J Women's Health. 2010;19:2098–217.
27. Smith-DiJulio K, Woods NF, Mitchell ES. Well-being during the menopausal transition and early postmenopause: A longitudinal analysis. Menopause. 2008;15:1095–102.
28. Woods NF, Mitchell ES, Percival DB, Smith-DiJulio K. Is the menopausal transition stressful? Observations of perceived stress from the Seattle Midlife Women's Health Study. Menopause. 2009;16:90–7.
29. Mitchell ES, Woods NF. Pain symptoms during the menopausal and early postmenopause: Observations from the Seattle Midlife Women's Health Study. Climacteric. 2010;13:467–78.
30. Woods NF, Mitchell ES, Smith-DiJulio K. Sleep symptoms during the menopausal transition and early postmenopause Observations from the Seattle Midlife Women's Health Study. Sleep. 2010;33:539–49.
31. Woods NF, Mitchell ES. Symptom interference with work and relationships during the menopausal transition and early postmenopause: Observations from the Seattle Midlife Women's Health Study. Menopause. 2011;18:654–61.
32. Mitchell ES, Woods NF. Cognitive symptoms during the menopausal transition and early postmenopause: Observations from the Seattle Midlife Women's Health Study. Climacteric. 2011;14:252–61.
33. Woods NF, Mitchell ES. Consequences of incontinence for women during the menopausal transition and early postmenopause: Observations from the Seattle Midlife Women's Health Study. Menopause. 2013;20:915–21.
34. Mitchell ES, Woods NF. Hot flush severity during the menopausal transition and early postmenopause: beyond hormones. Climacteric. 2015;18:536–44.
35. Development Core Team. R: A Language and Environment for Statistical Computing. Vienna, Austria: R Foundation for Statistical Computing, 2005. Available at: http://www.R-project.org. Accessed 13 June 2007.
36. Soules MR, Sherman S, Parrott E, Rebar R, Santoro N, Utian W, Woods NF. Executive summary: Stages of Reproductive Aging Workshop (STRAW). Fertil Steril. 2001;76:874–78.
37. Harlow SD for the ReSTAGE Collaboration (in alphabetical order), Cain K, Crawford S, Dennerstein L, Little R, Mitchell ES, Nan B, Randolph J, Taffe J, Yosef M. Evaluation of four proposed bleeding criteria for the onset of late menopausal transition. J Clin Endocrinol Metab. 2006;91:3432–8. [PMID: 16772350] PMCID:PMC1950694.
38. Harlow SD, Mitchell ES, Crawford S, Nan B, Little R, Taffe J, ReSTAGE Collaboration. The ReSTAGE Collaboration: Defining Optimal Bleeding Criteria for the Onset of Early Menopausal Transition. Fertility Sterility. 2008;89:129–40.
39. Harlow S, Cain K, Crawford S, Dennerstein L, Little R, Mitchell E, Nan B, Randolph J, Taffe J, Yosef M. Evaluation of four proposed bleeding criteria for the onset of late menopausal transition. J Clin Endocrinol Metabol. 2006;91(9):3432–8.
40. Smith-DiJulio K, Mitchell ES, Woods NF. Concordance of retrospective and prospective reporting of menstrual irregularity by women in the menopausal transition. Climacteric. 2005;8:390–7.
41. Brook RH, Ware Jr JE, Davies-Avery A, Stewart AL, Donald CA, Rogers WH, et al. Overview of adult health measures fielded in Rand's health insurance study, ch 6. Findings Conclusions Medical Care. 1979;17:16–55.
42. Woods NF, Mariella A, Mitchell ES. Depressed mood symptoms during the menopausal transition: Observations from the Seattle Midlife Women's Health Study. Climacteric. 2006;9:195–203.
43. Woods NF, Mitchell ES, Tao Y, Viernes HM, Stapleton PL, Farin FM. Polymorphisms in the Estrogen Synthesis and Metabolism Pathways and Symptoms during the Menopausal Transition: Observations from the Seattle Midlife Women's Health Study. Menopause. 2006;13:902–10.
44. Mitchell ES, Farin FM, Stapleton PL, Tsai JM, Tao EY, Smith-DiJulio K, Woods NF. Association of estrogen-related polymorphisms with age at menarche,

age at final menstrual period and stages of the menopausal transition. Menopause. 2008;15:105–11.

45.  Cray LA, Woods NF, Herting JR, Mitchell ES. Symptom clusters during the late reproductive stage through the early postmenopause: Observations from the Seattle Midlife Women's Health Study. Menopause. 2012;2012(19):864–9.

46.  Cray LA, Woods NF, Mitchell ES. Identifying symptom clusters during the menopausal transition: Observations from the Seattle Midlife Women's Health Study. Climacteric. 2013;16:539–49.

47.  Woods NF, Cray L, Mitchell ES, Herting JR. Endocrine biomarkers and symptom clusters during the menopausal transition and early postmenopause: observations from the Seattle Midlife Women's Health Study. Menopause. 2014;21:646–52.

48.  Woods NF, Mitchell ES. Staging reproductive aging: contemporary research applications of Staging Reproductive Aging Workshop and Staging Reproductive Aging Workshop + 10. Menopause. 2013;20:717–8.

49.  Taylor-Swanson L, Thomas A, Ismail R, Schnall JG, Cray L, Mitchell ES, Woods NF. Effects of traditional Chinese medicine on symptom clusters during the menopausal transition. Climacteric. 2015;18:142–56.

50.  Ismail R, Taylor-Swanson L, Thomas A, Schnall JG, Cray L, Mitchell ES, Woods NF. Effects of herbal preparations on symptom clusters during the menopausal transition. Climacteric. 2015;18:11–28.

51.  Thomas AJ, Ismail R, Taylor-Swanson L, Cray L, Schnall JG, Mitchell ES, Woods NF. Effects of isoflavones and amino acid therapies for hot flashes and co-occurring symptoms during the menopausal transition and early postmenopause: a systematic review. Maturitas. 2015;78:263–76.

52.  Woods NF, Mitchell ES, Schnall JG, Cray L, Ismail R, Taylor-Swanson L, Thomas A. Effects of mind-body therapies on symptom clusters during the menopausal transition. Climacteric. 2014;17:10–22.

53.  Woods NF, Berg J, Mitchell ES. Midlife Women's Health. In: Alexander I, Kostos-Polsten E, Mallard VJ, Fogel C, Woods NF, editors. Women's Health Care in Advanced Practice Nursing. New York: Springer Publishing; 2017. pp. 155-190.

# 6

# It is not just menopause: symptom clustering in the Study of Women's Health Across the Nation

Siobán D. Harlow[1*], Carrie Karvonen-Gutierrez[1], Michael R. Elliott[2], Irina Bondarenko[2], Nancy E. Avis[3], Joyce T. Bromberger[4], Maria Mori Brooks[5], Janis M. Miller[6] and Barbara D. Reed[7]

## Abstract

**Background:** Patterns of symptom clustering in midlife women may suggest common underlying mechanisms or may identify women at risk of adverse health outcomes or, conversely, likely to experience healthy aging. This paper assesses symptom clustering in the Study of Women's Health Across the Nation (SWAN) longitudinally by stage of reproductive aging and estimates the probability of women experiencing specific symptom clusters. We also evaluate factors that influence the likelihood of specific symptom clusters and assess whether symptom clustering is associated with women's self-reported health status.

**Methods:** This analysis includes 3289 participants in the multiethnic SWAN cohort who provided information on 58 symptoms reflecting a broad range of physical, psychological and menopausal symptoms at baseline and 7 follow-up visits over 16 years. We conducted latent transition analyses to assess symptom clustering and to model symptomatology across the menopausal transition (pre, early peri-, late peri- and post-menopausal). Joint multinomial logistic regression models were used to identify demographic characteristics associated with premenopausal latent class membership. A partial proportional odds regression model was used to assess the association between latent class membership and self-reported health status.

**Results:** We identified six latent classes that ranged from highly symptomatic (LC1) across most measured symptoms, to moderately symptomatic across most measured symptoms (LC2), to moderately symptomatic for a subset of symptoms (vasomotor symptoms, pain, fatigue, sleep disturbances and physical health symptoms) (LC3 and LC5) with one class (LC3) including interference in life activities because of physical health symptoms, to numerous milder symptoms, dominated by fatigue and psychological symptoms (LC4), to relatively asymptomatic (LC6). In pre-menopause, 10% of women were classified in LC1, 16% in LC2, 14% in LC3 and LC4, 26% in LC5, and 20% in LC6. Intensity of vasomotor and urogenital symptoms as well as sexual desire) differed minimally by latent class. Classification into the two most symptomatic classes was strongly associated with financial strain, White race/ethnicity, obesity and smoking status. Over time, women were most likely to remain within the same latent class as they transitioned through menopause stages (range 39–76%), although some women worsened or improved. The probability of moving between classes did not differ substantially by menopausal stage. Women in the highly symptomatic classes more frequently rated their health as fair to poor compared to women in the least symptomatic class.

(Continued on next page)

* Correspondence: harlow@umich.edu
[1]Department of Epidemiology, School of Public Health, University of Michigan, 1415 Washington Heights, Suite 6610 SPH I, Ann Arbor, MI 48109-2029, USA
Full list of author information is available at the end of the article

(Continued from previous page)

**Conclusion:** Clear patterns of symptom clustering were present early in midlife, tended to be stable over time, and were strongly associated with self-perceived health. Notably, vasomotor symptoms tended to cluster with sleep disturbances and fatigue, were present in each of the moderate to highly symptomatic classes, but were not a defining characteristic of the symptom clusters. Clustering of midlife women by symptoms may suggest common underlying mechanisms amenable to interventions. Given that one-quarter of midlife women were highly or moderately symptomatic across all domains in the pre-menopause, addressing symptom burden in early midlife is likely critical to ameliorating risk in the most vulnerable populations.

**Keywords:** Symptom clusters, Sleep, Pain, Fatigue, Vasomotor symptoms, Psychological symptoms, Menopause, Aging, Latent transition analysis

## Background

Studies of the menopausal transition have found that women who experience hot flashes are at increased risk of experiencing additional symptoms, such as anxiety, depression or sleep, both concurrently and longitudinally [1–4]. Woods [5] proposed that symptom clustering may suggest common underlying mechanisms, and may identify women at risk of adverse health outcomes or, conversely, more likely to experience healthy aging. Studies of breast cancer patients have reported clustering of depression, fatigue and sleep over time [6] and of fatigue, pain and psychological symptoms [7] Studies of cardiovascular disease suggest that symptom clustering differs by age, with younger patients reporting more symptoms and older patients reporting fewer but more diffuse symptoms [8]. Despite interest in menopausal symptoms, relatively few studies have evaluated symptom clustering among midlife in women [5, 9–17].

Research conducted in nonclinical populations of midlife women find that women report different symptom patterns, with clusters generally based on symptom intensity and sometimes on whether or not vasomotor symptoms cluster with other symptoms. Most previous studies in midlife women include symptoms defined a priori as being characteristic of menopause [9–17]. Cray and colleagues [9–11] conducted principal component and multilevel latent cluster analyses in the Seattle Women's Midlife Health Study (SWMHS) using data from a 3-day symptom diary of 19 symptoms from six pre-defined symptom groups (hot flashes, sleep, pain, mood, cognitive and tension). One analysis suggested similar factor structures across the stages of reproductive aging [11]. However, another identified three latent classes: low symptom, low hot flash/moderate symptoms and high hot flash/moderate symptoms [10], that varied by menopausal stage. Women were less likely to be in either of the two latent classes that included hot flashes when they were premenopausal. In the MsFLASH clinical trial, latent class analysis based on hot flash, insomnia, sleep, depressed mood, anxiety and pain symptoms identified 5 classes, 4 of which included hot flashes [12]. Mishra and Dobson [13] conducted factor analysis to identify symptom clusters of 17 general health and menopausal symptoms using data from the Australian Longitudinal Study of Women's Health (ALSWH). They identified four factors (somatic, urogynecological, vasomotor and physical). Longitudinal latent class analysis of each of the four symptom groups suggested that women clustered into patterns of mild, moderate, severe and very severe symptoms that remained consistent over time and across menopausal stages for all symptom groups except the vasomotor symptom group, which differed by the timing of change in severity scores.

Additional analyses of SWMHS suggest that symptom clustering was associated with both sex steroid hormones [9, 14] and cortisol levels [9]. A high symptom class was associated with decreased urinary cortisol levels while the high hot flash/aches/wakening class was associated with both higher urinary cortisol and lower urinary estrone levels [9]. A more recent analysis of symptom severity found that being in a class with severe hot flashes was associated with higher urinary follicle-stimulating hormone (FSH), lower urinary estrone and higher epinephrine levels but not with cortisol levels [14]. Greenblum and colleagues [15] using principal components analysis in a clinical sample identified three symptom clusters (psychological symptoms; weight gain and urinary incontinence; and, vaginal dryness and sleep disturbances), and reported that the vaginal dryness and sleep disturbance cluster was most strongly associated with self-reported quality of life.

Only a few studies have evaluated cross-cultural or race/ethnic differences in symptom profiles. The four country Decisions at Menopause Study (DAMES) found that hot flashes grouped with other symptoms differentially across countries [16]. Im and colleagues [17] reported race/ethnic differences in reporting of the number and severity of physical symptoms but only in the least symptomatic cluster. The MS-Flash study reported that Black women were more likely than White women to cluster in the severe hot flash, insomnia and pain cluster [12].

In the multiethnic Study of Women's Health Across the Nation (SWAN), we have examined associations between pairs of symptoms [1–3] and a triad of symptoms (sleep disturbances, depressed mood and sexual problems) [18] while Avis and colleagues [19] considered evidence for a menopausal syndrome. In the present paper, we used longitudinal data from SWAN to conduct latent transition analysis to assess symptom clustering as women transition through the menopause. Unlike most prior studies, which defined symptom groups a priori, we used a more agnostic, data-driven approach utilizing information on all reported symptoms to construct latent classes of symptoms and estimate how women move between these classes over time. Like Mishra and Dobson [13], our aim is to understand the broader symptom experience of midlife women and whether symptom clustering differs by menopausal status. We further assess whether demographic characteristics, including race/ethnicity, body size or smoking status were associated with specific symptom clustering and evaluate the association between symptom clustering and women's self-reported health status.

## Methods

This paper uses data from the longitudinal cohort study, the Study of Women's Health Across the Nation, details of which have been described elsewhere [20]. In brief, eligible women were identified through a cross-sectional screening survey at seven clinical sites and enrolled in the cohort study. Eligibility for the cohort study included residence in the geographic area of the clinical site, being age 42–52 years old, self-identification as White (at all sites) or as Black (at the southeastern Michigan, Boston, Chicago or Pittsburgh sites), Chinese (at the Northern California site), Japanese (at the Southern California site) and Hispanic (at the New Jersey site), the ability to speak English, Cantonese, Japanese or Spanish and ability to give verbal consent. In addition, women had to have an intact uterus, at least one menstrual period and not have used reproductive hormones in the past 3 months, and could not be pregnant or lactating at the time of enrollment. The study protocol was approved by the Institutional Review Boards at each study site. A total of 3302 women were enrolled in 1996/1997 and followed approximately annually thereafter with 12 clinic visits completed by 2012, at which time the study remained in contact with over 80% of surviving participants. All participants provided written, informed consent at each visit.

Each visit included interviewer-administered and self-administered questionnaires on a broad range of topics, including menstrual characteristics, socio-demographic characteristics, lifestyle and physical, psychological, and menopausal symptoms. Physical assessments included measurement of height and weight.

As the set of questions asked varied by visit, we sought to maximize the number of questions related to women's symptom profile while ensuring measurement consistency across multiple visits. Thus this analysis includes data derived from 58 questions included at the baseline visit, as well as follow-up visits 1, 2, 3, 6, 8, 10 and 12. A woman's first observed visit in each stage of reproductive aging (premenopausal, early-perimenopause, late-perimenopause and post-menopause) was selected for inclusion in this analysis. Given timing of the visits, women were not always observed at all stages. Data from an individual visit were excluded when information on more than 10 of the included symptoms was missing, after a hysterectomy or bi-lateral oophorectomy, or when menopausal stage could not be classified because of HT use. Based on these exclusions 13 women had no eligible observations, leaving 3289 women eligible for this analysis.

### Menopausal stage

Menopausal stage was defined based on women's self-reported menstrual characteristics at each visit. Women were classified as premenopausal if they had had a menstrual period in the previous 3 months and reported no change in menstrual regularity in the past 12 months; as early peri-menopausal if they reported decreased regularity in their menses in the past 12 months and had had a menstrual period in the previous 3 months; as late peri-menopausal if they had had no menses in the past 3–11 months; and, as postmenopausal if they had had no menses for the past 12 or more months. Surgical menopause was defined by report of either hysterectomy or bilateral oophorectomy. Women were censored at the time of surgical menopause ($n = 237$). At enrollment women were either pre- or early peri-menopausal. Of the 3289 women included in the analysis, 1761 were observed at least once in the premenopausal stage, 2777 in the early peri-menopausal stage, 927 in the late peri-menopausal stage, and 2222 in the early post-menopause.

### Symptoms

A total of 58 questions ascertained information on a broad range of symptoms. Although a number of these questions are items from existing scales intended to measure specific concepts (e.g., items from the CESD scale designed to measure depressive symptoms), this data-driven approach considers each item independently. This approach recognizes that women may differentially endorse specific questions in a scale and that examining the broader pattern of responses across large question sets may yield new insights. The questions included here were drawn from the SF-36 domains of role-physical, bodily pain, role-emotional, vitality and social functioning [21], the Center for Epidemiologic Studies Depression Scale (CES-D) [22, 23], the 4-item Cohen's Perceived Stress Scale [24] as well as a 14-item list of general symptoms assessed in SWAN and other studies of the menopausal transition including vasomotor symptoms, mood symptoms, somatic symptoms and vaginal dryness [25–27]. For the latter, women were asked how often within the past 2 weeks (ranging from not at all to daily) they experienced each symptom. Additional questions included items related to self-reported sleep quality (trouble falling asleep and staying asleep, waking early and perceived sleep quality) [28, 29], as well as questions on involuntary urine loss [30] and sexual desire [31].

*Self-Reported Health* was assessed by the question "Would you say your health in general is excellent, very good, good, fair or poor?" [21].

## Covariates

Race/ethnicity was self-defined and categorized as Black, Chinese, Japanese, Hispanic or White. Information on highest level of education attained (high school graduate/GED or less than high school versus at least some college), economic strain and smoking status (current, past, never) was obtained at baseline. Economic strain was assessed with the question "how hard is it to pay for basics (very hard, somewhat hard or not hard)?" Height and weight were measured without shoes, and in light indoor clothing. BMI, calculated as weight in kilograms divided by height in meters squared, was categorized as underweight ($<18.5$ kg/m$^2$), normal weight (18.5–24.9 kg/m$^2$), overweight (25.0–29.9 kg/m$^2$), or obese ($\geq30.0$ kg/m$^2$).

## Statistical analysis

Latent class analysis (LCA) [32] is a data reduction method for categorical variables akin to factor analysis for continuous variables. LCA estimates a probability $p_{ijk}$ of response to the *kth* category of the *jth* symptom for the *ith* latent class. For example, based on our analyses, the appetite symptom "I did not feel like eating; my appetite was poor" is described by 44.4% of women in latent class 1 (most symptomatic) as occurring "rarely or none of the time" (=1), 26.6% as "some or a little of the time" (=2), 17.5% as "occasionally or a moderate amount of the time" (=3), and 11.6% as "most or all of the time" (=4). In contrast, this symptom is described by 84.5% of women in latent class 6 (minimally symptomatic) as occurring "rarely or none of the time", 11.7% as "some or a little of the time", 2.9% as "occasionally or a moderate amount of the time", and 0.8% as "most or all of the time".

By assuming women belong to unobserved (latent) groupings of reported symptoms, in which symptom reports are assumed to be independent conditional on latent class, a data-driven clustering of symptoms can be determined. As an initial exploratory step we conducted latent class analyses [32] cross-sectionally at each menopausal stage to assess whether latent classes differed across the menopausal transition. Analyses were conducted first with all women and then with only those women observed in all of the four menopausal stages to evaluate whether the latent class structure was sensitive to lost-to-follow up. These exploratory analyses indicated that latent classes remained consistent over time and across menopausal stage when a fixed set of symptoms were included (data not shown).

Latent Transition analysis (LTA) extends LCA to a longitudinal data setting [33, 34]. We used LTA to determine how symptoms cluster and to estimate how women transition between the identified clusters across menopausal stages (SAS PROC LTA) [33]. At each menopausal stage (pre-menopause, early peri-menopause, late peri-menopause and post-menopause) women are assumed to belong to one of *C* unobserved ("latent") classes. Conditional on this latent class, each symptom is assumed to have a specific distribution, and again conditional on this latent class, all symptoms are assumed to be mutually independent. Along with clustering of symptoms into classes, LTA estimates a *C x C* transition matrix between latent classes for each time point. Based on the exploratory analysis above and to assist in interpretation, latent classes were kept constant across the time points.

The Bayesian Information Criterion (BIC) (which penalizes models with large numbers of latent classes to avoid overfitting), along with scientific judgement, was used to select the number of classes. Finally, since PROC LTA does not use multiple start points to ensure convergence of the LTA model, we introduced multiple start-points to ensure consistent estimation of the global maximum likelihood.

To summarize composition of latent classes (i.e., the distribution of symptomatology across the latent classes), we estimated average intensity of each symptom within each class. Since symptoms were measured on different scales (e.g. a few were dichotomous responses while others might have as many as six response levels), we standardized all symptom responses to a [0,1] scale, with 0 the most favorable category listed, and 1 being the worst. This symptom intensity for a given class was constructed as $P_{ij} = \sum_{k=1}^{K} p_{ijk}\left(\frac{k-1}{K-1}\right)$, where $i$ indexes the latent class, $j$ the symptom question and $k$ the category associated with the symptom question (where response options were consistently (re) ordered to run from "best" to "worst"). Thus $0 \leq P_{ij} \leq 1$, with *low intensity* values corresponding to latent classes in which women rarely reported problems with that symptom and *high intensity* values (near 1) corresponding to latent classes in which women often reported problems with that symptom. For example, using the appetite symptom and response probabilities for latent classes 1 and 6 presented above, the intensity is $P_{1,APPETITE} = 100 \times (.444 \times 0/3 + .266 \times 1/3 + .175 \times 2/3 + .116 \times 3/3) = 32.1$ for latent class 1 and $P_{6,APPETITE} = 100 \times (.845 \times 0/3 + .117 \times 1/3 + .029 \times 2/3 + .008 \times 3/3) = 6.6$ for latent class 6. These intensity measures are then summarized into a "heat map" corresponding to the measures of $P_{ij}$ to help interpret the symptom intensity distribution results of the latent classes produced by LTA. No a priori grouping of symptoms into specific domains was assumed. In order to enhance interpretation of the symptom distributions in each cluster, we ordered the symptoms in the heat map by intensity level across latent classes and grouped symptoms post hoc conceptually (e.g. sleep disturbance, pain, psychological).

Joint multinomial logistic regression was used to compute the odds of belonging to a given initial latent class relative to a reference initial latent class as a function of baseline covariates: age, obesity status, race/ethnicity, smoking status (current, past or never smoker), financial strain (very hard to pay for basics, hard to pay for basics, not hard to pay for basics), and education (high school graduate or less versus some college or more). A bootstrap was used to compute empirical confidence intervals for the final multivariable multinomial logistic regression on baseline latent classes.

In order to determine whether the latent classes were related to self-reported health (categorized as excellent, very good, good and fair or poor) at each time point, a four-level partial proportional odds regression model was fit using the estimated symptom latent class at each menopausal stage and menopausal status as predictors, adjusted for age, obesity status, race/ethnicity, smoking status, financial strain and education. This model was fit using SAS PROC NLMIXED with a subject-level random intercept to account for within-woman correlation across the four time points. Variation in uncertainty of the latent class assignment was addressed with entropy based design weights [34].

## Results

Women had a mean age of 45.7 years at baseline and a mean BMI of 27.2 kg/m². The study population was 28.3% Black, 47.0% White, 7.6% Chinese, 8.5% Hispanic, and 8.5% Japanese (Table 1). One-quarter of the women had a high school education or less and about one-third reported they found it somewhat or very hard to pay for basics. Less than half had ever smoked. At baseline, the majority of women reported they had very good or excellent health, but 13.2% rated themselves as having fair or poor health.

### Latent classes

The LTA identified 6 distinct latent classes. These classes were ordered based on the number and intensity of symptoms from 1 (most symptoms present and highest intensity) to 6 (least symptoms present and least intensity). Figure 1 provides the heat map showing symptom intensity of each symptom within each latent class. (Additional file 1 provides the full question item that corresponds with the shorter symptom labels provided

**Table 1** Baseline demographics of 3289 women in the analytic sample, Study of Women's Health Across the Nation (SWAN)

| | Total (N = 3289) | Per Cent |
|---|---|---|
| Study site | | |
| Michigan | 542 | 16.5% |
| Boston | 448 | 13.6% |
| Chicago | 456 | 13.9% |
| Davis | 459 | 14.0% |
| Los Angeles | 496 | 15.1% |
| New Jersey | 425 | 12.9% |
| Pittsburgh | 463 | 14.1% |
| Race/ethnicity | | |
| Black | 931 | 28.3% |
| White | 1546 | 47.0% |
| Chinese | 250 | 7.6% |
| Hispanic | 281 | 8.5% |
| Japanese | 281 | 8.5% |
| Education[a] | | |
| Some college or more | 2446 | 75.0% |
| High school or less | 814 | 25.0% |
| Smoking status[b] | | |
| Never | 1867 | 57.3% |
| Past | 824 | 25.3% |
| Current | 567 | 17.4% |
| How hard it is to pay for basics[c] | | |
| Very hard | 302 | 9.2% |
| Somewhat hard | 1002 | 30.7% |
| Not hard | 1965 | 60.1% |
| Self-rated health[d] | | |
| Excellent | 695 | 21.4% |
| Very good | 1179 | 36.3% |
| Good | 945 | 29.1% |
| Fair | 368 | 11.3% |
| Poor | 62 | 1.9% |

[a]29 Missing observations
[b]31 Missing observations
[c]20 Missing observations
[d]40 Missing observations

in the heat map.) Latent Class 1 (LC1) is highly symptomatic with high intensity ratings for most measured symptoms. Latent Class 2 (LC2) is similar to LC1, but with moderate intensity rating for most measured symptoms. Latent Classes 3–5 each include fewer moderate to high intensity symptoms than LC1 or LC2. Latent Class 3 (LC3) includes moderate intensity vasomotor, pain, fatigue, sleep and physical health symptoms sufficient to interfere in life activities, but fewer and lower intensity psychological symptoms. Like LC1 and LC2, Latent Class 4 (LC4) includes numerous symptoms but

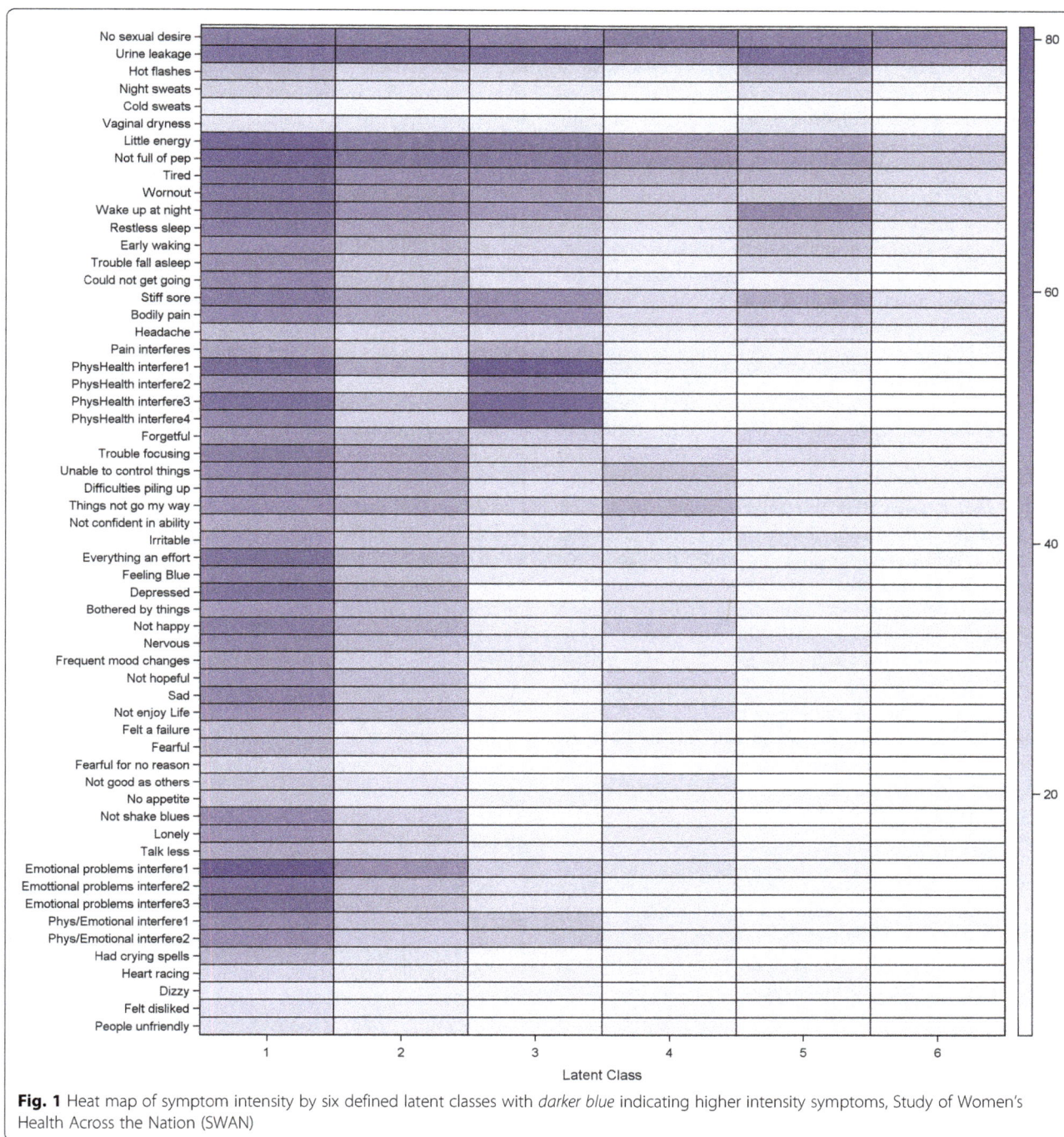

**Fig. 1** Heat map of symptom intensity by six defined latent classes with *darker blue* indicating higher intensity symptoms, Study of Women's Health Across the Nation (SWAN)

of milder intensity, dominated by fatigue and psychological symptoms. Latent Class 5 (LC5) is similar to LC3 but does not include the physical health interference items. Latent Class 6 (LC6) is relatively asymptomatic with only a few, mild symptoms mostly related to fatigue. Notably, vasomotor symptoms tended to cluster with sleep disturbances and fatigue and were present in each of the moderate to highly symptomatic clusters (LC1,2,3 and 5). This triad represents the most intense

symptoms only in LC5. Intensity of low sexual desire and urogenital symptoms differed little across classes.

**Probability of transition from latent class to latent class across reproductive stage**

In the pre-menopause, fully 26% of women were classified as moderately to highly symptomatic: 10% in the highly symptomatic LC1 and 16% in the moderately symptomatic LC2. Another 40% were classified as moderately symptomatic for a subset of measured symptoms: 14% in LC3 and 26% in LC5. Another 14% were classified as mildly symptomatic (LC4) while 20% were classified in relatively asymptomatic cluster (LC6).

Because transition probabilities did not differ significantly across menopausal stages ($X^2$ = 76.84 on 64 *df*, *p*-value = 0.13), transition probabilities were set to be constant over time. Table 2 provides the probability of women in a given class transitioning to the same or a different class from one menopausal stage to the next. Although symptoms improved and/or worsened for some women, most women remained in their same class at each subsequent time-point.

Figure 2 illustrates how the LC transition probabilities affect the movement of women from one class to another and the resultant proportion of women in each latent class at each stage of the menopausal transition. The width of the lines represents the probability of moving from class to class. Thus the wide vertical lines illustrate that women were most likely to remain in their same class as they transitioned through menopause. The thinner diagonal lines represent the lower probability of movement between classes, particularly more distant classes. By post-menopause, the probability of being in each latent class was 8% for the most highly symptomatic LC1, 16%, 12%, 15% and 26% for latent classes 2–5, respectively and 24% for the least symptomatic LC6. The biggest differences by menopausal stage can be seen in LC4 and LC5: 26% of premenopausal women were in class 4 compared to 15% by the post-menopause whereas 14% of premenopausal women were in LC5 compared to 26% by the post-menopause.

### Characteristics associated with latent class membership

Table 3 presents the fully adjusted model for the association of baseline sociodemographic factors, obesity status and smoking status with the probability of being in each latent class compared to being in the least symptomatic

LC6 (referent) at the premenopausal visit. After adjusting for all other covariates in the model, financial strain stands out as the variable most strongly and consistently related to symptoms. Having a somewhat or very hard time paying for basics was associated with over a five-fold and seventeen-fold increased odds, respectively, of being in the most symptomatic class (LC1) as well as with over a four-fold increased odds of being in the moderate symptom class (LC5) compared to women who did not report financial strain. Being obese was associated with a more than a two-fold odds of being in the highly symptomatic class (LC1) or the mildly symptomatic class (LC 5) : and with an 80% increase in the odds of being in the moderately symptomatic class (LC2) compared to non-obese women. Black women were one-half to one-third as likely to be in the more symptomatic clusters LC1 to LC3 than White women with similar characteristics, while Japanese were less likely to be in LC1 and Chinese women were less likely to be in LC2 than White women. Current smokers had a two and half fold increased odds and past smokers had a 75% increased odds of being in LC1 compared to never smokers. Older age at baseline was associated with slightly reduced odds of being in the more highly symptomatic LC1 and LC2, compared to younger women, although the confidence interval for the former includes 1.0. Level of education was not independently associated with latent symptom classes.

### Association between latent class membership and self-reported health status

Table 4 presents the regression coefficients for the association of self-reported health with menopausal stage and latent class membership adjusted for age, obesity, education, difficulty paying for basics, current smoking and race/ethnicity. (The distribution of self-reported health by menopausal status and latent class is provided in Additional file 2). Although, women in the late peri- and post- menopause were somewhat more likely to report being in fair to poor health compared to when they were premenopausal, women in the high to moderate symptomatic latent classes were much more likely to rate their health as fair to poor than women in the least symptomatic class. For example, based on the regression coefficients presented in Table 4, the odds of being in less than excellent health, less than very good health and less than good health were 3.56, 2.94 and 1.60 times higher for postmenopausal compared to premenopausal women, respectively. The comparable increased odds were 7.48, 8.21 and 9.73 times higher for women in LC1 compared to LC6. Figure 3 plots the odds ratios for each level of self-reported health by latent class to more clearly illustrate the magnitude of the association between LC and perceived health.

**Table 2** Latent class transition probabilities (latent classes numbered from maximal symptoms (1) to least symptoms (6)), Study of Women's Health Across the Nation(SWAN)

| Latent Class$_t$ | Probability of transition to latent class$_{t+1}$ | | | | | |
| | 1 | 2 | 3 | 4 | 5 | 6 |
|---|---|---|---|---|---|---|
| 1 | **0.55** | 0.26 | 0.04 | 0.10 | 0.03 | 0.03 |
| 2 | 0.12 | **0.47** | 0.12 | 0.14 | 0.13 | 0.01 |
| 3 | 0.04 | 0.14 | **0.39** | 0.11 | 0.23 | 0.10 |
| 4 | 0.04 | 0.13 | 0.07 | **0.44** | 0.20 | 0.11 |
| 5 | 0.01 | 0.08 | 0.09 | 0.07 | **0.62** | 0.13 |
| 6 | 0.01 | 0.00 | 0.06 | 0.06 | 0.11 | **0.76** |

(the diagonal, in bold, is the proportion of women who remain in the same latent class)

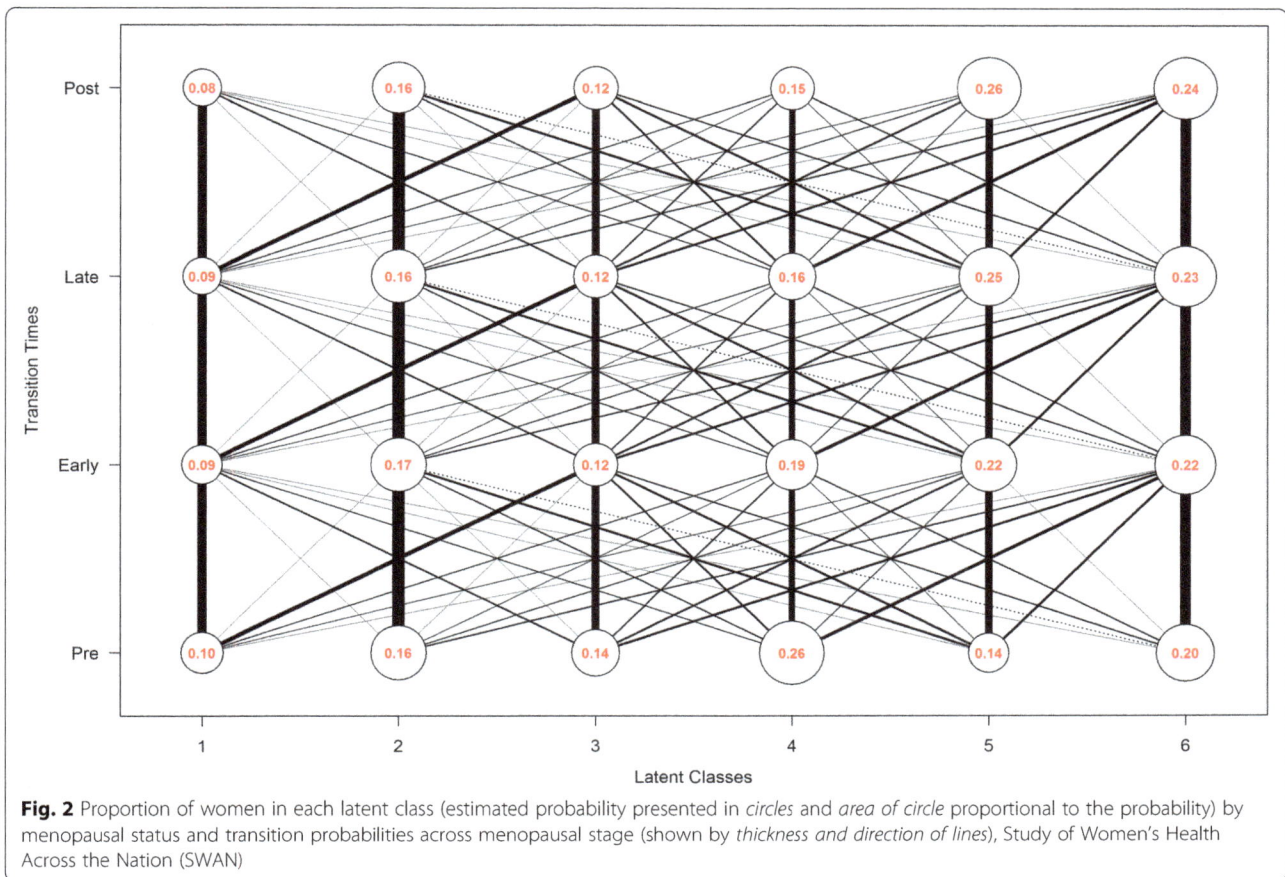

**Fig. 2** Proportion of women in each latent class (estimated probability presented in *circles* and *area of circle* proportional to the probability) by menopausal status and transition probabilities across menopausal stage (shown by *thickness and direction of lines*), Study of Women's Health Across the Nation (SWAN)

## Discussion

The evaluation of a broad range of physical and psychological symptom in a multi-ethnic cohort of midlife women contextualizes symptoms thought to be associated with menopause (e.g. hot flashes) within midlife women's overall symptom experience. We identified six latent symptom classes that ranged from highly or moderately symptomatic across all measured symptoms, to moderately symptomatic for a subset of symptoms (vasomotor, pain, fatigue, sleep and physical health), to mildly symptomatic predominately associated with fatigue and psychological symptoms, to minimally or asymptomatic. Notably, vasomotor symptoms tended to cluster with sleep disturbances and fatigue, but were the most intense symptoms within only one mildly symptomatic latent class. Other symptoms often associated with menopause – low sexual desire and urogenital symptoms – were also not unique to, or of differential intensity, across the latent classes. This finding suggests that women may perceive these symptoms differently from other symptom domains, or that their underlying physiologic or social correlates differ from the other symptoms measured here. Although some women worsened or improved over time, they tended to track within latent class and menopausal stage did not influence the probability of movement between latent classes. Notably, one-quarter of the women were highly or moderately symptomatic in the pre-menopause and latent class was strongly associated with women's self-perceived health.

These clustering patterns provide interesting insights into the aging and disablement processes. Sleep and fatigue symptoms, though mild, were present even in the least symptomatic cluster. As clusters became more symptomatic, sleep disturbance and fatigue symptoms worsened and pain symptoms emerged, becoming more prevalent and severe in the more symptomatic clusters. Psychological symptoms were prominent in just three of the six classes, but the two most highly symptomatic classes were characterized by having multiple, high/moderate intensity psychological symptoms.

The co-occurrence of sleep, fatigue and vasomotor symptoms has been reported by other studies [9] while SWAN has reported a triad of symptoms (sleep disturbances, depressed mood and sexual problems) associated with lower household incomes, less education and fair to poor self-rated health [18]. In the SWMHS, the high hot flash/aches/wakening cluster was associated with low estrone [9] while higher FSH and lower estradiol levels were associated with being in the severe hot flash cluster

**Table 3** Socio-demographic and lifestyle factors associated with premenopausal latent class ((latent classes numbered from most symptomatic (1) to less symptomatic (5), all compared to the least symptomatic (6, referent)), Study of Women's Health Across the Nation (SWAN)

| | Latent class (reference = LC6) | | | | |
| | 1 | 2 | 3 | 4 | 5 |
| | OR (95% CI) | OR (95% CI) | OR (95% CI) | OR (95% CI) | OR (95% CI) |
|---|---|---|---|---|---|
| Age | **0.94 (0.89, 1.00)**[a] | **0.92 (0.87, 0.98)** | 1.04 (0.96, 1.13) | 0.95 (0.88, 1.03) | 1.00 (0.94, 1.06) |
| Body mass index | | | | | |
| Obese | **2.34 (1.46, 3.74)** | **1.80 (1.11, 2.94)** | 1.25 (0.53, 2.95) | 1.05 (0.47, 2.35) | **2.64 (1.11, 6.25)** |
| Not obese | ref | ref | ref | ref | ref |
| Race/ethnicity | | | | | |
| Black | **0.54 (0.30, 0.97)** | **0.42 (0.24, 0.76)** | **0.38 (0.16, 0.92)** | 0.59 (0.31, 1.16) | 0.59 (0.32, 1.11) |
| White | ref | ref | ref | ref | ref |
| Chinese | 0.55 (0.18, 1.68) | **0.43 (0.19, 0.96)** | 0.36 (0.10, 1.29) | 1.20 (0.41, 3.52) | 0.73 (0.34, 1.53) |
| Hispanic | 1.16 (0.48, 2.81) | 0.94 (0.37, 2.37) | 0.26 (0.04, 1.82) | 0.66 (0.26, 1.65) | 1.55 (0.49, 4.94) |
| Japanese | **0.21 (0.06, 0.70)** | 0.66 (0.28, 1.57) | 0.37 (0.11, 12.80) | 0.99 (0.32, 3.09) | 0.58 (0.23, 1.42) |
| Smoking status | | | | | |
| Past | **1.75 (1.09, 2.80)** | 1.13 (0.66, 1.91) | 1.57 (0.81, 3.05) | 1.08 (0.66, 1.77) | 0.95 (0.55, 1.65) |
| Current | **2.53 (1.52, 4.22)** | 1.42 (0.89, 2.27) | 0.79 (0.38, 1.64) | 0.95 (0.50, 1.82) | 1.07 (0.61, 1.89) |
| Never | ref | ref | ref | ref | ref |
| How hard it is to pay for basics | | | | | |
| Very | **17.80 (8.50, 37.50)** | **4.85 (2.31, 10.20)** | 1.46 (0.40, 5.33) | **3.63 (1.59, 8.27)** | 1.72 (0.58, 5.04) |
| Somewhat | **5.75 (3.46, 9.58)** | **4.10 (2.66, 6.30)** | **2.01 (1.03, 3.92)** | **2.53 (1.38, 4.65)** | **2.01 (1.10, 3.70)** |
| Not at all | ref | ref | ref | ref | ref |
| Education | | | | | |
| HS or less | 1.54 (0.94, 2.51) | 1.04 (0.63, 1.73) | 0.56 (0.23, 1.35) | 1.05 (0.61, 1.82) | 0.77 (0.42, 1.42) |
| Some college | ref | ref | ref | ref | ref |

[a]Significant Odds Ratios are bolded

**Table 4** Association of latent class and menopausal status with self-reported health[a] (latent classes numbered from most symptomatic (1) to least symptomatic (6)), Study of Women's Health Across the Nation

| | Self-reported health Beta (95% CL) | | |
| | Less than excellent vs. excellent | Less than very good vs. very good or better | Fair/poor vs. good or better |
|---|---|---|---|
| Menopausal status | | | |
| Pre | ref | ref | ref |
| Early peri | 0.54 (0.32, .76) | 0.34 (0.14,0.54) | 0.12 (−0.15, 0.39) |
| Late peri | 1.34 (1.01, 1.67) | 0.89 (0.64, 1.14) | 0.39 (0.04, 0.74) |
| Post | 1.31 (1.07, 1.55) | 1.08 (0.88, 1.28) | 0.59 (0.32, 0.86) |
| Latent class | | | |
| 1 | 2.75 (2.20,3.30) | 3.02 (2.67, 3.37) | 3.58 (3.13, 4.03) |
| 2 | 1.99 (1.66, 2.32) | 2.05 (1.78, 2.32) | 2.14 (1.73, 2.55) |
| 3 | 1.80 (1.43, 2.17) | 2.09 (1.80, 2.38) | 2.43 (2.00, 2.86) |
| 4 | 1.06 (0.79, 1.33) | 1.06 (0.81, 1.31) | 0.91 (0.46, 1.36) |
| 5 | 1.14 (1.39, 2.05) | 0.92 (0.67, 1.17) | 0.78 (0.31, 1.25) |
| 6 | ref | ref | ref |

[a]Adjusted for obesity, education, difficulty paying for basics, current smoking, race/ethnicity and age

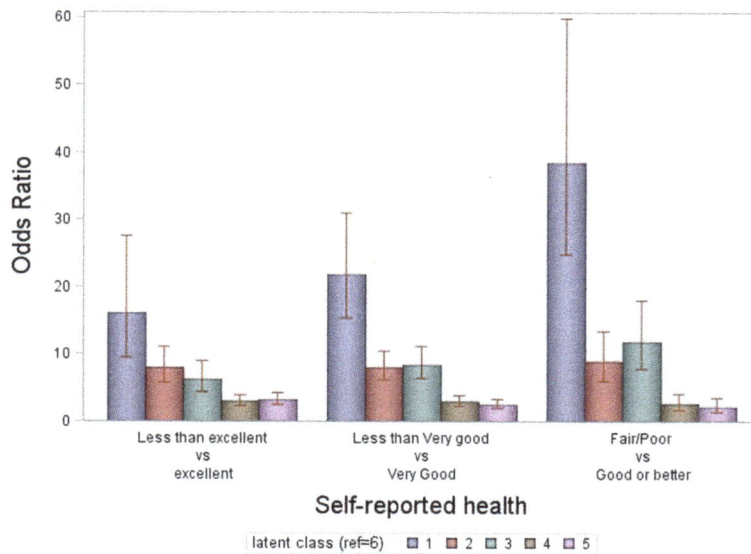

**Fig. 3** Adjusted Odds Ratios for different levels of self-reported health by latent class, Study of Women's Health Across the Nation (SWAN)

[14]. Future analyses of the SWAN data will assess the association between the identified symptom clusters and reproductive hormone levels.

Across previous studies, the number and content of factors/latent classes varies dependent on the number of women in the analytical sample, the number and types of symptoms considered, and the methodology used to identify clusters. For example, analyses from the SWMHS [9–11, 14] were based on a 3-day symptom diary that ascertained 47 symptoms, but the publications included fewer and a varied number of symptoms (i.e., 22, 19 or 15 symptoms or 5 indicator symptoms) and different subsets of the study population ($n = 103$ to 292 women). Nonetheless high/moderate symptom and low symptom profiles were evident in each analysis, with hot flashes often emerging more clearly in the low symptomatology clusters, as observed here.

The saliency of hot flashes in many studies may reflect their identification a priori as a study focus [10] or because the sample over-represented women who self-identified as having troublesome hot flashes [12]. The ALSWH included a broad range of symptoms in a population-based sample of women [13], identified vasomotor symptoms as one and uro-gynecological symptoms as another of four factors. However, the ALSWH study included a list of just 17 symptoms. In the present analysis, the triad of vasomotor symptoms, sleep disturbance and fatigue stood out uniquely only in an otherwise low symptomatic cluster (LC5), but were present in 5 of the 6 classes. Unlike the ALSWH, we found that intensity of low sexual desire and urogenital symptoms differed little across latent classes.

We found that the number and symptom content of the latent classes was consistent across menopausal

stage. Similar symptom factor structures across stages of reproductive aging have also been reported in the SWMHS [11]. In the ALSWH, severity of women's scores tended to remain stable over a 14-year period [13].

As might be expected, current and former smokers were more likely to be classified in the highly symptomatic cluster as were obese women. However, experiencing financial strain was the risk factor most strongly associated with being in the highly symptomatic clusters. Financial strain has been shown to be a major correlate of disability in SWAN [35] and other studies [36, 37]. Individuals with substantial financial limitations may be a particularly vulnerable group lacking health care access and related resources.

Only a few studies have evaluated cross-cultural or race/ethnic differences in symptom profiles. In the DAMES study [16], hot flashes did not cluster with other symptoms in the United States or Lebanon, but clustered with vaginal dryness and sexual symptoms in Spain and with general symptoms in Morocco. A multi-ethnic internet-based survey [17], observed differences by race/ethnicity only in the least symptomatic cluster: Black and White women reported more and greater severity of symptoms compared to Hispanic and Asian women. In contrast, the MS-Flash study reported that Black women were more likely than White women to cluster in the severe hot flash, insomnia and pain cluster [12]. In the present multi-ethnic study, after controlling for other covariates including financial strain, Black women but also Japanese and Chinese women were less likely to be classified in the most symptomatic latent classes.

Notably, one quarter of premenopausal women were highly or moderately symptomatic and experiencing numerous physical and psychological symptoms. Thus prior to beginning the menopausal transition a substantial proportion of women were highly symptomatic. Consistent with other studies examining the impact of high symptomatology on quality of life [7, 10], women in the high symptomatic cluster were most likely to perceive themselves in fair to poor health. The SWAN study population excluded women who experienced menopause earlier than their same age peers and women who were surgically menopausal. Given that earlier menopause and surgical menopause is associated with poorer health and mortality [38–41], participants were likely healthier than the general population of midlife women. Thus, this analysis may underestimate the proportion of women who are highly symptomatic as they enter the midlife, as further evidenced by the fact that older women at baseline tended to be in the less symptomatic latent classes. Further evaluation of symptom burden in the midlife may provide increased understanding of risk factors for the development of multiple morbidities and disability in later life. In the ALSWH, among women aged 76–81 years, multi-morbidity in the musculoskeletal/somatic, neurological/mental health and cardiovascular domains were each associated with poorer function as measured by Activities of Daily Living and the Instrumental Activities of Daily Living Scales [42].

This study has some limitations. As noted above, the SWAN cohort was left truncated and likely excluded women in poorer health [38]. Similarly, women who were lost to follow-up may have been in poorer health. Thus the burden of high symptomatology in midlife women may be underestimated. Although some bias may exist, retention in the SWAN cohort is fairly high (81% of the living participants at visit 12). Results from the latent class analyses were similar when we used complete cases and all cases, and the findings were robust across visits and menopausal status. Finally, assessment of urogenital symptoms as well as sexual desire was limited to only one question each and may not have fully ascertained women's symptom experience in these domains.

The study has several strengths. This analysis includes data from a community based and multiethnic cohort of over 2900 midlife women followed longitudinally, enabling us to evaluate the stability of latent classes and transition probabilities over time and across the stages of the menopausal transition in a large sample of women and to evaluate potential race/ethnic differences. As identification of latent class structure is dependent on the symptom domains included in the analysis and, to a lesser extent, on the number of symptoms allocated to a given domain, our inclusion of 58 symptom responses from a broad range of symptom domains, without a priori selection to highlight purported menopausal symptoms, enabled us to

characterize women's menopausal experience within their broader life and health experience.

## Conclusions

This paper illustrates that midlife women experience substantially different symptom burdens, that a large fraction of women report a significant symptom burden prior to the onset of the menopausal transition, that high and intense symptomatology across physical and psychological domains is strongly associated with financial strain, and that a high symptom burden influences women's perception of being in fair or poor health. Vasomotor symptoms cluster with sleep disturbances and fatigue, but are of unique salience to women's symptom burden only in a relatively small subset of women. Given that one-quarter of midlife women were already highly or moderately symptomatic in the pre-menopause, ensuring access to chronic disease preventive strategies in the early midlife is likely critical to ameliorating risk in the most vulnerable populations. Development of rigorous, evidence-based protocols for health and functional evaluations, inclusive of physical and mental health assessments as well as prevention and intervention guidance for women as they reach the midlife is likely warranted. Future studies should evaluate whether women with high symptomatology as they enter the midlife are at risk of premature mortality or earlier onset of disability, and whether low symptomatology at the onset of this life stage is a marker of healthy aging.

## Additional files

**Additional file 1:** Questions included in this analysis of symptom clusters and the corresponding labels used in the heat map.

**Additional file 2:** Distribution of self-reported health by latent class and menopausal status, study of women's health across the nation (SWAN).

**Additional file 3:** Institutional Review Board approval information for each study site.

**Acknowledgements**
SDH gratefully acknowledge use of the services and facilities of the Population Studies Center at the University of Michigan, funded by NICHD Center Grant R24 HD041028.
Clinical Centers: *University of Michigan, Ann Arbor – Siobán Harlow, PI 2011 – present, MaryFran Sowers, PI 1994–2011; Massachusetts General Hospital, Boston, MA – Joel Finkelstein, PI 1999 – present; Robert Neer, PI 1994–1999; Rush University, Rush University Medical Center, Chicago, IL – Howard Kravitz, PI 2009 – present; Lynda Powell, PI 1994–2009; University of California, Davis/Kaiser – Ellen Gold, PI; University of California, Los Angeles – Gail Greendale, PI; Albert Einstein College of Medicine, Bronx, NY – Carol Derby, PI 2011 – present, Rachel Wildman, PI 2010–2011; Nanette Santoro, PI 2004–2010; University of Medicine and Dentistry – New Jersey Medical School, Newark – Gerson Weiss, PI 1994–2004; and the University of Pittsburgh, Pittsburgh, PA – Karen Matthews, PI.*
NIH Program Office: *National Institute on Aging, Bethesda, MD – Chhanda Dutta 2016- present; Winifred Rossi 2012–2016; Sherry Sherman 1994–2012; Marcia Ory 1994–2001; National Institute of Nursing Research, Bethesda, MD – Program Officers.*

Central Laboratory: *University of Michigan, Ann Arbor – Daniel McConnell (Central Ligand Assay Satellite Services).*
Coordinating Center: *University of Pittsburgh, Pittsburgh, PA – Maria Mori Brooks, PI 2012 - present; Kim Sutton-Tyrrell, PI 2001–2012; New England Research Institutes, Watertown, MA - Sonja McKinlay, PI 1995–2001.*
Steering Committee: *Susan Johnson, Current Chair; Chris Gallagher, Former Chair*
We thank the study staff at each site and all the women who participated in SWAN.

## Funding
The National Institute of Aging and National Institute of Nursing Research program officers participated in the design of the SWAN study. They were not involved in the data analysis, interpretation of data or writing of this manuscript.
The Study of Women's Health Across the Nation (SWAN) has grant support from the National Institutes of Health (NIH), DHHS, through the National Institute on Aging (NIA), the National Institute of Nursing Research (NINR) and the NIH Office of Research on Women's Health (ORWH) (Grants U01NR004061; U01AG012505, U01AG012535, U01AG012531, U01AG012539, U01AG012546, U01AG012553, U01AG012554, U01AG012495). The content of this article is solely the responsibility of the authors and does not necessarily represent the official views of the NIA, NINR, ORWH or the NIH.

## Authors' contributions
SDH conducted the literature review and had primary responsibility for drafting the manuscript. SDH and CKG made substantial contributions to conception, design, acquisition and interpretation of the data as well as to the design of the data analysis. MRE made substantial contributions to and oversaw the data analysis, and contributed to the drafting of the manuscript. IB conducted the data analysis and contributed to drafting the manuscript. BDR, CKG, JB, JMM, MMB, NEA contributed to the critical revision of the manuscript for important intellectual content. All authors have read and approved the final manuscript.

## Competing interests
SD Harlow is Editor In Chief of this journal. As per the journal policy, peer review and all decisions regarding the manuscript were handled by an Associate Editor from a different institution, and SD Harlow was blinded to the peer review. MM Brooks receives a research grant from Gilead Sciences, Inc. The other authors have no competing interests.

## Author details
[1]Department of Epidemiology, School of Public Health, University of Michigan, 1415 Washington Heights, Suite 6610 SPH I, Ann Arbor, MI 48109-2029, USA. [2]Department of Biostatistics, School of Public Health, University of Michigan, Ann Arbor, USA. [3]Department of Social Sciences and Health Policy, Wake Forest School of Medicine, Winston-Salem, USA. [4]Departments of Epidemiology and Psychiatry, University of Pittsburgh, Pittsburgh, USA. [5]Department of Epidemiology, University of Pittsburgh, Pittsburgh, USA. [6]School of Nursing, University of Michigan, Ann Arbor, USA. [7]Department of Family Medicine, University of Michigan School of Medicine, Ann Arbor, USA.

## References
1. Gold E, Colvin A, Avis N, Bromberger J, Greendale GA, Powell L, Sternfeld B, Matthews K. Longitudinal analysis of vasomotor symptoms and race/ethnicity across the menopausal transition: study of women's health across the nation (SWAN). Am J Public Health. 2006;96:1226–35.
2. Kravitz HM, Ganz PA, Bromberger J, Powell LH, Sutton-Tyrrell K, Meyer PM. Sleep difficulty in women at midlife: a community survey of sleep and the menopausal transition. Menopause. 2003;10:19–28.
3. Bromberger JT, Kravitz HM, Wei HL, Brown C, Youk AO, Cordal A, Powell LH, Matthews KA. History of depression and women's current health and functioning during midlife. Gen Hosp Psychiatry. 2005;27:200–8.
4. Freeman E, Sammel M, Lin H, Gracia C, Kapoor S, Ferdousi T. The role of anxiety and hormonal changes in menopausal hot flashes. Menopause. 2005;12:258–66.
5. Woods NF. Symptom clusters and quality of life. Menopause. 2012;20:5–7.
6. Ho SY, Rohan KJ, Parent J, Tager FA, McKinley PS. A longitudinal study of depression, fatigue, and sleep disturbances as a symptom cluster in women with breast cancer. J Pain Symptom Manag. 2015;49:707–15.
7. Avis NE, Levine B, Marshall SA, Ip EH. Longitudinal examination of symptom profiles among breast cancer survivors. J Pain Symptom Manag. 2017;53:703–10.
8. DeVon HA, Vuckovic K, Ryan CJ, Barnason S, Zerwic JJ, Pozehl B, Schulz P, Seo Y, Zimmerman L. Symptomatic review of symptom clusters in cardiovascular disease. Eur J Cardiovasc Nurs. 2017;16:6–17.
9. Cray L, Woods NF, Mitchell ES. Symptom clusters during the late menopausal transitions stage: observations from the Seattle midlife women's health study. Menopause. 2010;17:972–7.
10. Cray LA, Woods NF, Herting JR, Mitchell ES. Symptom clusters during the late reproductive stage through early postmenopause: observations from the Seattle midlife women's health study. Menopause. 2012;19:864–9.
11. Cray LA, Woods NF, Mitchell ES. Identifying symptom clusters during the menopausal transition: observations from the Seattle midlife women's health study. Climacteric. 2013;16:539–49.
12. Woods NF, Hohensee C, Carpenter JS, Cohen L, Ensrud K, Freeman EW, Guthrie KA, Joffe H, LaCroix AZ, Otte JL. Symptom clusters among MsFLASH clinical trial participants. Menopause. 2016;23(2):158–65.
13. Mishra GD, Dobson AJ. Using longitudinal profiles to characterize women's symptoms through midlife: results from a large prospective study. Menopause. 2012;19:549–55.
14. Woods NF, Cray L, Mitchell ES, Herting JR. Endocrine biomarkers and symptom clusters during the menopausal transition and early postmenopause: observations from the Seattle midlife women's health study. Menopause. 2014;21:646–52.
15. Greenblum CA, Rowe MA, Neff DF, Greenblum JS. Midlife women: symptoms associated with menopause transition and early postmenopause quality of life. Menopause. 2013;20:22–7.
16. Sievert LL, Obermeyer CM, Saliba M. Symptom groupings at midlife: cross-cultural variation and association with job, home, and life change. Menopause. 2007;14:798–807.
17. Im EO, Ko Y, Chee E, Chee W. Cluster analysis of midlife women's sleep-related symptoms: racial/ethnic differences. Menopause. 2015;22:1182–9.
18. Prairie BA, Wisniewski SR, Luther J, Hess R, Thurston RC, Wisner KL, Bromberger JT. Symptoms of depressed mood, disturbed sleep, and sexual problems in midlife women: cross-sectional data from the study of women's health across the nation. J Womens Health. 2015;24:119–26.
19. Avis NE, Brockwell S, Colvin A. A universal menopausal syndrome? Am J Med. 2005;118(suppl 12B):S37–46.
20. Sowers M, Crawford S, Sternfeld B, et al. SWAN: a multicenter, multiethnic, community-based cohort study of women and the menopausal transition. In: Lobo RA, Kelsey J, Marcus R, editors. Menopause: biology and pathobiology. San Diego: Academic; 2000. p. 175–88.
21. Ware J. The SF-36 health survey manual and interpretation guide. New England medical center. Boston: The Health Institute; 1993.
22. Radloff LS. The CES-D scale: a self-report depression scale for research in the general population. Appl Psychol Meas. 1977;1:385–401.
23. Roberts RE. Reliability of the CES-D scale in different ethnic contexts. Psychiatry Res. 1980;2:125–34.
24. Cohen S, Kamarck T, Mermelstein R. A global measure of perceived stress. J Health Soc Behav. 1983;24:385–96.
25. Avis NE, McKinlay SM. A longitudinal analysis of women's attitudes toward the menopause: results from the Massachusetts women's health study. Maturitas. 1991;13:65–79.
26. Matthews KA, Wing RR, Kuller LH, Meilahn EN, Plantinga P. Influence of the perimenopause on cardiovascular risk factors and symptoms of middle-aged healthy women. Arch Intern Med. 1994;154:2349–55.
27. Neugarten BL, Kraines RJ. Menopausal symptoms in women of various ages. Psychosom Med. 1965;27:266–73.
28. Buysse DJ, Reynolds CF, Monk TH, Berman SR, Kupfer DJ. The Pittsburgh sleep quality index: a new instrument for psychiatric practice and research. Psychiatry Res. 1989;28:193–213.
29. Levine DW, Kripke DF, Kaplan RM, Lewis MA, Naughton MJ, Bowen DJ, Shumaker SA. Reliability and validity of the women's health initiative insomnia rating scale. Psychol Assess. 2003;15:137–48.

30. Sandvik H, Hunskaar S, Seim A, Hermstad R, Vanvik A, Bratt H. Validation of a severity index in female urinary incontinence and its implementation in an epidemiological survey. J Epidemiol Community Health. 1993;47:497–9.

31. Avis NE, Brockwell S, Randolph Jr JF, Shen S, Cain VS, Ory M, Greendale GA. Longitudinal changes in sexual functioning as women transition through menopause: results from the study of women's health across the nation. Menopause. 2009;16:442–52.

32. Clogg CC. Latent class models. In: Arminger G, Clogg CC, Sobel ME, editors. Handbook of statistical modeling for the social and behavioral sciences. New York: Plenum Press; 1995. p. 311–59.

33. Lanza ST, Dziak JJ, Huang L, Wagner AT, Collins LM. Proc LCA & Proc LTA users' guide (Version 1.3.2). The Methodology Center, Penn State: University Park; 2015. Available at https://methodology.psu.edu/sites/default/files/software/proclcalta/proc_lca_lta_1-3-2-1_users_guide.pdf. Accessed 22 Dec 2016.

34. Collins LM, Lanza ST. Latent class and latent transition analysis: with applications in the social, behavioral, and health sciences. New York: Wiley; 2013.

35. Karvonen-Gutierrez CA, Ylitalo KR. Prevalence and correlates of disability in a late middle-aged population of women. J Aging Health. 2013;25:701–17.

36. Szanton SL, Thorpe RJ, Whitfield K. Life-course financial strain and health in African-Americans. Soc Sci Med. 2010;71:259–65.

37. Matthews RJ, Smith LK, Hancock RM, Jagger C, Spiers NA. Socioeconomic factors associated with the onset of disability in older age: a longitudinal study of people aged 75 years and over. Soc Sci Med. 2005;61:1567–75.

38. Gold EB, Bromberger J, Crawford S, Samuels S, Greendale GA, Harlow SD, Skurnick J. Factors associated with age at natural menopause in a multiethnic sample of midlife women. Am J Epidemiol. 2001;153:865–74.

39. Snowdon DA, Kane RL, Beeson WL, Burke GL, Sprafka JM, Potter J, Iso H, Jacobs Jr DR, Phillips RL. Is early natural menopause a biologic marker of health and aging? Am J Public Health. 1989;79:709–14.

40. Jacobsen BK, Heuch I, Kvale G. Age at natural menopause and all-cause mortality: a 37-year follow-up of 19,731 Norwegian women. Am J Epidemiol. 2003;157:923–9.

41. Wu X, Cai H, Kallianpur A, Gao YT, Yang G, Chow WH, Li HL, Zheng W, Shu XO. Age at menarche and natural menopause and number of reproductive years in association with mortality: results from a median follow-up of 11.2 years among 31,955 naturally menopausal Chinese women. PLoS ONE [Electronic Resource]. 2014;9(8):e103673.

42. Jackson CA, Jones M, Tooth L, Mishra GD, Byles J, Dobson A. Multimorbidity patterns are differentially associated with functional ability and decline in a longitudinal cohort of older women. Age Ageing. 2015;44:810–6.

# 7

# Changes in androstenedione, dehydroepiandrosterone, testosterone, estradiol, and estrone over the menopausal transition

Catherine Kim[1]*⬛, Siobàn D. Harlow[2], Huiyong Zheng[2], Daniel S. McConnell[2] and John F. Randolph Jr.[3]

## Abstract

**Background:** Previous reports have noted that dehydroepiandrosterone-sulfate (DHEAS) increases prior to the final menstrual period (FMP) and remains stable beyond the FMP. How DHEAS concentrations correspond with other sex hormones across the menopausal transition (MT) including androstenedione (A4), testosterone (T), estrone (E1), and estradiol (E2) is not known. Our objective was to examine how DHEAS, A4, T, E1, and E2 changed across the MT by White vs. African-American (AA) race/ethnicity.

**Methods:** We conducted a longitudinal observational analysis of a subgroup of women from the Study of Women's Health Across the Nation observed over 4 visits prior to and 4 visits after the FMP ($n = 110$ women over 9 years for 990 observations). The main outcome measures were DHEAS, A4, T, E1, and E2.

**Results:** Compared to the decline in E2 concentrations, androgen concentrations declined minimally over the MT. T ($\beta$ 9.180, $p < 0.0001$) and E1 ($\beta$ 11.365, $p < 0.0001$) were higher in Whites than in AAs, while elevations in DHEAS ($\beta$ 28.80, $p = 0.061$) and A4 ($\beta$ 0.2556, $p = 0.052$) were borderline. Log-transformed E2 was similar between Whites and AAs ($\beta$ 0.0764, $p = 0.272$). Body mass index (BMI) was not significantly associated with concentrations of androgens or E1 over time.

**Conclusion:** This report suggests that the declines in E2 during the 4 years before and after the FMP are accompanied by minimal changes in DHEAS, A4, T, and E1. There are modest differences between Whites and AAs and minimal differences by BMI.

**Keywords:** Dehydroepiandrosterone-sulfate, Androstenedione, Testosterone, Estrone, Menopause

## Background

The menopausal transition (MT) represents a marked shift in women's sex steroid profile, of which changes in estradiol (E2) are the best studied [1]. On average, women's E2 concentrations begin to change more rapidly about 2 years prior to the final menstrual period (FMP) and stabilize several years after the FMP [2]. The rapidity of decline and average E2 levels may be predicted by race/ethnicity and body mass index (BMI) at

the beginning of the transition [3, 4]. The most pronounced differences occur between African-American (AA) and White women, the former group having more gradual changes than the latter group [4]. Presumably in part due to adipose tissue production of E2, women with higher BMI have more gradual changes than women with lower BMI [3, 4].

The adrenal gland is the primary source of dehydroepiandrosterone-sulfate (DHEAS) and androstenedione (A4) and also contributes to circulating testosterone (T) [5]. Aromatase catalyzes A4 and T into estrogens, i.e. A4 into estrone (E1) and T into estradiol (E2). Previous reports have suggested that, prior to the FMP, adrenal DHEAS production increases even as

* Correspondence: cathkim@umich.edu
[1]Departments of Medicine and Obstetrics & Gynecology, University of Michigan, 2800 Plymouth Road, Building 16, Room 430W, Ann Arbor, MI 48109, USA
Full list of author information is available at the end of the article

peripheral E2 decreases [6–10]. As adrenal sex hormones exist in equilibrium with ovarian sex hormones in the peripheral circulation, it is plausible that adrenal hormone metabolism also changes over the MT [11]. This is consistent with the hypothesis that increasing adrenal sex hormone production and aromatization may be concurrent with decreasing ovarian estrogen production [12]. It is also possible that DHEAS production may also eventually decline over time resulting lower peripheral A4 and E1 concentrations.

Few longitudinal studies examine changes in a comprehensive array of adrenal sex hormones across the MT. Since concentrations of circulating DHEAS increase in the 5th decade of life [6–10] and concentrations among women in their 8th decade of life are low [13], DHEAS must decline in the postmenopause. However, it is uncertain when in the postmenopause this might occur. In addition, few reports examine concentrations of A4 or E1 during the MT and whether ratios of A4:E1 change over the MT, consistent with changes in aromatase activity or consistent with increased A4 production and concomitant increases in aromatization. No reports examine whether E1 concentrations change across the MT. In addition, studies have not examined whether these patterns differ by BMI, as has been reported for E2, or between Whites and AAs.

Therefore, using data from the Study of Women's Health Across the Nation (SWAN), we characterized serum adrenal and ovarian sex steroid changes over the MT. We assessed concentrations of DHEAS, A4, T, E2, and E1 annually in the 4 years before and the 4 years after the FMP. We assessed whether concentrations changed in relation to the FMP during this time period and whether patterns differed between White and AA race/ethnicity, and BMI. We hypothesized that concentrations of DHEAS and A4 would increase slightly over the 4 years prior to and after the FMP, consistent with augmented adrenal androgen production. We hypothesized that AA women would be less likely to have adrenal sex hormone changes over the MT, as previous reports have suggested that AA women have less fluctuation in DHEAS concentrations than White women [4]. We also hypothesized that women with higher BMI would be more likely to have more gradual increases in DHEAS and A4 over the MT, since previous SWAN reports have suggested that women with higher BMI have more gradual declines in E2 than women with lower BMI [3].

## Methods

The study protocol of SWAN has been described previously: briefly, eligibility criteria for the SWAN cohort study enrollment included the following: age 42–52 years,

no surgical removal of uterus and/or both ovaries; not currently using exogenous hormone medications that were known to affect ovarian function; at least one menstrual period as well as one of the following five other racial/ethnic groups. These groups included women who were White, AA, Chinese and Japanese, and Hispanic. A total of 3302 women were recruited. Institutional review boards approved the study protocol at each site; signed, written informed consent was obtained from all participants. The current study included a subsample of White and AA women who met inclusion criteria. We focused upon these 2 racial/ethnic groups as they had sufficient numbers of subjects with a documented final menstrual period (FMP) and complete hormone data for 4 years before and after the FMP, they were the largest number of participants in SWAN, the largest racial/ethnic differences in sex steroids have previously been observed between these 2 populations, and funds restricted examination of other racial/ethnic groups [3].

Other inclusion criteria included having a BMI of 22–30 kg/m$^2$, a natural FMP i.e. no history of hysterectomy or oophorectomy, no exogenous hormone therapy use, and at least 9 sequential annual samples spanning 4 years before and 4 years after the FMP, for a total of 110 women with 990 observations. Compared to White participants in SWAN generally, White women in the current report were similarly aged at baseline, were more likely to report excellent or very good self-reported health, and had similar smoking status. Compared to AA participants who did not meet inclusion criteria, AA women in the current report had similar age, self-rated health, and smoking status. Due to the inclusion criteria designed to limit outliers of BMI, both White and AA women in the current report had lower BMI than women who did not meet inclusion criteria.

Annual fasting blood samples were collected. Two attempts were made to collect a follicular phase sample. When follicular phase samples were not available or when a woman stopped menstruating, a random fasting sample was collected within 90 days of the baseline recruitment date. All serum hormones were measured at the CLASS/RSP Central Laboratory at the University of Michigan (Ann Arbor, MI). A4 was measured using a commercially available enzyme-linked immunosorbent assay (ELISA) from Diagnostic Systems Laboratories (DSL). The assay measures analyte concentrations from 0.1 to 10 ng/mL with a minimum detectable concentration of 0.1 ng/mL, and a sensitivity of 0.03 ng/mL. The inter-assay coefficient of variation (CV) is 3.9% at 0.98 ng/mL and 3.0% at 6.1 ng/mL. The intra-assay CV is 2.1% at 0.98 ng/mL, 1.3% at 6.1 ng/mL. DHEAS was measured using an automated, ACS:180-based chemiluminescent assay developed in the CLASS laboratory and based upon the Bayer Diagnostics ACS:180. The detection level of this assay is approximately 1.9 μg/dL. The intra-assay CV is 8.02% (*n* = 261) and inter-assay CV is 11.34% (53.32 μg/dL, *n* = 37) and 9.74% (250.21 μg/dL, n = 37). The CLASS laboratory modified the ACS:180 total testosterone chemiluminescent assay to measure with greater precision samples in the low ranges found in women in the peri- and postmenopause. To accomplish this, sample volume was increased while evaluating the consequences of this change on volumes of subsequent reagents. The limit of detection of this assay is <5.15 ng/dL. The limit of quantification (lowest reported value) is set at the lowest standard, 5.15 ng/dL. The intra-assay CV is 11.78% (24.4 ng/dL, *n* = 30), 4.6% (191.2 ng/dL, n = 30) and 9.1% (414.2 ng/dL, n = 30). The inter-assay CVs are 11.34% (53.3 ng/dL, *n* = 37) and 9.7% (250.2 ng/dL, n = 37). E1 was measured using a commercially available ELISA from DSL. This method features a wide dynamic standard range of 0.05 to 90 ng/mL, and a minimum detectable concentration of 0.01 ng/mL. Inter-assay CVs were 12.7% at 1.2 ng/mL and 10.8% at 9.2 ng/mL, and intra-assay CVs were 6.7% at 1.2 ng/mL and 2.9% at 9.2 ng/mL. E2 concentrations were measured using the Estradiol-6 III immunoassay performed on the ADVIA Centaur instrument (Siemens HealthCare Diagnostics). Inter-assay CVs are 11.0% (102.9 pg/mL) and 7.0% (225.9 pg/mL) and 3.8% (615.9 pg/mL). Intra-assay CVs are 3.9% (102.9 pg/mL), 5.0% (225.9 pg/mL) and 1.4% (615.9 pg/mL). Follicle stimulating hormone (FSH) was measured with a two-site chemiluminescence (sandwich) immunoassay with a minimum detectable concentration of 0.3 mIU/mL. Inter- and intra-assay CVs are 8.1% and 3.5%, respectively.

### Statistical analyses

For the purposes of this analysis, BMI was analyzed in tertiles (< 25 kg/m$^2$, 25–26.9 kg/m$^2$, >27 kg/m$^2$) and by White vs. AA race/ethnicity. Distributions of DHEAS, A4, T, E2, and E1 were examined at each year in relation to time before and after the FMP. Population hormone trajectories in relation to FMP and covariates were analyzed using linear mixed models. Piecewise linear mixed models were applied to test the rate of changes at each stage, i.e., pre-menopause (2 years before FMP), transition stage (+/− 2 years around FMP), and post-menopause (2 years after FMP). [2, 14, 15] For presentation in Figs. 1 and 2, data were stratified by race/ethnicity and BMI (normal vs. overweight and by tertile of BMI). In order to determine whether race/ethnicity or BMI was associated with serum hormone concentrations, we created semiparametric stochastic mixed models that accounted for the multiple repeated measures in women and adjusted for the time from the FMP. [16] Hormone distributions were also examined after log-transformation; log transformation did not alter the pattern of the results with the exception of E2, so non-transformed values are presented for other sex

hormones. Racial/ethnic differences in SHBG were also examined, but differences were minimal (results not shown). All analyses were performed with SAS Windows 9.2 (SAS Institute, Cary NC).

### Results

Thirty-four AA and 76 White women were included. Participant characteristics are shown in Table 1. Forty-seven (42%) of women had BMIs of 22–24.9 kg/m$^2$ vs. 30 (27%) of women who had BMIs 25.0–26.9 kg/m$^2$ vs. 33 (30%) who had BMIs 27.0–30.0 kg/m$^2$. Women had lower median FSH concentrations at 4 years prior to their FMP (21.4 IU/L) compared to 4 years after their FMP (125.7 IU/L), consistent with the transition from premenopause to postmenopause.

Figure 1 displays the average concentrations of sex hormones across the FMP for White and AA women for each year of the MT. Declines in log E2 concentrations were the most marked out of all of the sex hormone changes in both Whites and AAs, but E2 declines were not accompanied by increases in E1 concentrations. The ratio of E1:A4 remained fairly constant across the MT. Table 2 shows median values for sex hormones at 4 years prior the FMP, the year of the FMP, and 4 years after the FMP for Whites and AAs, and Table 3 shows the association between race/ethnicity and hormone concentration after adjustment for FMP and repeated measures within women. Hormone concentrations were generally higher in Whites than AAs, although only T and E1 met criteria for significance and log E2 concentrations were similar between Whites and AAs.

Figure 2 shows the average concentration trajectories of sex hormones across the MT for women by BMI tertile. Table 2 shows median values for sex hormones at 4 years prior the FMP, the year of the FMP, and 4 years after the FMP by BMI tertile. BMI tertile was not associated with differences in DHEAS, A4, or E1 at different times in relation to the FMP. Table 4 shows the association between BMI as a continuous variable and hormone concentration after adjustment for FMP and repeated measures within women. Although BMI as a continuous variable was associated with slightly higher T concentrations, this association was of borderline statistical significance (*p* = 0.051). Otherwise, higher BMI was not associated with higher hormone concentrations.

### Discussion

In a longitudinal analysis spanning 8 years across the MT, DHEAS concentrations were stable across the MT [6, 7]. We also note that A4, T, and E1 concentrations remain relatively stable as long as 4 years after the FMP. Moreover, the ratios of E1 and A4 remained fairly constant across the MT. Although A4 and E1 declined slightly, these changes did not mirror the dramatic declines in E2

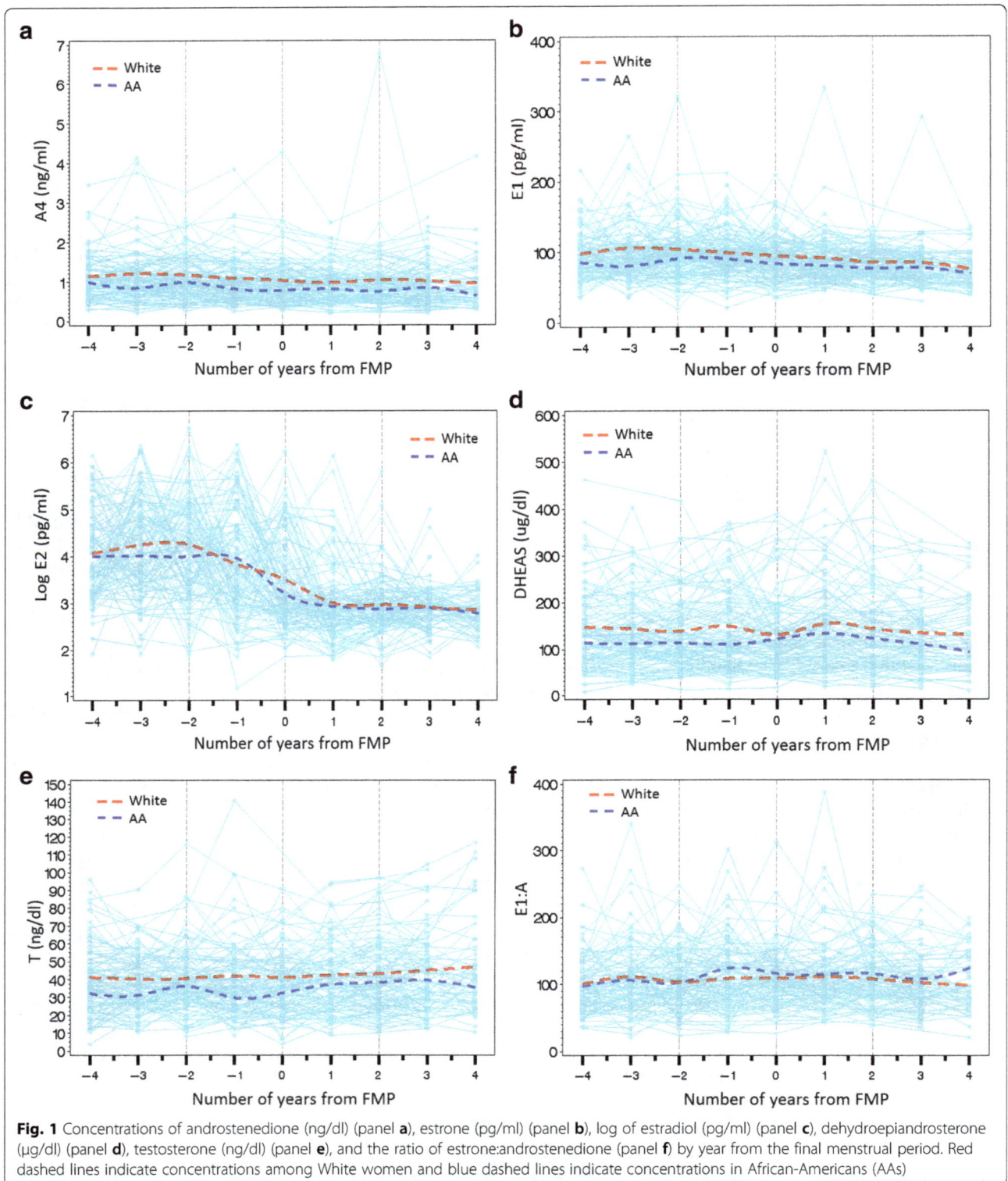

**Fig. 1** Concentrations of androstenedione (ng/dl) (panel **a**), estrone (pg/ml) (panel **b**), log of estradiol (pg/ml) (panel **c**), dehydroepiandrosterone (µg/dl) (panel **d**), testosterone (ng/dl) (panel **e**), and the ratio of estrone:androstenedione (panel **f**) by year from the final menstrual period. Red dashed lines indicate concentrations among White women and blue dashed lines indicate concentrations in African-Americans (AAs)

production. We also found that AAs had slightly lower sex hormone concentrations than Whites. The racial/ethnic differences were likely not due to BMI, as the nature and rate of decline in DHEAS, A4, and E1 were similar by BMI.

Our results are consistent with previous reports that suggest that a rise in DHEAS concentrations prior to menopause is concurrent with the declines in peripheral levels of other sex steroids, as well as reports that note declines in

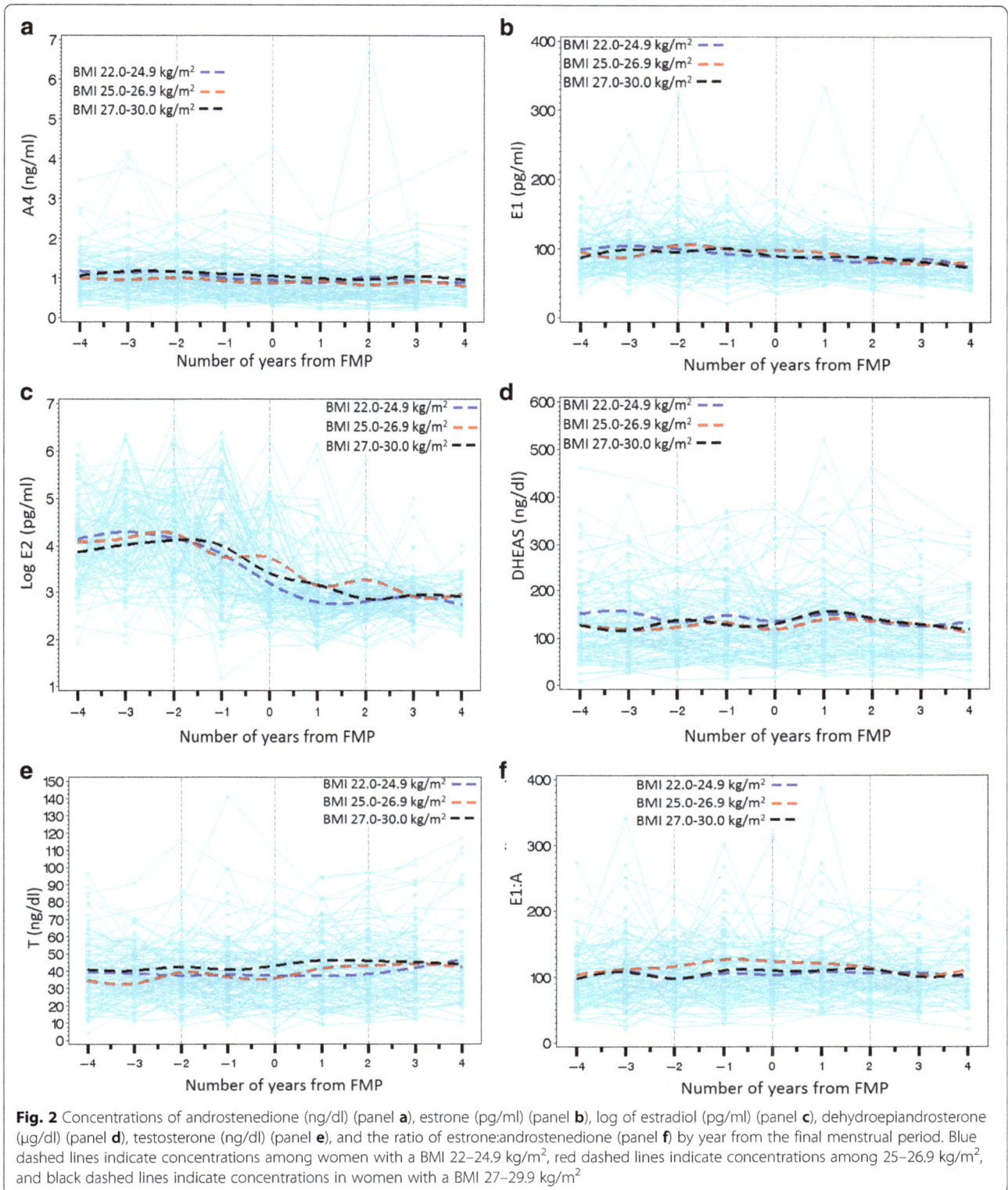

**Fig. 2** Concentrations of androstenedione (ng/dl) (panel **a**), estrone (pg/ml) (panel **b**), log of estradiol (pg/ml) (panel **c**), dehydroepiandrosterone (μg/dl) (panel **d**), testosterone (ng/dl) (panel **e**), and the ratio of estrone:androstenedione (panel **f**) by year from the final menstrual period. Blue dashed lines indicate concentrations among women with a BMI 22–24.9 kg/m², red dashed lines indicate concentrations among 25–26.9 kg/m², and black dashed lines indicate concentrations in women with a BMI 27–29.9 kg/m²

DHEAS after the FMP [6–10]. Our report is novel in its inclusion of AAs, the breadth of sex hormones examined, the longitudinal analysis of androgens timed to the FMP, and the length of time spanning the MT.

With the marked decline in ovarian estrogen production in the postmenopause, the adrenal gland becomes a particularly important source of sex steroids, chiefly androgens. DHEA produced by the ovary and the adrenal gland

**Table 1** Characteristics of the study population by race/ethnicity

| | White women (n = 76) | African-American women (n = 34) |
|---|---|---|
| Age at baseline (years) | 46.36 (2.47) | 45.96 (2.05) |
| Age at final menstrual period (years) | 52.03 (2.52) | 51.96 (1.97) |
| Self-reported health (n, %) | | |
| Excellent | 29 (38.67%) | 4 (12.50%) |
| Very good | 36 (48.00%) | 9 (28.13%) |
| Good | 8 (10.67%) | 15 (46.88%) |
| Fair/Poor | 2 (2.67%) | 4 (12.50%) |
| Body mass index (kg/m$^2$) | 25.61 (2.18) | 25.71 (2.01) |
| Baseline smoking status (n,%) | | |
| Never | 40 (52.63%) | 20 (60.61%) |
| Past | 26 (34.21%) | 7 (21.21%) |
| Current | 10 (13.16%) | 7 (21.21%) |

is aromatized peripherally via A4 to bioactive estrogens such as E1. The adrenal gland is also an important source of T which is aromatized to E2. Adrenal-ovarian sex hormone production, conversion to other hormones, and clearance have been postulated to exist in equilibrium [6]. However, longitudinal studies testing this hypothesis are few. Previous reports in SWAN have noted that the majority of women had slight increases in DHEAS prior the FMP followed by declines after the FMP [6, 7], raising the possibility that increased production of DHEAS and/or conversion to other androgens could be a contributor to women's increased androgenicity postmenopause.

Our report extends this prior work: we confirm a modest perimenopausal increase in DHEAS levels, stable T concentrations, and minimal declines in A4 up to 4 years after the FMP. Additionally, since DHEAS and A4 changes do not mirror each other over the transition, it is unlikely that the fluctuations in DHEAS are due to increased peripheral conversion into A4. Similarly, as E1:A4 ratios were stable over time, it is also unlikely that aromatization of A4 to E1 changes significantly over the MT, assuming that A4 production remains the same, although it is possible that both A4 production and aromatization increased concomitantly. Other reports have not reported changes in DHEAS, A4, and T across the menopause. In a cohort of 59 Norwegian women, Overlie and colleagues noted that A4 levels corresponded with both E1 and E2 levels, consistent with the shift from ovarian to adrenal sex hormone production in the postmenopause. However, A4 levels declined in the premenopause, and no significant changes were observed in DHEAS [17]. In a cohort of Swedish women, Rannevik and colleagues also observed that A4 correlated with postmenopausal E1 and E2 concentrations, but concentrations of DHEAS and A4 declined minimally [18].

Our report and previous SWAN studies may have found modest perimenopausal elevations in DHEAS due to larger sample size and our ability to follow women over a longer period of time prior to and after the FMP. Thus, changes in the estrogen/androgen ratio are driven by declines in circulating estrogens, and this relative increase in androgenicity may drive some of the phenotypic changes characteristic of later menopause, such as increased hirsutism [19]. Although speculative, it is possible that such effects are exerted at the tissue level, due to the differential binding of A4 and E2 [20]. Changes in the estrogen/androgen ratio may also be driven by the adrenal response to changing LH concentrations: studies in humans have noted the presence of luteinizing hormone (LH) receptors in the adrenal cortex [21], and mouse models note increases in LH receptors in response to increasing LH levels [22], thus explaining how the adrenal gland might increase sex hormone production even as ovarian response to LH declines.

Previous publications have also reported racial/ethnic differences in androgens, although the direction of reported associations is inconsistent. In a cross-sectional study, Spencer and colleagues noted that even after adjustment for age, BMI, and insulin resistance, AA women had lower DHEAS, A4, and T concentrations than White women [23]. In contrast, Kim and colleagues noted minimal differences in a glucose-intolerant population [24]. Thus, the source of racial/ethnic differences in DHEAS, A4, E1, and T remain speculative. Previous analyses using SWAN data have noted that AAs had the lowest overall DHEAS levels and lowest rates of decline with chronologic age [6, 7]. In those reports, concentrations of A4 were not examined, and thus it was unclear whether racial/ethnic differences in DHEAS concentrations were due to increased adrenal androgen production vs. decreased metabolism of DHEAS into A4. Our report suggests that racial/ethnic differences in A4 metabolism are unlikely to contribute to racial/ethnic differences in DHEAS concentrations.

Previous reports have also suggested that weight may be a significant modifier of adrenal sex hormone production, possibly by affecting E2 concentrations, which in turn might lead to compensatory increases in E1. However, we did not find significant effect modification by tertile of BMI for the sex hormones examined in this report. Our report agrees with that of population-based studies examining cross-sectional associations between DHEAS, A4, and BMI in postmenopausal women [25, 26]. Although E2 and T correlate with waist circumference and BMI in women, the association between BMI and other sex hormones has been relatively weak. One explanation for our conflicting results is that we examined non-obese women within a narrow range of BMI. It is also possible that BMI and waist circumference do not reflect adipose tissue

**Table 2** Median (interquartile range) serum hormone levels of women 4 years prior to their final menstrual period (FMP), at the time of their FMP, and 4 years after their FMP ($n = 110$)

| | 4 years prior to FMP | Year of the FMP | 4 years after the FMP |
|---|---|---|---|
| DHEAS (µg/dl) | 127.5 (100.4) | 108.2 (89.1) | 98.6 (105.9) |
| African-American | 103.2 (82.4) | 104.8 (113.5) | 98.2 (66.7) |
| White | 130.2 (109.7) | 109.6 (79.2) | 102.1 (123.3) |
| p-value | 0.116 | 0.583 | 0.156 |
| BMI 22.0–24.9 kg/m$^2$ | 133.0 (118.2) | 108.2 (92.8) | 125.1 (128.8) |
| BMI 25.0–26.9 kg/m$^2$ | 110.0 (63.1) | 110.3 (58.2) | 98.2 (70.6) |
| BMI 27.0–30.0 kg/m$^2$ | 107.2 (69.3) | 84.4 (110.8) | 95.6 (56.8) |
| p-value | 0.316 | 0.730 | 0.772 |
| A4 (ng/ml) | 1.03 (0.67) | 0.84 (0.58) | 0.70 (0.59) |
| African-American | 1.03 (0.72) | 0.75 (0.33) | 0.61 (0.38) |
| White | 1.01 (0.71) | 0.91 (0.65) | 0.78 (0.62) |
| p-value | 0.338 | 0.066 | 0.075 |
| BMI 22.0–24.9 kg/m$^2$ | 1.10 (0.70) | 0.86 (0.57) | 0.77 (0.59) |
| BMI 25.0–26.9 kg/m$^2$ | 0.99 (0.59) | 0.83 (0.52) | 0.70 (0.61) |
| BMI 27.0–30.0 kg/m$^2$ | 0.94 (0.53) | 0.81 (0.64) | 0.68 (0.58) |
| p-value | 0.348 | 0.800 | 0.883 |
| T (ng/dl) | 35.9 (24.8) | 36.3 (21.0) | 38.3 (24.4) |
| African-American | 34.6 (18.7) | 30.9 (20.0) | 33.6 (26.2) |
| White | 36.7 (30.2) | 38.7 (20.2) | 38.8 (29.6) |
| p-value | 0.095 | 0.020 | 0.111 |
| BMI 22.0–24.9 kg/m$^2$ | 37.8 (32.8) | 36.3 (22.1) | 38.8 (24.8) |
| BMI 25.0–26.9 kg/m$^2$ | 31.2 (18.2) | 36.2 (20.5) | 40.1 (29.9) |
| BMI 27.0–30.0 kg/m$^2$ | 36.4 (19.7) | 37.2 (28.3) | 37.7 (24.2) |
| p-value | 0.418 | 0.566 | 0.831 |
| E2 (pg/ml) | 53.0 (74.8) | 21.6 (39.8) | 16.6 (8.0) |
| African-American | 53.5 (65.5) | 18.7 (10.3) | 16.6 (14.9) |
| White | 51.6 (79.8) | 24.4 (54.8) | 16.6 (7.9) |
| p-value | 0.741 | 0.155 | 0.692 |
| BMI 22.0–24.9 kg/m$^2$ | 59.5 (99.0) | 18.8 (27.4) | 14.4 (5.3) |
| BMI 25.0–26.9 kg/m$^2$ | 41.7 (123.8) | 21.0 (127.6) | 18.1 (7.0) |
| BMI 27.0–30.0 kg/m$^2$ | 51.6 (46.6) | 24.3 (32.9) | 17.5 (9.2) |
| p-value | 0.533 | 0.166 | 0.090 |
| E1 (pg/ml) | 89.4 (39.4) | 87.0 (38.6) | 69.9 (31.0) |
| African-American | 77.8 (44.5) | 85.4 (34.5) | 64.8 (30.6) |
| White | 93.4 (38.4) | 88.4 (40.4) | 72.7 (29.9) |
| p-value | 0.069 | 0.232 | 0.369 |
| BMI 22.0–24.9 kg/m$^2$ | 97.0 (42.3) | 86.9 (45.9) | 67.9 (23.9) |
| BMI 25.0–26.9 kg/m$^2$ | 94.4 (41.8) | 100.0 (42.0) | 82.8 (42.9) |
| BMI 27.0–30.0 kg/m$^2$ | 80.5 (26.7) | 80.3 (34.2) | 65.5 (34.5) |
| p-value | 0.111 | 0.317 | 0.633 |

**Table 3** Associations between race/ethnicity and hormone levels from semiparametric stochastic mixed models, beta-coefficient (standard error) and p-value

|  | Beta-coefficient (standard error) | p-value |
|---|---|---|
| DHEAS (µg/dl) | 28.80 (15.34) | 0.061 |
| A4 (ng/ml) | 0.2556 (0.1315) | 0.052 |
| T (ng/dl) | 9.180 (1.652) | <0.00001 |
| ln E2 | 0.0764 (0.0695) | 0.272 |
| E1 (pg/ml) | 11.365 (0.7306) | <0.00001 |
| E1:A4 | −6.527 (7.040) | 0.354 |

Reference group is African-American women; a beta-coefficient greater than 0 indicates higher sex hormone levels in white women

deposition, as examination of associations between visceral adiposity and sex steroids using radiographic imaging has found stronger associations [27].

Strengths of the current report include the longitudinal design, inclusion of AAs, examination of a comprehensive list of adrenal sex hormones, high assay sensitivity for low androgen concentrations, and observation for 9 years during the MT for 990 observations. Limitations include a limited sample size, and thus small fluctuations in hormone concentrations may not have been detected. Our ability to adjust for confounders, particularly racial-ethnic differences in adipose tissue deposition, was also limited. It is possible that self-rated health and smoking status contributed to racial/ethnic differences along with unmeausured confounders, but we had limited power to adjust for these possibilities. We did not use LC/MS for measurement of E2 concentrations, which are low after the FMP; however, our objective was to show relative change over the MT, rather than to establish a definitive absolute value for E2. Finally, we did not conduct adrenal and ovarian vein sampling, and thus cannot definitively distinguish between ovarian and adrenal production of androgens and estrogens.

## Conclusions

Our report supports the importance of adrenal androgens as the primary source of estrogens in the postmenopause

**Table 4** Associations between body mass index (BMI) and hormone levels from semiparametric stochastic mixed models, beta-coefficient (standard error) is the unit hormone increase per kg/m$^2$

|  | Beta-coefficient (standard error) | p-value |
|---|---|---|
| DHEAS (µg/dl) | 0.0000 (0.0000) | 1.00 |
| A4 (ng/ml) | −0.0026 (0.0289) | 0.929 |
| T (ng/dl) | 0.7359 (0.3758) | 0.051 |
| ln E2 | 0.0230 (0.0151) | 0.128 |
| E1 (pg/ml) | −0.3466 (0.912) | 0.704 |
| E1:A4 | 0.0274 (1.5409) | 0.354 |

and the increased androgenicity of the postmenopausal hormonal milieu. It is also possible that ovarian production of E1 remains even as E2 declines. Modest increases in DHEAS concentrations are not accompanied by measurably increased levels of A4, T, or E1. Concentrations of these hormones appear to be lower in AAs than White women in the perimenopause, and these racial/ethnic differences are unlikely due to BMI. Examination of the mechanisms for lower DHEAS, A4, and T concentrations in AA women is needed, particularly prior the FMP when declines in other sex hormones occur. Examination of whether these differences contribute to vasomotor symptoms or altered risk of chronic disease risk by race/ethnicity, particularly in other groups besides Whites and AAs, is needed.

### Abbreviations
A4: Androstenedione; AAs: African-Americans; BMI: Body mass index; DHEAS: Dehydroepiandrosterone sulfate; E1: Estrone; E2: Estradiol; FMP: Follicle stimulating hormone; FSH: Follicle stimulating hormone; LC/MS: Liquid chromatography mass spectrometry; LH: Luteinizing hormone; MT: Menopausal transition; T: Testosterone

### Acknowledgments
We thank the study staff at each site and all the women who participated in the Study of Women's Health Across the Nation (SWAN). This publication was supported in part by the National Center for Research Resources and the National Center for Advancing Translational Sciences, National Institutes of Health through UCSF-CTSI Grant UL1 RR024131.

### Authors' contributions
CK interpreted the data regarding hormone distributions and wrote the manuscript. HZ performed the analysis, interpreted the data, and revised the manuscript. DM performed the assays and revised the manuscript. SH collected the data, guided the analyses, and revised the manuscript. JR guided the analyses and revised the manuscript. All authors read and approved the final manuscript.

### Funding
The Study of Women's Health Across the Nation (SWAN) has grant support from the National Institutes of Health (NIH), Department of Health and Human Services, through the National Institute on Aging (NIA), the National Institute of Nursing Research (NINR) and the NIH Office of Research on Women's Health (ORWH) (Grants U01NR004061, U01AG012505, U01AG012535, U01AG012531, U01AG012539, U01AG012546, U01AG012553, U01AG012554, and U01AG012495). The content of this manuscript is solely the responsibility of the authors and does not necessarily represent the official views of the NIA, NINR, ORWH, or the NIH.

### Competing interests
The authors declare that they have no competing interests.

### Author details
[1]Departments of Medicine and Obstetrics & Gynecology, University of Michigan, 2800 Plymouth Road, Building 16, Room 430W, Ann Arbor, MI 48109, USA. [2]Department of Epidemiology, University of Michigan, Ann Arbor, MI, USA. [3]Department of Obstetrics & Gynecology, University of Michigan, Ann Arbor, MI, USA.

## References

1. Santoro N, Randolph J Jr. Reproductive hormones and the menopause transition. Obstet Gynecol Clin N Am. 2011;38:455–66.

2. Sowers M, Zheng H, McConnell D, Nan B, Harlow S, Randolph J Jr. Estradiol rates of change in relation to the final menstrual period in a population-based cohort of women. J Clin Endocrinol Metab. 2008;93(10):3847–52.

3. Randolph J Jr, Zheng H, Sowers M, Crandall C, Crawford S, Gold E, et al. Change in follicle-stimulating hormone and estradiol across the menopausal transition: effect of age at the final menstrual period. J Clin Endocrinol Metab. 2011;96(3):746–54.

4. Tepper P, Randolph J, McConnell D, Crawford S, El Khoudary S, Joffe H, et al. Trajectory clustering of estradiol and follicle-stimulating hormone during the menopausal transition among women in the study of Women's health across the nation. J Clin Endocrinol Metab. 2012;97(8):2872–80.

5. Davison S, Bell R, Donath S, Montalto J, Davis S. Androgen levels in adult females: changes with age, menopause, and oophorectomy. J Clin Endocrinol Metab. 2005;90(7):3847.

6. Lasley B, Santoro N, Randolph J Jr, Gold E, Crawford S, Weiss G, et al. The relationship of circulating dehydroepiandrosterone, testosterone, and estradiol to stages of the menopausal transition and ethnicity. J Clin Endocrinol Metab. 2002;87(8):3760–7.

7. Crawford S, Santoro N, Laughlin G, Sowers J, McConnell D, Sutton-Tyrrell K, et al. Circulating dehydroepiandrosterone sulfate concentrations during the menopausal transition. J Clin Endocrinol Metab. 2009;94(8):2945–51.

8. Lasley B, Chen J, Stanczyk F, El Khoudary S, Gee N, Crawford S, et al. Androstenediol complements estrogenic bioactivity during the menopausal transition. Menopause. 2012;19(6):650–7.

9. McConnell D, Stanczyk F, Sowers M, Randolph J Jr, Lasley B. Menopausal transition stage-specific changes in circulating adrenal androgens. Menopause. 2012;19(6):658–63.

10. Lasley B, Crawford S, Laughlin G, Santoro N, McConnell D, Crandall C, et al. Circulating dehydroepiandrosterone sulfate levels in women with bilateral salpingo-oophorectomy during the menopausal transition. Menopause. 2011;18(5):494–8.

11. Lasley B, Crawford S, McConnell D. Adrenal androgens and the menopausal transition. Obstet Gynecol Clin N Am. 2011;38(3):467–75.

12. Lobo R, Pickar J, Stevenson J, Mack W, Hodis H. Back to the future: hormone replacement therapy as part of a prevention strategy for women at the onset of menopause. Atherosclerosis. 2016;254:282–90.

13. Cappola A, O'Meara E, Guo W, Bartz T, Fried L, Newman A. Trajectories of dehydroepiandrosterone sulfate predict mortality in older adults: the cardiovascular health study. J Gerontol A Biol Sci Med Sci. 2009;64(12):1268–74.

14. Randolph J Jr, Sowers M, Bondarenko I, Harlow S, Luborsky J, Little R.

Change in estradiol and FSH across the early menopausal transition: effects of ethnicity and age. J Clin Endocrinol Metab. 2004;89(4):1555–61.

15. Sowers M, Zheng H, McConnell D, Nan B, Harlow S, Randolph J Jr. Follicle stimulating hormone and its rate of change in defining menopause transition stages. J Clin Endocrinol Metab. 2008;93(10):3958–64.

16. Zhang D, Lin X, Raz J, Sowers M. Semiparametric stochastic mixed models for longitudinal data. J Am Stat Assoc. 1998;93(442):710–9.

17. Overlie I, Moen M, Morkrid L, Skjaeraasen J, Holte A. The endocrine transition around menopause–a five year prospective study with profiles of gonadotropins, estrogens, androgens, and SHBG among healthy women. Acta Obstet Gynecol Scand. 1999;78(7):642–7.

18. Rannevik G, Jeppsson S, Johnell O, Bjerre B, Laurell-Borulf Y, Svanberg L. A longitudinal study of the perimenopausal transition: altered profiles of steroid and pituitary hormones, SHBG and bone mineral density. Maturitas. 2008;61(102):67–77.

19. Shifren J, Gass M. North American Menopause Society recommendations for clinical Care of Midlife Women Working Group. The North American Menopause Society recommendations for clinical care of midlife women. Menopause. 2014;21(10):1038–62.

20. Miller K, Al-Rayyan N, Ivanova M, Mattingly K, Ripp S, Klinge C, et al. DHEA metabolites activate estrogen receptors alpha and beta. Steroids. 2013;78(1):15–25.

21. Pabon J, Li X, Lei Z, Sanfilippo J, Yussman M, Rao C. Novel presence of luteinizing hormone/chorionic gonadotropin receptrs in human adrenal glands. J Clin Endocrinol Metab. 1996;81(2397–400.

22. Lasley B, Crawford S, McConnell D. Ovarian adrenal interactions during the menopausal transition. Minerva Ginecol. 2013;65(6):641–51.

23. Spencer J, Klein M, Kumar A, Azziz R. The age-associated decline of androgens in reproductive age and menopausal black and white women. J Clin Endocrinol Metab. 2007. epub ahead of print.

24. Kim C, Golden S, Mather K, Laughlin G, Kong S, Nan B, et al. Racial/ethnic differences in sex hormone levels among postmenopausal women in the diabetes prevention program. J Clin Endocrinol Metab. 2012;97(11):4051–60.

25. Kische H, Gross S, Wallaschofski H, Volzke H, Dorr M, Nauck M, et al. Clinical correlates of sex hormones in women: the study of health in Pomerania. Metabolism. 2016;65(9):1286–96.

26. Daan N, Jaspers L, Koster M, Broekmans F, de Rijke Y, Franco O, et al. Androgen levels in women with various forms of ovarian dysfunction: associations with cardiometabolic features. Hum Reprod. 2015;30(10):2376–86.

27. Mongraw-Chaffin M, Anderson C, Allison M, Ouyang P, Szklo M, Vaidya D, et al. Association between sex hormones and adiposity; qualitative differences in women and men in the multi-ethnic study of atherosclerosis. J Clin Endocrinol Metab. 2015;100:E596–600.

# 8

# Contraception pathway: application for midlife women

Chi-Son Kim, Deanna Tikhonov*, Lena Merjanian and Adrian C. Balica

## Abstract

**Objective:** To create a system where evidence based medicine can be applied to accommodate every woman's needs by designing a contraceptive pathway that can be utilized by any healthcare provider, regardless of the patient's age, and to offer appropriate counseling in order to maximize patient outcomes, especially for the midlife woman.

**Methods:** United States Medical Eligibility Criteria for Contraceptive Use, 2016 (US MEC) was used as the framework for these recommendations for a contraceptive care pathway that can be incorporated into care for midlife women.

**Discussion:** By utilizing a total office approach that includes the scheduler, receptionist, medical assistant, nurse and health care provider as members of a team, the entire spectrum of the patient population in need of contraception from teenagers to midlife can be captured. Specifically for midlife women the need for an effective form of contraception may be overlooked as fecundity declines in this age group. This paper will highlight the use of this pathway for midlife women.

**Keywords:** Contraception in midlife women, Unintended pregnancy, Contraceptive pathway

## Background

In 2011, 45% of the 6.1 million pregnancies were unintended in the United States (U.S.) [1]. Fortunately the overall unintended pregnancy rate has declined over the recent years from 54% in 2008 to 45% in 2011 [1]. Nevertheless, about half are still unintended, emphasizing the importance of appropriate contraceptive counseling. Specifically, the group that is often overlooked when discussing contraception is midlife women. Many of the choices in family planning for this group of patients may not be ideal for them due to comorbidities that put them at an increased risk for poor health outcomes, such as cardiovascular disease or chronic hypertension.

Despite a number of new and innovative options approved by the FDA over the last fifteen years, many have not directly addressed the needs of the midlife woman. Healthcare providers are struggling not only with recommending the most effective form of contraception, but also with overcoming social biases and myths about midlife women. The most significant bias concerns a woman's diminished fertility which can cause the

* Correspondence: Dt488@rwjms.rutgers.edu
Department of Obstetrics, Gynecology and Reproductive Sciences, Rutgers Robert Wood Johnson Medical School, 125 Paterson Street, New Brunswick, NJ 08901, USA

provider to overlook the potential risk for an unplanned pregnancy [2]. It is important that all women of reproductive age, through one year past their last normal menstrual period be given contraceptive counseling if they are at risk for unintended pregnancy.

To best address the needs of the midlife woman, as well as all reproductive- aged women, we created a contraceptive pathway that can be utilized by any healthcare provider to identify a woman's specific needs, regardless of her age, and to offer appropriate counseling in order to maximize patient outcomes. Obstetrician/gynecologists, family practice providers, pediatricians, advanced practice nurses, nurse midwives and primary care providers can apply this pathway to meet the specific needs of their patient population. This clinical pathway, is a structured care plan to detail essential steps in the care of the patient with a specific clinical problem, such as the midlife woman [3]. Both clinical staff and providers are involved in the pathway to ensure a smooth process for the patient to obtain the most effective and appropriate method. Based on a patient's age and medical history this pathway can be tailored to meet their contraceptive needs. Standardized delivery of clinical care has become central in evidence based medical practice.. The development of a clinical pathway is an example of a strategy created to reduce variation in clinical care, but still take into account patient differences [2].

A key component of the clinical pathway presented in this article is the ability to utilize the entire office staff creating a clinical care team in order to individualize care and deliver it seamlessly [4]. The team includes the schedulers, receptionists, medical assistants, LPNs and RNs, and healthcare providers. Patient care teams have become a cornerstone in patient centered care illustrated within the Veterans Affairs clinics using Patient Aligned Care Teams or PACT [5]. Effective contraceptive counseling requires not only access to the latest evidence based medicine, but also having a team understand each woman's needs and circumstances, providing seamless coordination [4]. For example, in a scenario involving a midlife patient who smokes 1 pack of cigarettes per day and who has migraine headaches, her options may be limited. A contraceptive pathway can be applied to accommodate this woman's needs, so that the best contraceptive choice is made. In addition, health care providers from various specialties can utilize the same pathway improving contraceptive access for the patient regardless of where she receives her care, therefore enhancing patient safety.

## Methods

We will describe our clinical pathway and how to utilize it when caring for midlife women. The contraceptive clinical pathway we suggest encompasses the United States Medical Eligibility Criteria for Contraceptive Use, 2016 (US MEC) guidelines [6]. The US MEC was created by the CDC to guide healthcare providers in counseling women, men, and couples about contraceptive choices [6]. Although midlife women are included, those women without a menses for one year, indicating menopause, are excluded [7].

## Overview

To use this pathway, every patient encounter should be viewed as an opportunity to discuss contraceptive options. The clinical care team will be involved throughout the process to coordinate women's contraceptive care. As seen in Fig. 1, the contraceptive care pathway starts with the patient scheduling an appointment with a scheduler who will assess if she is interested in a birth control method and provide her with a resource for contraceptive information to review prior to her appointment. This component of the care pathway creates a great opportunity for the patient to learn about her contraceptive options and potentially narrow her choices prior to the visit. When the patient arrives to the office, the receptionist will provide a birth control questionnaire for her to complete. This action by the receptionist enhances the flow of the visit because the questionnaire begins to tailor the contraceptive options for which the

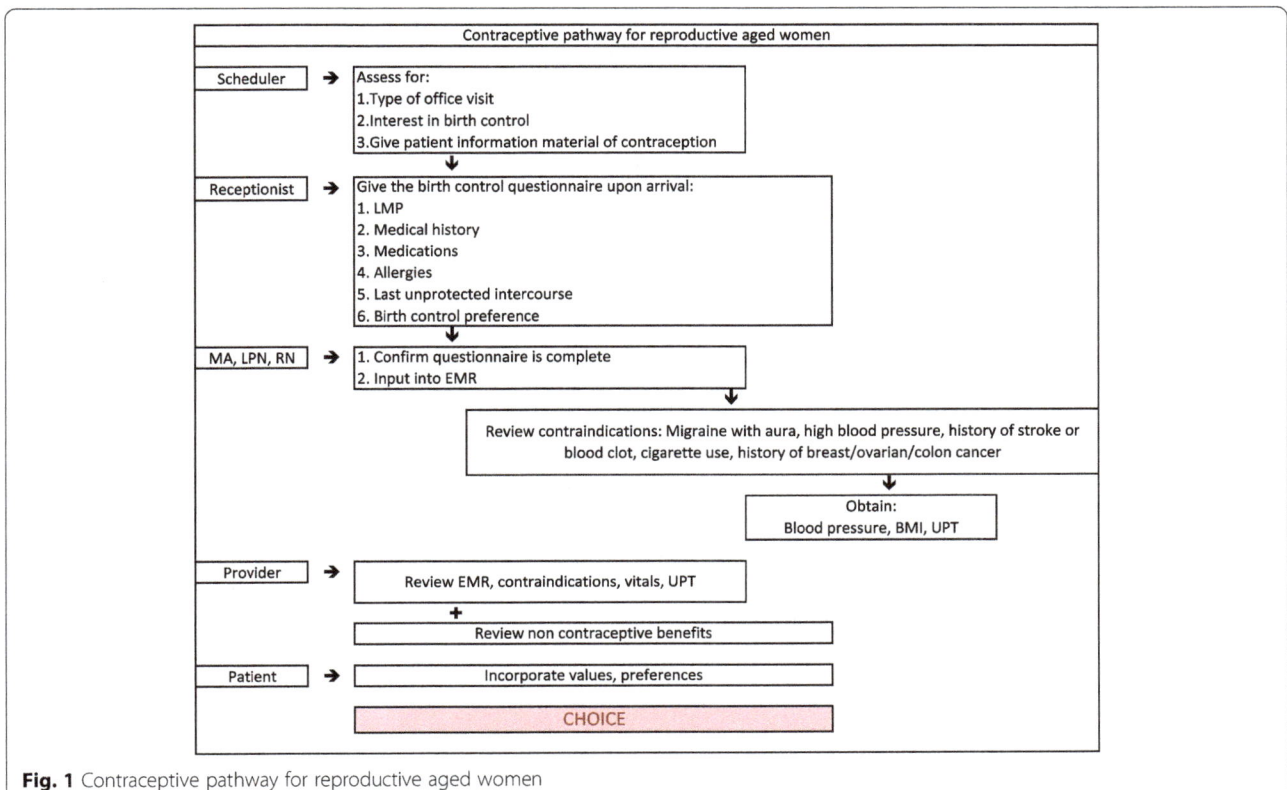

**Fig. 1** Contraceptive pathway for reproductive aged women

patient is eligible. The medical/nursing staff will confirm the questionnaire is complete, input the information into the electronic medical record, and obtain vital signs from the patient. They will also utilize a checklist, which assesses for contraindications, as outlined in Figs. 1 and 2. After these activities are completed, the health care provider will review the patient's electronic medical record and meet with the patient. The pathway ends with the counseling and contraceptive choice determined in conjunction by the patient and healthcare provider. Figure 2 illustrates the application of the contraceptive care pathway to a woman who is 42 years old and has a history of tobacco use. Clinicians using this care pathway can take into account varying needs and circumstances of each age group, referring to the U. S. Medical Eligibility Criteria for Contraceptive Use shown in Fig. 3.

For optimal care, phone or patient portal follow up is performed at three months and one year by a nurse to identify the following outcomes: contraceptive failures that lead to pregnancy, continued use of contraceptive method, patient satisfaction with the method, and adverse events that may have caused discontinuation of method. The outcomes will be recorded by the nurse

and compared to patients within the practice who are not using this contraceptive pathway to note the difference in outcomes. The clinical care team will meet for huddles throughout the follow up process to review the outcomes being revealed and discuss any challenges they have encountered using the contraceptive clinical pathway. These data will be used as an educational tool for quality improvement to determine if the utilization of this pathway improves unintended pregnancy rates, compliance with birth control method, and improves patient safety.

The contraceptive clinical pathway specifically benefits midlife women because it reminds the clinical care team of the importance of addressing contraceptive needs and reassessing for contraindications in women who may not believe they can become pregnant and have comorbidities. It also allows for better opportunity to discuss contraceptive change. For example, a 42 year old woman who is found to have a blood pressure of 170/100 during her well woman exam, may have been using combined oral contraceptive pills for several years and ask for a refill to continue. The contraceptive pathway ensures that her contraindications will be reviewed and allows for a dialogue between the patient and provider to reach the

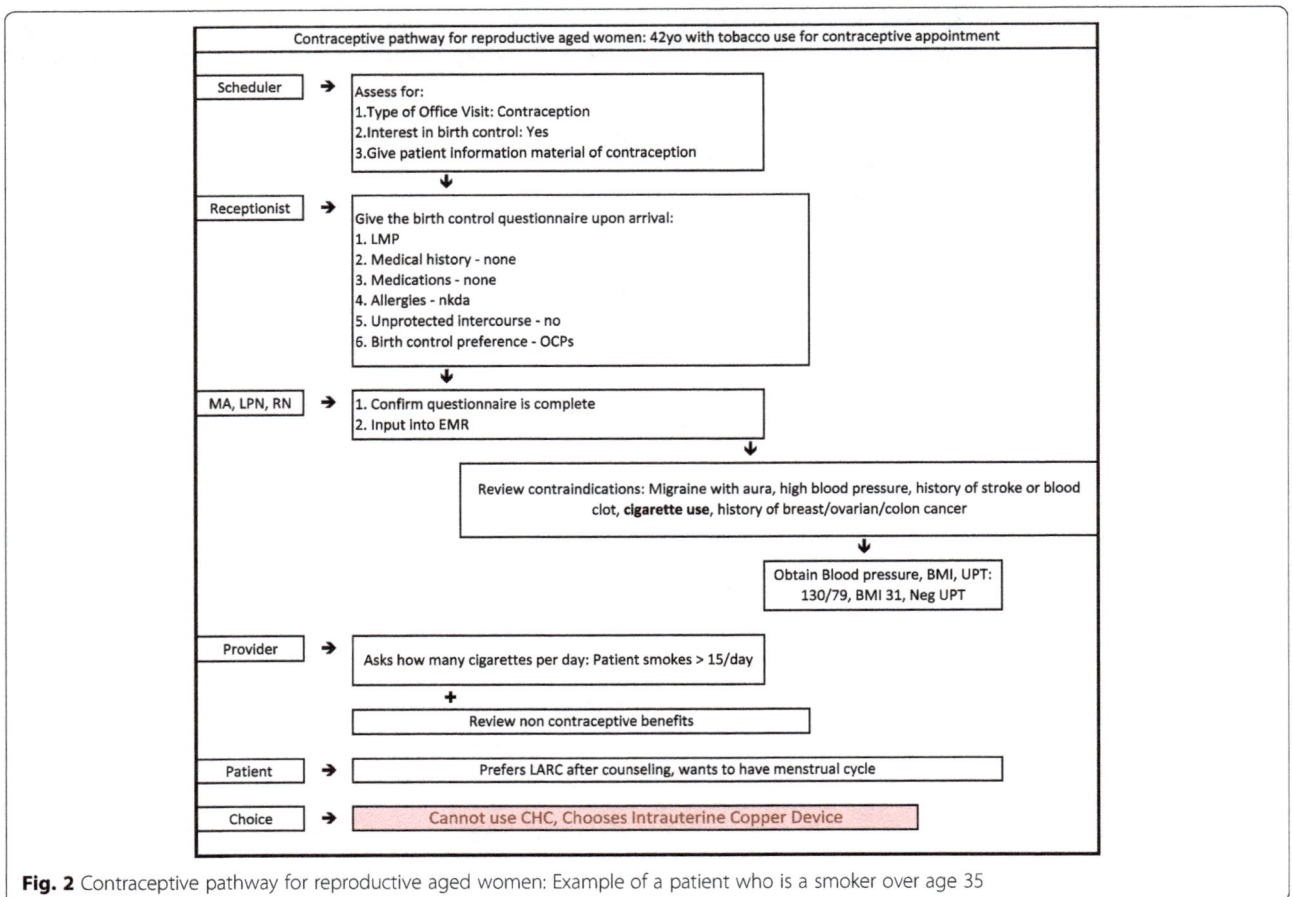

Fig. 2 Contraceptive pathway for reproductive aged women: Example of a patient who is a smoker over age 35

**Contraceptive Options from Adolescence to Perimenopause**

| Contraceptive method | Age <20 | Age 20-40 | Age 40-45 | Age >45 | Smoker < 35 y/o | Smoker > 35 y/o | | Risk factors for atherosclerotic cardiovascular disease* | Migraine | |
|---|---|---|---|---|---|---|---|---|---|---|
| Cu-IUD | Yes | Yes | Yes | Yes | Yes | Yes | | Yes | Yes | |
| LNG-IUD | Yes | Yes | Yes | Yes | Yes | Yes | | Yes | Yes | |
| Implant | Yes | Yes | Yes | Yes | Yes | Yes | | Yes | Yes | |
| Progesterone only pill | Yes | Yes | Yes | Yes | Yes | Yes | | Yes | Yes | |
| DMPA | Yes | Yes | Yes | Yes | Yes | Yes | | caution | Yes | |
| CHC | Yes | Yes | Yes | Yes | Yes | < 15 cigarettes caution | >15 cigarettes No | caution, multiple risk factors No | Without aura, Yes | With aura, No |

**Key**

| Category 1 | Category 2 | Category 3 | Category 4 |
|---|---|---|---|

Category 1 refers to no restrictions to use the contraceptive method, Category 2 refers to advantages generally outweigh the risks to use the method, Category 3 refers to risks usually outweigh the advantages to use the method, and Category 4 refers to conditions represent an unacceptable health risk if the method is used.
Cu-IUD: Intrauterine copper device
LNG-IUD: Levonorgestrel intrauterine device
DMPA: Depo-Provera
CHC: Combined hormonal contraceptives
*Risk factors for atherosclerotic cardiovascular disease include older age, hypertension, smoking, diabetes, low HDL, and high LDL or triglycerides.

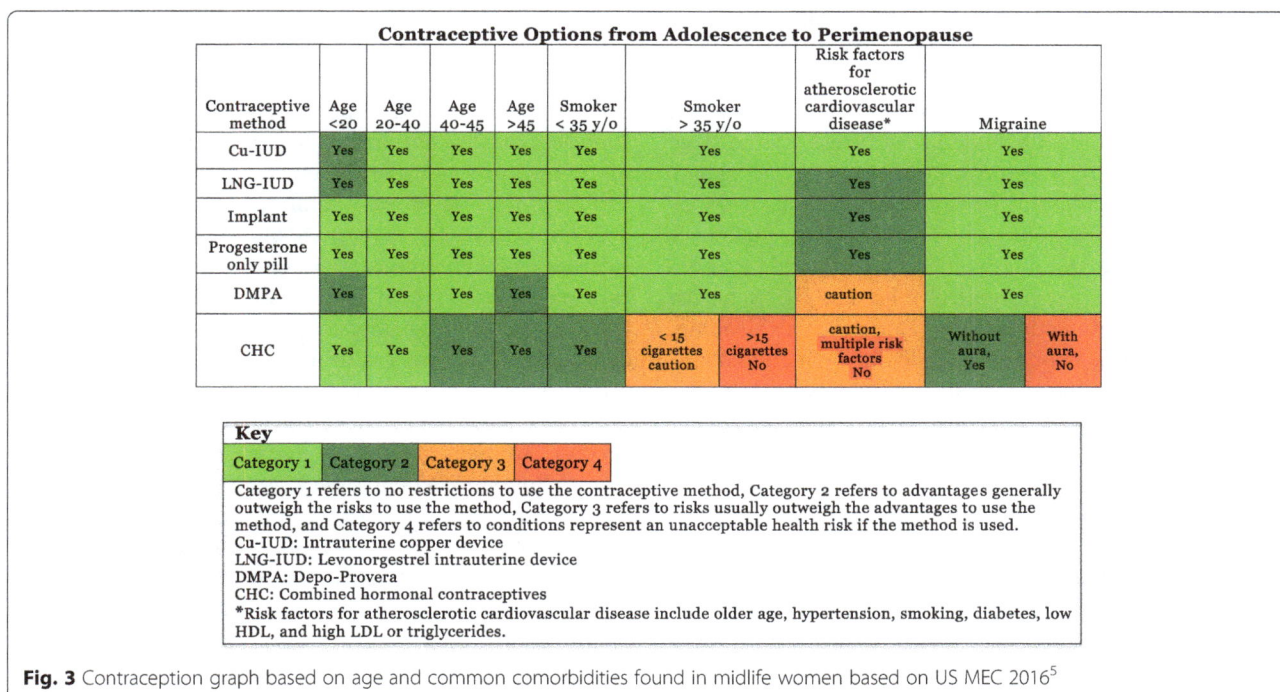

**Fig. 3** Contraception graph based on age and common comorbidities found in midlife women based on US MEC 2016[5]

safest most acceptable method for the patient. Specific points geared to midlife women that practitioners should focus on include [7]:

1. future pregnancy desires, including whether they will pursue ART
2. risk for sexually transmitted infections if she has recently terminated a committed relationship
3. medical conditions including cardiovascular disease, stroke, VTE, liver disease, gall bladder symptoms
4. gynecologic conditions such as fibroid uterus, heavy menstrual bleeding, endometriosis
5. lifestyle factors such as smoking, obesity, and frequent air travel

## Discussion

The challenge in contraceptive management for midlife women differs from that for other reproductive aged women. Pregnancy rates have increased for women aged 30 and older since the late 1990s, especially for those aged 40 and over. This trend is mainly due to delayed first and second births, but there are also unplanned and unintended pregnancies [1]. The data suggest that the unintended pregnancy rate for women 35 and older is 16%, accompanied by the incidence of abortion increasing from 1998 to 2008 [1, 8]. Regarding contraception, U.S. women in this age group have a higher prevalence of sterilization when compared to Canada and the United Kingdom (UK) [8]. The need for an effective form of contraception may be overlooked in midlife

women since fecundity is diminished in this age group [7]. In addition, with increase in irregular cycles, ovulation is less predictable, making techniques such as the rhythm method difficult to use effectively. Potential clinical and social consequences of an unintended pregnancy for midlife women are usually more detrimental to their health and their fetus' health as well, when compared to younger reproductive-aged women. Risks associated with pregnancy in women over 40 include miscarriage, aneuploidy, maternal morbidity and mortality, and neonatal complications including preterm delivery [9].

Although age alone is not a contraindication for any specific contraceptive method, it should again be emphasized that midlife women often have comorbidities that must be considered when deciding on a form of contraception. The USMEC categorizes eligibility for use of different contraception into four categories: Category 1-no restriction (method can be used); Category 2-advantages generally outweigh theoretical or proven risks; Category 3-theoretical or proven risks usually outweigh the advantages; and Category 4- unacceptable health risk (method not to be used) [6]. The common comorbidities that midlife women should be routinely screened for include: hypertension, obesity, uncontrolled diabetes, ischemic heart disease, and multiple risk factors for cardiovascular disease (smoking, obesity, diabetes, hyperlipidemia, and hypertension) [6]. For this age group, despite these increased risk factors, the benefit of using most contraceptives outweigh the risk of unintended pregnancy.

Starting with the most effective birth control method, long acting reversible contraceptives (LARCs) include the copper IUD, the levonorgestrel-releasing IUD, and the subdermal etonogestrel implant. There are different non-contraceptive health benefits for these methods as well. The copper IUD also can be used as an emergency contraceptive, in addition to reducing the risk of endometrial cancer. This method is hormone free, making it an ideal option for midlife women with multiple comorbidities [10]. The levonorgestrel-releasing IUD's health benefit includes reduction in heavy menstrual bleeding, including bleeding associated with leiomyoma and adenomyosis, hence improving quality of life [9, 11] In the UK, the levonorgestrel-releasing IUD also is approved for endometrial hyperplasia protection during estrogen therapy [9]. The subdermal implant causes variable bleeding pattern, but it has been shown to reduce dysmenorrhea [9].

The combined hormonal contraceptives (CHC) are available as daily pills, a monthly vaginal ring, and weekly transdermal patch. Indications and contraindications are similar for all combined hormonal methods for all age groups [12]. Current guidelines suggest use of combined hormonal contraceptives in midlife women without contraindications [6]. CHCs not only provide contraceptive benefits but also offer cycle regularity, treatment of vasomotor symptoms, protection against bone loss, and reduced risk of ovarian and endometrial cancer [11, 13].

Barrier methods including the male and female condom, are forms of contraception that can be used by most people regardless of age or comorbidities. Furthermore, they are the only methods that also provide protection against sexually transmitted infections. Research has noted that sexually transmitted infections are still a prevalent issue among midlife women and are often underestimated among this population [7].

## Conclusions

On average, U.S. women have two children. This means that a woman will spend about three years of her life trying to conceive, being pregnant or postpartum. The rest of a woman's life is then spent on avoiding unintended pregnancy [1]. Of women aged 15–44 who have ever had sexual intercourse, 99% of them have used at least one contraceptive method [10]. Appropriate contraceptive counseling, leading to the use of most effective method of contraception and adherence is crucial, and should always include the midlife woman. Despite misconceptions that certain contraceptive methods cannot be used in certain age groups, we highlight that age alone is not a contraindication to most birth control methods [6].

Additionally, midlife can be seen as a difficult time for contraceptive management among providers as patients may have comorbidities or patients may not view contraception as an important need with their declining fecundity. However, unintended pregnancy among older women has far worse implications for a woman's health than utilizing a contraceptive method in most circumstances. It also is important to note most contraceptive methods have non-contraceptive health benefits that could be of value to the midlife patient.

Contraceptive counseling should include specific considerations for midlife women. Our clinical contraceptive care pathway is a tool to be used in conjunction with USMEC to guide healthcare providers. The goal of the contraceptive pathway is to incorporate a total office approach using a clinical care team that is patient- driven. Individual preferences and medical history are taken into account to help navigate evidence-based medicine in helping midlife women, as well as all other reproductive-aged women, choose the most effective and appropriate form of contraception. This pathway strives to let clinicians integrate the USMEC in contraceptive care.

**Acknowledgements**
Not applicable.

**Funding**
Not applicable.

**Authors' contributions**
CSK was the major contributor in writing the manuscript. DT contributed to the initial draft of this manuscript, editing and did the background research. LM performed background research. AB performed final editions. All authors read and approved the final manuscript.

**Competing interests**
Not applicable.

**References**
1.  Finer LB, Zolna MR. Declines in unintended pregnancy in the United States, 2008-2011. N Engl J Med. 2016;374:843–52.
2.  Buchert AR, Butler GA. Clinical pathways: driving high-reliability and high-value care. Pediatr Clin N Am. 2016;63(2):317–28.
3.  Seehusen DA. Clinical pathways: effects on practice, outcomes, and costs. Am Fam Physicians. 2010;82(11):338–9.
4.  Breaking the contraceptive barrier: techniques for effective contraceptive consultations. Association of reproductive health professionals. 2008. http://www.arhp.org/Publications-and-Resources/Clinical-Proceedings/Breaking-the-Contraceptive-Barrier.
5.  U.S Department of Veterans Affairs. What is PACT? VA Healthcare-VISN 4. 2015. https://www.visn4.va.gov/VISN4/CEPACT/what_is_pact.asp.
6.  Center for Disease Control and Prevention. United states medical eligibility criteria (US MEC) for contraceptive use, 2016. https://www.cdc.gov/reproductivehealth/contraception/usmec.htm.
7.  Shifren JL, Gas MLS. The North American Menopause Society Recommendations for Clinical Care of Midlife Women. 2014;21(10):1038–62.
8.  The ESHRE Capri Workshop Group. Female contraception over 40. Hum Reprod Update. 2009;15(6):599–612.
9.  Allen RH, Cwiak CA, Kaunitz AM. Contraception in women over 40 years of age. CMAJ. 2013;185(7):565–73.
10. Daniels K, Mosher WD, Jones J. Contraceptive methods women have ever used: United States, 1982-2010. National health statistics report. 2013 No 62.
11. Hardman SM, Gebbie AE. The contraception needs of the perimenopausal woman. Best prac res clin obstet gynaecol. 2014;28(6):903–15.
12. Curtis KM, Jatlaoui TC, Tepper NK, Zapata LB, Horton LG, Jamieson DJ, Whiteman MK. US Selected Practice Recommendations for Contraceptive Use. 2016. https://www.cdc.gov/mmwr/volumes/65/rr/pdfs/rr6504.pdf.

# 9

# Depressed mood during the menopausal transition: is it reproductive aging or is it life?

Ellen Sullivan Mitchell[1] and Nancy Fugate Woods[2*]

## Abstract

**Background:** Although there has been noteworthy attention to both depressed mood symptoms and majordepressive disorder during the menopausal transition (MT), recently investigators have questioned whether there is an over-pathologizing of the MT by emphasizing hormonal effects on depression and deflecting attention from the everyday conditions of women's lives as they relate to depressed mood. In addition, fluctuation of mood over short periods of time may not be captured by measures of depressed mood symptoms such as the CESD, especially when administered using a reference period such as a week or more. The purpose of this study was to examine the association of menopausal transition factors, health-related factors, stress factors, social factors and symptoms with repeated measures of depressed mood reported for a 24 h period.

**Methods:** Seattle Midlife Women's Health Study participants ($n = 291$, 6977 observations) provided data from 1990 to 2013 including annual questionnaires, symptom diaries and urine specimens assayed for hormones several times per year. Multilevel modeling was used to test bivariate and multivariable models accounting for depressed mood severity.

**Results:** In individual models with age as the measure of time, being in early postmenopause, exercising more, and being partnered were associated with less severe depressed mood; greater perceived stress, having a history of sexual abuse, difficulty getting to sleep, early awakening, and awakening at night were each associated with higher depressed mood severity. In a multivariable model ($n = 234$, 6766 observations), being older, being in the early postmenopause, exercising more, being partnered, were associated with less severe depressed mood; reporting greater perceived stress, history of sexual abuse, difficulty getting to sleep and early awakening were associated with more severe depressed mood.

**Conclusions:** Clinicians need to consider the context in which midlife women experience the menopausal transition and mood symptoms as well as hormonal transitions during this part of the lifespan.

**Keywords:** Depressed mood, Menopausal transition stages, Early postmenopause, Urinary estrone, Health-related factors, Stress factors, Social factors, Abuse history, Sleep disruption symptoms

## Background

Gender differences in reports of depressed mood, as well as episodes of major depressive disorder, have prompted investigators to examine periods of biological variability in women's lives, such as phases of the menstrual cycle, pregnancy and postpartum, and the menopausal transition (MT), as windows of vulnerability [1, 2]. Progress in understanding stages of reproductive aging has provided a framework for understanding biological variability during the menopausal transition and early postmenopause as related to depression and depressed mood [3–7].

Longitudinal studies of community-based cohorts experiencing transitions of reproductive aging, including the Melbourne Midlife Women's Health Project (MMWHP) [8], the Study of Women's Health Across the Nation SWAN) [9], the Penn Ovarian Aging Study (POAS) [10], and the Seattle Midlife Women's Health Study (SMWHS) [11] included data on a variety of measures of depressed

* Correspondence: nfwoods@uw.edu
[2]Biobehavioral Nursing and Health Informatics, University of Washington, Seattle, USA
Full list of author information is available at the end of the article

mood symptoms from multi-ethnic community-based cohorts of women studied annually (some more frequently) for 20 years or longer. These studies have revealed a pattern of increasing depressed mood symptoms during the menopausal transition. Massachusetts Women's Health Study investigators had documented an increase in depressive symptoms, measured by the Center for Epidemiologic Studies Depression Scale (CES-D), especially among women who experienced a lengthy MT [12]. SWAN investigators found that dysphoric mood symptoms, measured by 4 mood symptoms, increased during early MT [13]. The Harvard Study of Moods and Cycles investigators found an elevated odds ratio (2.5) of experiencing depressive symptoms (CES-D) during the MT vs premenopause (late reproductive stage) [14] and POAS investigators reported elevated odds ratios of 1.5 to 5.4, depending on women's past history of depression [15, 16]. In addition, evidence supports a decrease in negative mood as women transition to early postmenopause. MMWHP investigators found an improvement in negative mood, measured by 10 negative adjectives, during the late MT stage and a decrease in negative mood as women progressed to PM [17]. POAS investigators found that reaching the final menstrual period (FMP) played a pivotal role in reduced prevalence of depressive symptoms (CES-D) [18].

Patterns of increasing incidence of major depressive disorder mirror those of depressed mood symptoms. SWAN investigators studying major depressive disorder found an increase in prevalence of new depression during the MT and early PM [19, 20].

Given the relationship seen between reproductive aging stages and depressed mood, it is tempting to attribute this association to hormonal changes. Investigations of the relationship of estrogen, testosterone, DHEAS, inhibin B, LH and FSH levels and variability to depressed mood have yielded a lack of definitive conclusions, likely attributable to variability in the endocrine measures, their timing and frequency, variability in the depressed mood measure and various analytic strategies used to assess hormone effects [21]. Nonetheless, there is some evidence implicating some hormones: POAS investigators found evidence for effects of increased levels of estradiol, FSH, decreased levels of inhibin B and LH, and greater estradiol, LH, and FSH variability on depressive symptoms (CES-D) [16, 17]. SWAN investigators found effects of both testosterone levels and their increase during the MT on depressive symptoms, but no associations between FSH or estradiol levels and their changing levels with depressive symptoms or with major depressive disorder [22, 23]. MMWHP investigators found declining estradiol levels were associated with depressive symptoms in a sample of women studied primarily during the PM [24].

The SMWHS team analyzed factors influencing depressive symptoms measured annually with the CES-D, finding no significant relationships with urinary estrone,

FSH, testosterone, or cortisol [25, 26]. Instead, depressive symptoms were a function of age (being younger) and being in late MT stage when the severity of depressive symptoms increased. Hot flashes, life stress, family history of depression, history of postpartum blues, sexual abuse history, BMI, and use of antidepressants were also related to depressive symptoms. Age at entry into and duration of late MT stage were unrelated to depressive symptoms. These findings suggest that factors accounting for depressive symptoms earlier in the life span, as well as contemporary stressors, influenced depressive mood symptoms during the MT.

Although there has been noteworthy attention to both depressed mood symptoms and major depressive disorder during the MT, recently investigators have questioned whether there is an over-pathologizing of the MT by emphasizing hormonal effects on depression and deflecting attention from the everyday conditions of women's lives as they relate to depressed mood [27]. In addition, fluctuation of mood over short periods of time may not be captured by measures of depressed mood symptoms such as the CESD, especially when administered using a reference period such as a week or more. Indeed, investigators have recently used ecological momentary assessment, a data capture technique involving repeated sampling made close in time to the experience in naturalistic environments [28]. Moore and colleagues found that among adults 65 years of age and older, sensitivity to change of the same symptoms of depressed mood, anxiety, and mindfulness varied across two different assessment methods: ecological momentary assessment (EMA) and traditional paper and pencil measures. Indeed, results indicated greater sensitivity of the ecological momentary assessment measures of depression, anxiety, and mindfulness in response to a mindfulness-based stress response intervention than a control intervention when the same symptoms were reported using the same items administered by EMA and by paper and pencil measures with a one week reference period.

The SMWHS team had obtained a single symptom measure of depressed mood, defined as an emotional state experienced over the past 24 h (reference period was today), on multiple occasions throughout multiple years of the study. Overnight urine samples were provided on the same day as the depressed mood rating and assayed for a variety of endocrine measures (e.g. urinary estrone-3-glucuronide (E1G)) [25]. The purpose of the analyses reported here was to test a longitudinal model of the effects of MT factors (menopausal transition stages, estrone, FSH), health-related factors (alcohol use, BMI, amount of exercise), stress factors (perceived stress, history of sexual abuse), social factors (partner status, number of live births), and symptoms (hot flashes and sleep symptoms) on depressed mood severity reported for a 24 h period. (See Fig. 1). We hypothesized that depressed mood would be positively related to perceived stress, history of sexual abuse, hot flashes, sleep symptoms, BMI, alcohol use, and FSH levels, and negatively related to age, being in the early postmenopausal stage, estrone levels, amount of exercise, being partnered, and number of live births.

## Methods

### Design

The data for these analyses are from a longitudinal study of the MT, the Seattle Midlife Women's Health Study (SMWHS), described in greater detail elsewhere [29]. Women entered the cohort between 1990 and early 1992 when most were not yet in the MT or were in the early stages of the transition to menopause. Eligibility for the parent study included ages 35–55, at least one ovary, a period within the previous 12 months, not pregnant or lactating and able to speak and read English. Screening all households within selected multiethnic neighborhoods in Seattle (11,222 households) yielded 820 women eligible for the study and 508 were able to participate in an interview during the recruitment window. After completing an initial in-person interview ($n = 508$) administered by a trained Registered Nurse interviewer, participants ($n = 390$) began providing data annually by questionnaire, menstrual calendar, and health diary. The health diary included a symptom checklist that included depressed mood and other symptoms, as well as indicators of health behaviors and stress. Diary data were obtained on days 5, 6 and 7 of the menstrual cycle and a first morning voided urine specimens was collected on day 6. The women provided urine specimens 8 to 12 times per year for endocrine assays (from late 1996 through 2000), and then quarterly for 2001–2005. These data were in addition to an annual health questionnaire and menstrual calendars.

### Sample

Eligible participants for this study ($N = 291$) were those who contributed ratings of depressed mood severity from the health diaries beginning in 1990 and were in either the late reproductive, early or late MT stages, or within 5 years from FMP at data collection during the course of the study. Women not eligible for this study either did not keep a daily diary or were not able to be classified into one of the eligible stages due to hormone use, inadequate calendar data, hysterectomy, chemotherapy or radiation therapy.

Women eligible for inclusion had a mean age of 41.5 (SD = 4.3) years at the beginning of the study, 15.9 years of education (SD = 2.8), and a median family income of $38,200 (SD = $15,000). Most (87%) were currently employed, 71% married or partnered, 22% divorced or separated or widowed, and 7% never married or partnered. They described their racial/ethnic identity as African American (7%), Asian American (9%), and White (82%). Women included in these analyses were similar with respect to employment status, marital status, and age to those who were ineligible. The only significant differences between those who were included and those who were not were higher incomes, greater likelihood to be White, and more years of education than those in the study. (See Table 1). Data obtained on any occasion when the woman was using hormones were excluded.

### Measures

Measures used in these analyses include: age; MT-related factors (MT stages, urinary estrone and urinary FSH); health-related factors (BMI, alcohol use and amount of exercise); stress factors (perceived stress and history of sexual abuse), social factors (number of live births and partner status), symptoms (hot flash severity and sleep symptoms) and depressed mood severity.

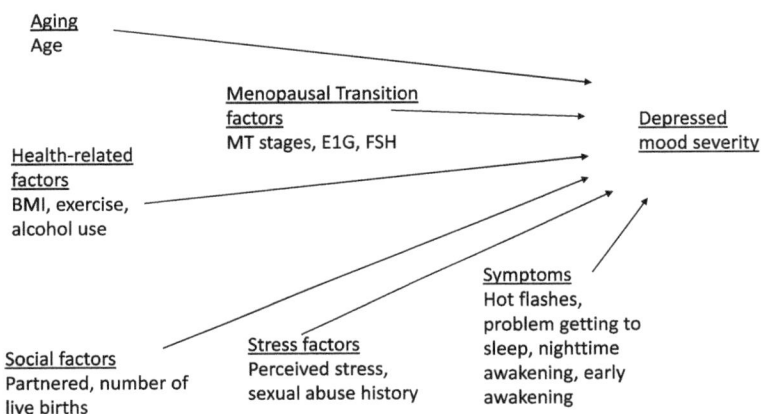

**Fig. 1** Factors influencing depressed mood severity during the menopausal transition and early postmenopause

**Table 1** Sample characteristics at start of study (1990–1991) of the eligible and ineligible women in the mixed effects modeling analyses of depressed mood severity

| Characteristic | Eligible Women (n = 291) Mean (SD) | Ineligible Women (n = 217) Mean (SD) | p value* |
|---|---|---|---|
| Age (years) | 41.5 (4.3) | 42.0 (5.0) | 0.18 |
| Years of education | 15.9 (2.8) | 15.3 (3.0) | 0.03 |
| Family income ($) | 38,200 (15,000) | 35,200 (17,600) | 0.04 |
| BMI wt kg/ht. m² | 25.3 (5.4) | 27.1 (7.2) | 0.002 |
| Exercise (min/week) | 187.8 (286.9) | 179.0 (368.5) | 0.76 |
| Characteristic | N (Percent) | N (Percent) | p value** |
| Currently employed | | | 0.42 |
| Yes | 254 (87.3) | 184 (84.8) | |
| No | 37 (12.7) | 33 (15.2) | |
| Race/ethnicity | | | 0.001 |
| African American | 20 (6.9) | 38 (17.5) | |
| Asian /Pacific Islander | 27 (9.3) | 16 (7.4) | |
| White | 238 (81.8) | 153 (70.5) | |
| Other (Hispanic, Mixed) | 6 (2.1) | 10 (4.6) | |
| Marital Status | | | 0.20 |
| Married/partnered | 278 (71.1) | 141 (65.0) | |
| Divorced/widowed/not partnered | 63 (21.7) | 62 (28.6) | |
| Never married/ partnered | 21 (7.2) | 14 (6.5) | |
| Alcohol Use | | | 0.001 |
| Yes | 264 | 174 | |
| No | 26 | 42 | |

*Independent t-test
**Chi-square test

### Depressed mood severity

Depressed mood severity was assessed in the health diary using one item that asked women to rate the severity of their feeling "depressed/sad or blue" on a scale where 1 indicated not present, 2 mild, 3 moderate and 4 extreme. The reference period was for "today". This single item has been validated in the PROMIS measures [30–32].

### Menopausal transition-related factors

Menopausal transition-related factors included MT stages as well as urinary estrone glucuronide and FSH. Using menstrual calendar data, women not taking any type of estrogen or progestin were classified according to stages of reproductive aging: late reproductive, early MT, late MT, or early PM, based on staging criteria developed by Mitchell, Woods and Mariella [11] and validated by the Re-STAGE collaboration [3–5]. The names of stages match those recommended at the Stages of Reproductive Aging Workshop (STRAW) [6]. The time before the onset of persistent menstrual irregularity during midlife was labeled the late reproductive stage when cycles were regular. Early stage was defined as persistent irregularity of 7 or more days absolute difference between any two consecutive menstrual cycles during the calendar year, with no skipped periods. Late stage was defined as persistent skipping of one or more menstrual periods. A skipped period was defined as 60 or more consecutive days of amenorrhea during the calendar year [3–5]. Persistence means the event, an irregular cycle or skipped period, reoccurred one or more times in the subsequent 12 months. Onset of early MT stage was the date of Day 1 for the bleeding segment when the irregularity criterion was first met. Onset of late stage was the date of Day 1 of the first bleeding segment with skipping. Final menstrual period was identified retrospectively after one year of amenorrhea without any known explanation. The first day of the FMP is synonymous with the term menopause and was used to determine age of onset of FMP. Early PM refers to the years within five years of the FMP.

### Urinary assays

Urinary assays were performed in our laboratories using a first-voided morning urine specimen provided on day 6 of the menstrual cycle, if menstrual periods were identifiable. For women with no bleeding or spotting or extremely erratic flow, a consistent date each month was used. Women abstained from smoking, caffeine use, and exercise before the urine collection. All assays were adjusted for urinary creatinine which was assayed in urine specimens using the method of Jaffe [33]. More assay details are reported elsewhere [34].

### Urinary estrone glucuronide ($E_1G$)

Urinary estrone glucuronide ($E_1G$) was selected to assess estrogens because it is stable, can be reliably measured without special preparation, and is highly correlated with serum estradiol levels [35–40]. Urinary $E_1G$ was measured by a competitive enzyme immunoassay (EIA) that cross-reacts 83% with estradiol glucuronide and less than 10% with free estrone, estrone sulfate, estriol glucuronide, estradiol and estriol [35]. The assay is described in detail elsewhere [41].

### Urinary FSH

Urinary FSH was assayed using Diagnostic Products Corporation (DPC) Double Antibody FSH Kit, using a radioimmunoassay (RIA) was designed for the quantitative measurement of FSH in serum and urine [42]. The procedure is described in detail elsewhere [41].

### Health-related factors

Health-related factors included women's use of alcohol, amount of exercise and BMI. Women were asked to indicate in the daily health diary whether or not they drank alcohol on that day (coded as 0 for no and 1 for yes). They estimated their exercise in response to the question: how many total minutes of non-work related exercise did you do today? (walking, running, biking, swimming, aerobics, sports, work out, gardening, yard work). In addition, height and weight were reported annually from which the BMI was calculated (wtkg/htm$^2$).

### Stress factors

Stress factors included perceived stress and history of sexual abuse. Perceived stress was assessed in the diary with a question "how stressful was your day?" that women rated from 1 (not at all) to 6 (extremely, a lot). Brantley, Waggoner, Jones, & Rappaport found that a global stress rating and the sum of stress ratings across multiple dimensions correlated significantly ($r = .35$, $p < .01$) [43] Sexual abuse history was assessed by asking "Have you ever been sexually assaulted, abused, or molested?" These data were obtained in 1999–2002. Also, beginning in 1996 and through the end of the study, women were asked "during the past year did you experience any sexual abuse or sexual assault?" A cumulative variable was created to represent any history of sexual abuse or assault and coded as 1 for yes and 0 for no at each data point.

### Social factors

Number of live births and partner status were assessed yearly from two items in the annual health questionnaire as were income and employment status. Race/ethnicity was established by self-report at beginning of the study.

### Symptoms

Hot flashes severity and sleep symptoms were assessed in the diary with single items that women rated from 0, not present to 4, extreme. Sleep symptoms included difficulty getting to sleep, awakening during the night, and early morning awakening.

### Analyses

To determine which covariates in the conceptual model (Fig. 1) had a significant effect when examined individually, bivariable mixed effects modeling was used. Finally, to test the multivariable model to determine which predictors had a significant effect on depressed mood severity over time, those individual variables from the bivariate analyses with a significance of $p \leq 0.1$ were entered together in a multivariable mixed effects model [42–47].

Before testing the conceptual model, an initial series of statistical models tested age alone as a predictor of depressed mood severity to learn whether a random intercept, fixed slope model or a random intercept, random slope model was the best fit. It was first postulated that overall levels of depressed mood severity would differ from woman to woman (random intercept), but the scores would change with age in a common manner (fixed slope). The second statistical model extended the first to postulate that each woman had a different mean level of depressed mood severity and rate of change (random intercept, random slope). The best fitting model (fixed slope or random slope) was determined by using the maximum likelihood estimation with Akaike Information Criterion (AIC) [48].

Using the best fitting model, individual covariates were added iteratively to test the effect on depressed mood severity over time. Because these analyses were for exploration and to stimulate further mechanistic studies, a $p$ value of $\leq 0.10$ was used as the criterion of significance for the univariate model and $\leq 0.05$ for the final model. Different numbers of women and observations occurred with each covariate tested because the analysis required pairing observations of the outcome and predictor variables at each time point. In all analyses, age was centered at the group mean to enable the interpretation of the effect of age on depressed mood severity.

### Results

Participants whose data were included in these analyses reported moderate levels of symptoms, with awakening during the night and problems getting to sleep, depressed mood, early awakening, and hot flashes in decreasing order of average severity. There were large standard deviations. Also 34% of these participants reported a history of sexual abuse. (See Table 2).

With age as a measure of time, a random intercept, random slope model was used to test separately each covariate in the model for effect on depressed mood. Being in the early PM was significantly and negatively associated with depressed mood as was reporting a higher amount of exercise. In addition, perception of stress, history of sexual abuse, and each of the three sleep symptoms were associated with an increase in depressed mood. Being partnered was negatively associated with depressed mood. Age, estrone and FSH levels, BMI, alcohol intake, number of live births, and hot flash severity were not associated significantly with depressed mood. (See Table 3).

When the significant factors ($p \leq 0.1$) from the univariate analysis listed above were included in a multivariate model, perceived stress, history of sexual abuse, problem getting to sleep, and early awakening significantly predicted an increase in depressed mood while increased age, being in the early postmenopause, greater amount of exercise and being partnered were associated with a decrease in depressed mood. (See Table 4).

## Discussion

In a multivariable model, depressed mood severity reported for a 24 h period was not associated with age, MT markers (reproductive aging stages, levels of estrone or FSH), or symptoms of hot flashes or awakening at night. Instead, factors reflecting the context of women's lives, including perceived stress, history of sexual abuse, being partnered, amount of exercise, and sleep symptoms (early awakening, problem getting to sleep), were associated with severity of depressed mood.

In the analyses presented here, depressed mood severity reported for a 24 h period was not related to any of the MT markers. Although prior research has provided limited evidence linking endocrine changes and the MT stages to depressive symptoms and also to episodes of major depressive disorder among women with no prior history of depression, Freeman's recent review concluded that the contribution of the changing endocrine milieu to the development of depressive symptoms was small [21]. She reminded us that only a minority of women experience debilitating depressive symptoms during this part of the lifespan and that hormonal change is not the only factor to consider in disentangling the complex pathways to depression.

There was not a significant relationship between hot flashes and depressed mood over the past 24 h in the diary-based data reported here. In contrast, Freeman's review [21] indicated that although the association between hot flashes and depressive symptoms predominantly measured with the CES-D was confirmed, the direction of the relationship was unclear and evidence for a relationship between hot flashes and major

depressive disorder was much less clear. Although hot flashes predicted negative mood on the next day in SWAN daily diary data, negative mood did not predict hot flashes on the subsequent day [49]. On the other hand, studies evaluating the risk of women with high levels of depressive symptoms (CES-D) indicated that depressive symptoms were likely to precede hot flashes among women who had not experienced either type of symptoms earlier in life [50, 51]. Women with consistently high levels of depressive symptoms in the SMWHS (CES-D) were more likely to experience hot flashes than those without more severe depressive symptoms [50]. Among POAS participants, 24% without high depressive symptoms (CES-D) or hot flashes at baseline reported depressive symptoms before reporting hot flashes over a 10 year follow up period, but only 8% reported hot flashes before reporting depressive symptoms [51].

Sleep symptoms and depressed mood co-occur frequently among midlife women. Indeed, use of poor sleep as one indicator of clinical depression makes it difficult to determine whether there is a causal relationship between the two symptoms. Awakening during the night was the only sleep symptom significantly related to MT stages in the SMWHS [52], but in the analyses reported here, both trouble getting to sleep and early awakening were associated with depressed mood over the past 24 h, while awakening during the night was not. Self-reported difficulty sleeping was associated with next-day negative mood in SWAN participants [49]. Burleson and colleagues tracked midlife women over 36 weeks during which they experienced the highest weekly frequency of vasomotor symptoms. They found that sleep problems occurring on one day predicted next-day negative mood (mean of 8 negative adjectives) more robustly than did vasomotor symptoms [53].

In a review of studies of sleep and the MT, Shaver [54] concluded that although the MT is associated with poor sleep beyond that anticipated with aging, perceptions of sleep are likely to be influenced by an emotional overlay on symptom reporting. Depressed mood and poor sleep are likely to be related in bidirectional ways [55]. Thus attention to mood as a factor contributing to sleep problems as well as sleep problems contributing to mood experiences is warranted. Induced poor sleep has been associated with more negative mood, but effects of improved sleep on mood during the MT remain to be examined. Induced poor sleep has been associated with more negative mood, but effects of improved sleep on mood during the MT remain to be examined. To date, a single clinical trial of cognitive behavioral therapy for insomnia delivered by telephone to women who were experiencing the menopausal transition or early postmenopause revealed that the treatment effect, when compared to a menopause education control, had the

**Table 2** Sample characteristics at start of study (1990–1991) of the eligible women in the mixed effects modeling analyses of depressed mood severity

| Characteristic | Eligible Women Mean (SD) |
| --- | --- |
| Depressed mood severity (0–4) | 0.41 (0.63) |
| Hot flashes (0–4) | 0.11 (0.41) |
| Problem getting to sleep (0–4) | 0.32 (0.67) |
| Awakening during the night (0–4) | 0.57 (0.87) |
| Early morning awakening (0–4) | 0.34 (0.66) |
| Perceived stress (1–6) | 2.77 (1.09) |
| Characteristic | N (Percent) |
| History of sexual abuse (N = 233) | |
| Yes | 80 (34%) |
| No | 153 (66%) |

**Table 3** Random effects models for depressed mood severity with age as predictor ($\beta_2$) and with individual covariates ($\beta_3$)

| Predictor | Mean Values (p values) | | | Standard Deviations | | | Number | |
|---|---|---|---|---|---|---|---|---|
| | $\beta_1^a$ | $\beta_2^a$ | $\beta_3^a$ | $\sigma_1^b$ | $\sigma_2^b$ | $\sigma_\varepsilon^b$ | Women | Observations |
| Age (47.7) | 0.51 | <0.001 (0.84) | – | 0.49 | 0.03 | 0.60 | 291 | 6977 |
| Menopausal Transition Factors | | | | | | | | |
| MT-stage | 0.52 (<.001) | 0.005 (0.25) | | 0.49 | 0.03 | 0.60 | 291 | 6977 |
| Early | | | 0.02 (0.56) | | | | | |
| Late | | | −0.006 (0.88) | | | | | |
| Early PM | | | −0.10 (0.05) | | | | | |
| Estrone (1.3) | 0.62 (<.001) | −0.01 (0.04) | −0.03 (0.32) | 0.50 | 0.04 | 0.60 | 131 | 4908 |
| FSH (1.1) | 0.58 (<.001) | −0.01 (0.04) | −0.02 (0.23) | 0.50 | 0.04 | .060 | 131 | 4996 |
| Health-related factors | | | | | | | | |
| BMI (26.0) | 0.37 (<.001) | <0.001 (0.97) | 0.005 (0.20) | 0.49 | 0.03 | 0.60 | 291 | 6977 |
| If drinks alcohol | 0.51 (<.001) | <0.001 (0.84) | −0.001 (0.97) | 0.49 | 0.03 | 0.60 | 291 | 6977 |
| Amount of exercise | 0.54 (<.001) | 0.001 (0.69) | −0.001 (<.001) | 0.49 | 0.03 | 0.60 | 291 | 6977 |
| Social factors | | | | | | | | |
| If partnered | 0.58 (<.001) | <0.001 (0.87) | −0.11 (0.002) | 0.49 | 0.03 | 0.60 | 291 | 6977 |
| Number of live births | 0.51 (<.001) | <0.001 (0.83) | −0.002 (0.93) | 0.49 | 0.03 | 0.60 | 291 | 6977 |
| Stress | | | | | | | | |
| Perceived Stress | 0.06 (0.10) | 0.008 (0.02) | 0.18 (<.001) | 0.47 | 0.03 | 0.58 | 291 | 6977 |
| History of sexual abuse | 0.42 (<.001) | <0.001 (0.82) | 0.25 (<.001) | 0.47 | 0.03 | 0.60 | 234 | 6766 |
| Symptoms | | | | | | | | |
| Hot flashes | 0.50 (<.001) | <0.001 (0.88) | 0.003 (0.78) | 0.49 | 0.03 | 0.60 | 291 | 6977 |
| Problem getting to sleep | 0.42 (<.001) | −0.0003 (0.91) | 0.24 (<.001) | 0.44 | 0.03 | 0.59 | 291 | 6977 |
| Early awakening | 0.44 (<.001) | −0.003 (0.41) | 0.13 (<.001) | 0.47 | 0.03 | 0.59 | 291 | 6977 |
| Awaken at Night | 0.43 (<.001) | −0.002 (0.50) | 0.11 (<.001) | 0.47 | .03 | 0.59 | 291 | 6977 |

[a] $\beta_1$, $\beta_2$, $\beta_3$ are the fixed effects (group averages) for the intercept, slope and covariate
[b] $\sigma_1$, $\sigma_2$, $\sigma_\varepsilon$ are the random effects (variability) for the intercept, slope and residual error

greatest treatment effects on hot flashes for women who had higher depression scores at baseline. Further analyses examining treatment effects on depressed mood are in process (McCurry, personal communication).

Perceived stress and stressful life events during MT have been associated with depressed mood in other cohorts [14, 23, 56]. SWAN investigators studied women's experiences of stressful and very stressful life events. Using a scale of 18 items women rated as most stressful, they found that women in the MT experiencing two or more very stressful life events since the last study visit (usually a one year period) reported the highest depressive mood score [23]. More recently Gordon and colleagues found that reports of very stressful life events experienced by women in the MT during the six months before study baseline were associated with depressive symptoms (CES-D) over a year later [56]. Very stressful life events included only the following six events: divorce or separation from a partner, serious illness or death of a close family member or close friend, a major worsening in one's financial status or major chronic financial

problems, being physically attacked or having one's life threatened, being sexually abused or assaulted, and being arrested for a serious crime or having a mate or close relative arrested for a serious crime [57]. Gordon and colleagues proposed that estradiol variability may have enhanced emotional sensitivity to these very stressful events that influenced depressed mood in this sample of midlife women 45–60 years of age [56, 58, 59].

The experience of sexual abuse has been included among very stressful life events in earlier studies and also associated with depressive symptoms in an earlier SMWHS investigation using the CES-D [25] as well as in the analyses of reports of depressed mood severity reported here. Sexual abuse history has not been associated with depressed mood in other cohorts of women during the MT. Nonetheless, Allsworth and colleagues found that history of sexual abuse or physical violence was associated with the timing of the MT [60] and violence history with high FSH and low estradiol during the perimenopause (MT), suggesting a plausible relationship of sexual abuse to endocrine perturbation [61].

**Table 4** Final random effects model for depressed mood (diary) with age as predictor and significant psychosocial and hormonal covariates entered simultaneously ($N = 234$; Observations = 6766)

|  | Beta Coefficient | Standard Error/ Standard Deviation | $p$ value |
|---|---|---|---|
| Fixed effects |  |  |  |
| $\beta_1$ intercept | 0.05 | 0.05 | 0.34 |
| $\beta_2$ Age (−47.7) years | 0.01 | 0.004 | 0.02 |
| $\beta_3$ Menopausal Transition Stage |  |  |  |
| Early Stage | 0.02 | 0.03 | 0.57 |
| Late Stage | −0.01 | 0.04 | 0.77 |
| Early PM | −0.10 | 0.05 | 0.03 |
| $B_4$ Perceived Stress | 0.16 | 0.008 | <.001 |
| $B_5$ History sexual abuse | 0.18 | 0.06 | 0.002 |
| $B_6$ Amount exercise | − < 0.001 | 0.0002 | 0.004 |
| $B_7$ Problem getting to sleep | 0.19 | 0.01 | <.001 |
| $B_8$ Early Awakening | 0.05 | 0.01 | <.001 |
| $B_9$ Awakening at night | 0.02 | 0.01 | 0.09 |
| $B_{10}$ If partnered | −0.11 | 0.03 | 0.001 |
| Random effects |  |  |  |
| $b_1$ Intercept $\sigma_1$ |  | 0.39 |  |
| $b_2$ Age (−47.7) years $\sigma_2$ |  | 0.02 |  |
| $b_\varepsilon$ residual $\sigma_\varepsilon$ |  | 0.57 |  |

Factors that protect women from experiences of depressed mood include those considered part of one's health promotion practices, such as engaging in physical activity and being in positive relationships. Sternfield and colleagues found that midlife women participating in an exercise trial experienced less severe depressive symptoms than controls when measured by PHQ-8 [62]. Being in a relationship with a partner may serve as either a risk or protective factor depending on the nature of the relationship [25, 63]. In analyses reported here, being partnered had protective effects on depressive symptoms. It is likely that the nature of the relationship influences the experience of depressed mood: SWAN participants who reported stressful relationships with partners were likely to experience more depressive symptoms [63].

Limitations of this study include relatively small numbers of women who provided urine specimens for hormonal assays ($N = 131$) compensated for in part by the intensive measurement on multiple occasions, yielding over 4,900 data points. SWAN provided data from a larger number of women from multiple sites in the US with annual measures for most variables, including a daily hormone study involving nearly 1,000 women. In addition, the proportion of women in SMWHS with low levels of education and income and a low proportion of women of color limit our ability to generalize the results broadly. SWAN and the POAS included a much more representative population of women.

## Conclusions

In conclusion, given the frequent and coincident measures of depressed mood and endocrine levels available for our analyses, it is likely that estrone and FSH did not play a major role in depressed mood severity reported for the same 24 h period. Nonetheless, others have found relationships when analyses were focused on the MT stages or endocrine values and when using measures of MDD or more severe depressive symptoms such as those included in the CES-D and a longer reference period. In addition, the results reported here afforded an examination of the relationships among depressed mood, urinary estrone and FSH levels, and perceived stress, hot flashes and sleep symptoms obtained for the same 24 h time period as recorded in a health diary, conditions that have not been available to many other investigators. We conclude that it is important for clinicians to consider the relationship of depressed mood to everyday life, even during the MT when it is tempting to attribute depressed mood to endocrine variability. These findings bear replication in larger populations of women and those in which ethnic/racial variability is maximized.

**Abbreviations**
FMP: final menstrual period; FSH: follicle-stimulating hormone; MT: menopausal transition; PM: Postmenopause; SMWHS: Seattle Midlife Women's Health Study; STRAW: Staging Reproductive Aging Workshop

**Funding**
National Institute of Nursing Research R01-NR 04141; NINR P30 NR 04001; University of Washington Research Intramural Funding Program.

**Authors' contributions**
NFW and ESM both contributed to writing the manuscript and both authors read and approved the final manuscript.

**Authors' information**
NFW and ESM: Study design and principal investigator of the Seattle Midlife Women's Health Study. Over the course of the entire study NFW and ESM rotated roles as principal investigator.

**Competing interests**
The authors declare they have no competing interests.

**Author details**
[1]Family and Child Nursing, University of Washington, Seattle, USA.
[2]Biobehavioral Nursing and Health Informatics, University of Washington, Seattle, USA.

**References**

1. Pratt LA, Brody DJ. Depression in the U. S. household population, 2009–2012. NCHS Data Brief. 2014;172:1–8.

2. Deecher D, Andree TH, Sloan D, Schechter LE. From menarche to menopause: exploring the underlying biology of depression in women experiencing hormonal changes. Psychoneuro. 2008;33:3–17.

3. Harlow SD, Cain K, Crawford S, Dennerstein L, Little R, Mitchell ES, Nan B, Randolph JF Jr, Taffe J, Yosef M. Evaluation of four proposed bleeding criteria for the onset of late menopausal transition. J Clin Endocrinol Metab. 2006;91:3432–8.

4. Harlow SD, Mitchell ES, Crawford S, Nan B, Little R, Taffe J, ReSTAGE Collaboration. The ReSTAGE collaboration: defining optimal bleeding criteria for onset of early menopausal transition. Fertil Steril. 2008;89:129–40.

5. Harlow SD, Crawford S, Dennerstein L, Burger HG, Mitchell ES, Sowers MF, ReSTAGE Collaboration. Recommendations from a multi-study evaluation of proposed criteria for staging reproductive aging. Climacteric. 2007;10:112–9.

6. Soules MR, Sherman S, Parrott E, Rebar R, Santoro N, Utian W, Woods NF. Executive summary: stages of reproductive aging workshop (STRAW). Fertil Steril. 2001;76:874–8.

7. Harlow SD, Gass M, Hall JE, Lobo R, Maki P, Rebar RW, Sherman S, Sluss PM, de Villiers TJ. Executive summary of STRAW+10: addressing the unfinished agenda of staging reproductive aging. Climacteric. 2012;15:105–14.

8. Dennerstein L, Dudley EC, Hopper JL, Guthrie JR, Burger HG. A prospective population-based study of menopausal symptoms. Obstet Gynecol. 2000;96:351–8.

9. Sowers M, Crawford S, Sternfeld B, Morganstein D, Gold E, Greendale G, Evans D, Neer R, Matthews K, Sherman S, Lo A, Weiss G, Kelsye J. SWAN: a multicenter, multiethnic community-based cohort study of women and the menopausal transition. In: Lobo R, Kelsey J, Marcus R, editors. Menopause: biology and pathobiology. San Diego: Academic Press; 2000. p. 175–88.

10. Freeman EW, Sammel MD, Lin H, Gracia ER, Pien GW, Nelson DB, Sheng L. Symptoms associated with menopausal transition and reproductive hormones in midlife women. Obstet Gynecol. 2007;110:230–40.

11. Mitchell ES, Woods NF, Mariella A. Three stages of the menopausal transition from the Seattle midlife Women's health study: toward a more precise definition. Menopause. 2000;7:334–49.

12. Avis NE, Brambilla D, McKinlay SM, Vass K. A longitudinal analysis of the association between menopause and depression. Ann Epidemiol. 1994;4:214–20.

13. Bromberger JT, Assmann SF, Avis NE, et al. Persistent mood symptoms in a multiethnic community cohort of pre-and perimenopausal women. Am J Epidemiol. 2003;158(4):347–56.

14. Soares CN, Almeida OP. Depression during the perimenopause. Arch Gen Psychiatry. 2001;58:306.

15. Freeman EW, Sammel MD, Liu L, Gracia CR, Nelson DB, Hollander L. Hormones and menopausal status as predictors of depression in women in transition to menopause. Arch Gen Psychiatry. 2004;61:62–70.

16. Freeman EW, Sammel MD, Lin H, Nelson DB. Associations of hormones and menopausal status with depressed in mood in women with no history of depression. Arch Gen Psychiatry. 2006;63:375–82.

17. Dennerstein L, Guthrie JR, Clark M, Leher P, Henderson VW. A population-based study of depressed mood in middle-aged, Australian-born women. Menopause. 2004;11:563–8.

18. Freeman EW, Sammel MD, Boorman DW, Zhang R. Longitudinal pattern of depressive symptoms around natural menopause. JAMA Psychiatr. 2014;71:36‾43.

19. Bromberger JT, Kravitz HM, Chang YF, Cyranowski JM, Brown C, Matthews KA, et al. Major depression during and after the menopausal transition: Study of Women's Health Across the Nation (SWAN). Psychol Med. 2011;41:1879–88.

20. Bromberger JT, Kravitz HM, Matthews K, Youk A, Brown C, Feng W, et al. Predictors of first lifetime episodes of major depression in midlife women. Psychol Med. 2009;39:55–64.

21. Freeman EW. Depression in the menopause transition: risks in the changing hormone milieu as observed in the general population. Women's Midlife Health. 2015;1:2. https://doi.org/10.1186/s40695-015-002-y.

22. Bromberger JT, Schott LL, Kravitz HM, Sowers M, Avis NE, Gold EB, et al. Longitudinal change in reproductive hormones and depressive symptoms across the menopausal transition: results from the study of Women's health across the nation (SWAN). Arch Gen Psychiatry. 2010;67:598–607.

23. Bromberger JT, Matthews KA, Schott LL, Brockwell S, Avis NE, Kravitz HM, et al. Depressive symptoms during the menopausal transition: the study of Women's health across the nation (SWAN). J Affect Disord. 2007;103:267–72.

24. Ryan J, Burger HG, Szoeke C, Lehert P, Ancelin ML, Henderson VW, et al. A prospective study of the association between endogenous hormones and depressive symptoms in postmenopausal women. Menopause. 2009;16:509–17.

25. Woods NF, Smith-DiJulio K, Percival DB, Tao EY, Mariella A, Mitchell ES. Depressed mood during the menopausal transition and early postmenopause: observations from the Seattle midlife Women's health study. Menopause. 2008;15:223–32.

26. Woods NF, Smith-DiJulio K, Percival DB, Tao EY, Taylor HJ, Mitchell ES. Symptoms during the menopausal transition and early postmenopause and their relation to endocrine levels over time: observations from the Seattle midlife Women's health study. J Women's Health. 2007;110:230–40.

27. Judd FK, Hickey M, Bryant C. Depression and midlife: are we overpathologising the menopause? J Affect Disord. 2012;136:199–211.

28. Moore R, Depp CA, Wetherell JL, Lenze E. Ecological momentary assessment versus standard assessment instruments for measuring mindfulness, depressed mood, and anxiety among older adults. J Psychiatr Res. 2016;75:116–23.

29. Woods NF, Mitchell ES. The Seattle midlife Women's health study: a longitudinal prospective study of women during the menopausal transition and early postmenopause. Women's Midlife Health. 2016;2:6. https://doi.org/10.1186/s40695-016-0019-x.

30. Bjorner J, Rose M, Gandek B, Stone A, Junghaenel D, Ware JJ. Difference in method of administration did not significantly impact item response: an IRT-based analysis from the patient-reported outcomes measurement information system (PROMIS) initiative. Qual Life Res. 2013;23:212–27.

31. Cella D, Yount S, Rothrock N, Gershon R, Cook K, Reeve B, et al. The Patient-Reported Outcomes Measurement Informatino System (PROMIS): progress of an NIH Roadmap cooperative group during its first two years. Med Care. 2007;45:S3e11.

32. Reeve B, Hays RD, Bjorner JB, Cook KF, Crane PK, Teresi JA, et al. Psychometric evalution and calibration of health-related quality of life item banks: plans for the Patient-Reported Outcomes Measurement Informatino System (PROMIS). Med Care. 2007;45:S22e31.

33. Taussky HH. A microcolorimetric determination of creatinine in urine by the Jaffe reaction. J Biol Chem. 1954;208:853–61.

34. Woods NF, Smith-DiJulio K, Percival DB, Tao EY, Taylor HJ, Mitchell ES. Symptoms during the menopausal transition and early post menopause and their relation to endocrine levels over time: observations from the Seattle midlife Women's health study. J Women's Health. 2007;16:667–77.

35. Denari JH, Farinati Z, Casas PR, Oliva A. Determination of ovarian function using first morning urine steroid assays. Obstet Gynecol. 1981;58:5–9.

36. Stanczyk FZ, Miyakawa I, Goebelsmann U. Direct radioimmunoassay of urinary estrogen and pregnanediol glucuronides during the menstrual cycle. Am J Obstet Gynecol. 1980;137:443–50.

37. O'Connor KA, Brindle E, Holman DJ, Klein NA, Soules MR, Campbell KL, Kohen F, Munro CJ, Shofer JB, Lasley BL, Woods JW. Urinary estrone conjugate and pregnanediol 3-glucuronide enzyme immunoassays for population research. Clin Chem. 2003;49:1139–48.

38. Baker TE, Jennison KIM, Kellie AE. The direct radioimmunoassay of oestrogen glucuronides in human female urine. Biochem J. 1979;177:729–38.

39. Ferrell RJ, O'Connor KA, Holman DJ. Monitoring the transition to menopause in a five year prospective study: aggregate and individual changes in steroid hormones and menstrual cycle lengths with age. Menopause. 2005;12:567–77.

40. O'Connor KA, Brindle E, Shofer JB, Miller RC, Klein NA, Soules MR, Campbell KL, Mar C, Handcock MS. Statistical correction for non-parallelism in a urinary enzyme immunoassay. J Immunoass Immunochem. 2004;25:259–78.

41. Woods NF, Mitchell ES. Pathways to depressed mood for midlife women: observations from the Seattle midlife Women's health study. Res Nurs Health. 1997;20:119–29.

42. Qui Q, Overstreet JW, Todd H, Nakajima ST, Steward DR, Lasley BL. Total urinary follicle stimulating hormone as a biomarker for detection of early pregnancy and peri implantation spontaneous abortion. Environ Health Perspect. 1997;105:862–6.

43. Brantley PJ, Waggoner CD, Jones GN, Rappaport NB. A daily stress inventory: development, reliability, and validity. J Behav Med. 1987;10:61–74.

44. Pinheiro J, Bates D, DebRoy S, Sarkar D, R Core Team. nlme: Linear and nonlinear mixed effects models, R package version 3.1. 2107:1–131. https://CRAN.R-project.org/package=nlme.

45. R Development Core Team. R: A Language and Environment for statistical computing. Vienna: R Foundation for Statistical Computing; 2005. http://www.R-project.org.

46. Sarkar D. Lattice: multivariate data visualization with R. http://lattice.r-forge.r-project.org/.

47. Pinheiro J, Bates D. Mixed-effects models in S and S-PLUS. NY: Springer; 2000.

48. Hox J. Multilevel analysis: techniques and applications. Mahwah: Lawrence Erlbaum Associates; 2002.

49. Gibson CJ, Thurston RC, Bromberger JT, Kamarck T, Matthews KA. Negative affect and vasomotor symptoms in the study of Women's health across the nation daily hormone study. Menopause. 2011;18:1270–7.

50. Woods NF, Mitchell ES. Patterns of depressed mood in midlife women: observations from the Seattle midlife Women's health study. Res Nurs Health. 1996;19:11–123.

51. Freeman EW, Sammel MD, Lin H. Tempral association of hot flashes and depression in the transition to menopause. Menopause. 2009;16:728–34.

52. Woods N, Mitchell ES. Sleep symptoms during the menopausal transition and early menopause: observations from the Seattle midlife Women's health study. Sleep. 2010;33(4):539–49.

53. Burleson MH, Todd M, Trevathan WR. Daily vasomotor symptoms, sleep problems, and mood: using daily data to evaluate the domino hypothesis in middle-aged women. Menopause. 2010;17:87–95.

54. Shaver JL, Woods NF. Sleep and menopause: a narrative review. Menopause. 2015;22:899–915.

55. Kahn M, Sheppes G, Sadeh A. Sleep and emotions: bidirectional links and underlying mechanisms. Int J Psychophysiol. 2013;89:218–28.

56. Gordon JL, Rubinow DR, Eisenlohr-Moul TA, Leserman J, Girdler SS. Estradiol variability, stressful life events, and the emergence of depressive symptomatology during the menopausal transition. Menopause. 2016;23:257–66.

57. Mugavero MJ, Raper JL, Reif S, Whetten K, Leserman J, Thielman NM, Pence BW. Overload: impact of incident stressful events on antiretroviral medication adherence and virologic failure in a longitudinal, multisite human immunodeficiency virus cohort study. Psychosom Med. 2009;71:920–6.

58. Woods NF, Mitchell ES, Percival DB, Smith-DiJulio K. Is the menopausal transition stressful? Observations of perceived stress from the Seattle midlife Women's health study. Menopause. 2009;16(1):90–7.

59. Freeman WE, Sammel MD, Boorman DW, Zhang R. Longitudinal pattern of depressive symptoms around natural menopause. JAMA Psychiatry. 2014;71:36–43.

60. Allsworth JE, Zierler S, Krieger N, Harlow BL. Ovarian function in late reproductive years in relation to lifetime experiences of abuse. Epidemiology. 2001;12(6):676–81.

61. Allsworth JE, Zierler S, Lapane KKL, Krieger N, Hogan JW, Harlow BL. Longitudinal study of the inception of perimenopasue in relation to lifetime history of sexual or physical violence. J Epidemiol Community Health. 2004;58:938–43.

62. Sternfeld B, Guthrie KA, Ensrud KE, et al. Efficacy of exercise for menopausal symptoms: a randomized controlled trial. Menopause. 2014;21:330–8. PMCID: PMC3353828

63. Lanza di Scalea T, Matthews KA, Avis NE, Thurston RC, Brown C, Harlow S, Bromberger JT. Role stress, role reward, and mental health in a multiethnic sample of midlife women: results from the study of Women's health across the nation (SWAN). J Women's Health (Larchmt). 2012;21(5):481–9.

# 10

# The role of smoking in the relationship between intimate partner violence and age at natural menopause

Gita D. Mishra[1]*(iD), Hsin-Fang Chung[1], Yalamzewod Assefa Gelaw[1] and Deborah Loxton[2]

## Abstract

**Background:** Age at natural menopause (ANM) is considered as a biologic marker of health and ageing. The relationship between intimate partner violence (IPV) and ANM is currently unknown, and whether smoking plays a role in this relationship is unclear. The aim of this study was to examine the association between IPV and ANM and to quantify the effect mediated through smoking.

**Methods:** Data were drawn from the 1946–51 cohort of the Australian Longitudinal Study on Women's Health, a prospective cohort study first conducted in 1996. History of IPV (yes or no) was self-reported at baseline. ANM was confirmed by at least 12 months of cessation of menses where this was not a result of medical interventions such as bilateral oophorectomy or hysterectomy and categorised as <45 (early menopause), 45–49, 50–51, 52–53, and ≥54 years. Regression models and mediation analyses based on the counterfactual framework were performed to examine the relationship between IPV and ANM and to quantify the proportion mediated through smoking (never, past, current <10, 10–19 and ≥20 cigarettes/day).

**Results:** Of 6138 women in the study with natural menopause, 932 (15%) reported a history of IPV and 429 (7.0%) had an early ANM (before age 45 years). Women with IPV were more likely to smoke and be heavy smokers (Odds Ratio: 2.77, 95% CI 2.19–3.51). Women with IPV were also at increased risk of early menopause (ANM <45 years) (Relative Risk Ratio: 1.36, 95% CI 1.03–1.80) after accounting for education level, income difficulties, age at menarche, parity, body mass index, and perceived stress, compared to the reference group (women without IPV and ANM at 50–51 years). This relationship was attenuated after adjusting for smoking (Relative Risk Ratio: 1.20, 95% CI 0.90–1.59). Mediation analysis showed that cigarette smoking explained 36.7% of the association between IPV and early menopause (ANM <45 vs. ≥45 years).

**Conclusion:** Cigarette smoking substantially mediated the relationship between IPV and early menopause. Findings suggest that as part of addressing the impact of IPV, timely interventions that result in cessation of smoking will partly mitigate the increased risk of early menopause.

**Keywords:** Age at natural menopause, Intimate partner violence, Mediation, Smoking

## Background

While the exact definition of intimate partner violence (IPV) varies between countries, the World Health Organization (WHO) defines IPV as physical violence, sexual violence, stalking and psychological aggression (including coercive acts) by a current or former intimate

* Correspondence: g.mishra@uq.edu.au
[1]School of Public Health, The University of Queensland, Herston Road, Herston, Brisbane, QLD 4006, Australia
Full list of author information is available at the end of the article

partner [1]. In 2013, the WHO multi-country study report documented the global prevalence of physical and/or sexual IPV was 30.0% (95% CI 27.8–32.2%), with the highest levels (approximately 37%) reported in the WHO African, Eastern Mediterranean and South-East Asia Regions [2, 3]. However, IPV against women can occur in all settings, age and socioeconomic groups [4] and is increasingly recognised as a pattern of behaviour that has both immediate and long term consequences for health and well-being [2, 5, 6]. The impact related to reproductive health for women who have experienced some form of IPV includes unintended and/or unwanted pregnancy, abortion, sexually transmitted diseases, cervical cancer and vaginal discharge [2, 6, 7]. The prevalence of smoking is also more likely to be higher among women who have experienced IPV [8–10].

Findings from Australia suggests that IPV is responsible for 8% of overall disease burden for women discussed as selected risks to health [11, 12]. An 11-year population-based study of mid-aged Australian-born women showed IPV was significantly associated with poorer mental and sexual health status [13], and analysis of data from the Australian Longitudinal Study on Women's Health (ALSWH) demonstrated mental and physical health deficits attributable to IPV that lasted the length of the 16 year study period [14]. A study in Victoria measuring the impact of IPV on the health of women reported that IPV accounted for 2.9% of the total disease and burden for women of all ages [15].

The age at natural menopause (ANM), which marks the cessation of menses, acts as a biomarker for reproductive ageing. The timing of ANM is also linked to a range of cardiovascular and metabolic conditions in later life [16], such as earlier ANM and increased risk of ischemic stroke [17]. While a range of factors is linked to the timing of ANM, smoking is one of the most well-established risk factors for earlier menopause [18]. Our earlier cross-sectional analysis of baseline ALSWH data indicated that smoking and postmenopausal status were associated with IPV among women aged 45–50 years [7]. However, 41% of women in the sample had not yet reached menopause, and the nature of the data precluded longitudinal analysis. Furthermore, the underlying mechanism by which IPV might act to drive early menopause was not identified. To date, there have been no studies that clearly identify links between IPV and ANM. Given that cigarette smoking is associated with both IPV and ANM, the aim of this study is to examine if IPV is associated with ANM and to investigate the role of cigarette smoking as a potential mediator of ANM by using a counterfactual framework for mediation analyses.

## Methods

### Study design and population

The Australian Longitudinal Study on Women's Health (ALSWH) is an ongoing population-based cohort study of factors affecting the health and well-being of Australian women born in 1921–26, 1946–51, and 1973–78. Women were randomly selected from the national Medicare dataset, which covers all citizens and permanent residents of Australia. Women were first surveyed in 1996 and were followed every 2–4 years using self-completed questionnaires. Full details of the study design, recruitment and response rates have been reported elsewhere [19, 20]. The study protocols were

approved by the Human Research Ethics Committees of the University of Newcastle and University of Queensland, Australia. Informed consent was obtained from all participants at each survey.

The present study focused on the 1946–51 cohort, which was first surveyed in 1996 when the women were aged 45 to 50 years (Survey 1, $n = 13,714$), and then in 1998 (Survey 2, $n = 12,338$), 2001 (Survey 3, $n = 11,226$), 2004 (Survey 4, $n = 10,905$), 2007 (Survey 5, $n = 10,638$), 2010 (Survey 6, $n = 10,011$) and 2013 (Survey 7, $n = 9151$). ANM was determined for 7635 women who reported to have natural menopause (not a result of medical interventions) and recorded their age at menopause over the study period. Among these women, 1497 were excluded due to missing baseline data on history of IPV ($n = 44$), smoking status ($n = 236$) and relevant covariates including education level ($n = 46$), income difficulties ($n = 36$), body mass index (BMI) ($n = 223$), perceived stress ($n = 26$), number of children ($n = 179$), and age at menarche ($n = 707$). Therefore, data from 6138 women were included in the analyses.

### Main outcome and exposure variables

Age at menopause was determined from responses to the question "if you have reached menopause, at what age did your periods completely stop?" asked in Survey 2 to Survey 6. ANM was confirmed by at least 12 months of cessation of menses where this was not a result of medical interventions such as surgical menopause due to bilateral oophorectomy or hysterectomy. If the ANM was reported at multiple surveys, data reported at the last available survey were used. ANM was treated as a continuous variable and was categorised as <45 (early menopause), 45–49, 50–51, 52–53 and ≥54 years [21].

IPV was defined from responses to the question at baseline "have you ever been in a violent relationship with a partner/spouse?" and categorised women as with or without a history of IPV. Women were also asked a question at Survey 5 "if you have ever lived with a violent partner or spouse, in which years did you experience violence?" Nearly 90% of the women reported they had experienced IPV before 1996 (baseline), which would indicate that the majority of victims had their first IPV experience before midlife.

### Smoking and covariates

Smoking status was reported at baseline and categorised as never, past smoker, and current smoker with <10, 10–19 and ≥20 cigarettes per day. Other baseline covariates included area of residence (categorised as urban and rural/remote), education level (no formal qualifications, less than high school/high school, trade/certificate/diploma and university or higher), difficulty on income management (easy/not bad/some difficult and difficult/

impossible), marital status (married/de facto, separated/ divorced, widowed and single), age at menarche (≤11, 12, 13, 14 and ≥15 years) and number of children (parity) (0, 1, 2–3 and ≥4 children). BMI was computed as self-reported weight (kg) divided by the square of height (m) and categorised as underweight (<18.5 kg/m$^2$), normal weight (18.5–24.9 kg/m$^2$), overweight (25–29.9 kg/m$^2$) and obese (≥30 kg/m$^2$). Perceived stress levels at baseline were assessed by asking participants to rate how stressed they had been in the last 12 months for the following life domains: own health, health of other family members, work/employment, living arrangements, study, money, relationship with parents, relationship with partner/spouse, relationship with children, relationship with other family members. The performance of this preceived stress scale was demonstrated with internal reliability and construct validity [22, 23]. The range of summary stress scores was from 0 to 4. Higher scores indicate more perceived stress. The scores were categorised as not at all stressed (0), somewhat stressed (<1), moderately stressed (1 to <2), very stressed (2 to <3) and extremely stressed (3 to 4). In our analysis, we dichotomised stressed status as absence (scores <1) and presence (scores ≥1).

## Statistical analysis

Participant characteristics at baseline were described according to the history of IPV (yes or no) and five categories of ANM (<45, 45–49, 50–51, 52–53 and ≥54 years). Descriptive statistics were presented as percentages for categorical data and the median (interquartile range) for continuous data. Chi-squared tests and regression models were used to examine the differences between groups.

To examine the contribution of smoking to the IPV and ANM relationship, the causal diagram presented in Fig. 1 was formulated. IPV was hypothesised to affect ANM both directly and indirectly, in which smoking acted as a mediator. Interactions between IPV and smoking categories on ANM were tested and taken into

account if significant. Education level, income difficulties, and age at menarche were the background confounders. High parity, obesity, and stress could be the consequence of IPV [24, 25], thus they were not considered as confounders in the causal diagram. To test these hypotheses, two complementary approaches were used. First, a series of logistic and linear regression models were performed to examine the relationship between IPV and ANM. Multinomial logistic regression models with five categories of outcome for ANM were used to estimate relative risk ratio (RRR) and 95% confidence interval (CI) with age 50–51 as the reference. Linear regression models were used to examine the association with ANM as a continuous outcome. Sequential multivariable regression models were built following multiple adjustment plans by adjusting for education level (Model 1), income difficulties (Model 2), age at menarche (Model 3), parity (Model 4), BMI (Model 5), stress status (Model 6), and subsequently further adjusting for smoking status (Model 7). Attenuated associations between IPV and ANM were expected after adjustment for smoking status, which would indicate a potential mediating role of smoking. Factors that were associated with IPV but did not affect the association between IPV and ANM included area of residence and marital status, thus they were not included in our models.

Second, we performed a formal mediation analysis by using the counterfactual approach [26, 27]. Using the counterfactual framework allows for decomposition of the total effect of IPV on ANM into natural direct and indirect effects mediated through smoking, even in models with non-linearities (e.g. when ANM and smoking are considered as a binary variable) and interactions (e.g. when the effect of IPV is worsened by smoking) [26, 27]. The mediation analysis was performed by fitting a logistic regression model for the binary outcome (ANM <45 and ≥45 years) and a linear regression model for ANM as a continuous outcome; fitting a linear or logistic regression model for the continuous mediator

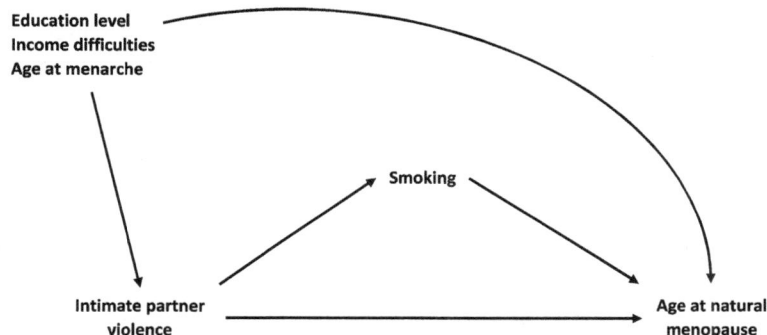

**Fig. 1** Directed acyclic graph for mediation analysis of the relationships between intimate partner violence (exposure), smoking (mediator) and age at natural menopause (outcome)

(treating the ordinal variable for smoking status as continuous) or binary mediator (dicotomised as current and non-current smoking) [28]. Models were adjusted for education level, income difficulties, and age at menarche. Interactions between IPV and smoking were not statistically significant from our preliminary regression analyses (p for interaction >0.4), thus no exposure-mediator interaction was included in our models. From these combined models, we obtained odds ratios (ORs) of natural direct effect (OR$^{NDE}$), natural indirect effect (OR$^{NIE}$) and total effect (OR$^{TE}$) for the binary outcome, while for the linear outcome, we derived parameter estimates of $\beta^{NDE}$, $\beta^{NIE}$ and $\beta^{TE}$. The proportion mediated through mediator was calculated on the risk difference scale. The proportion mediated was calculated as [OR$^{NDE}$ (OR$^{NIE}$ − 1)] / [OR$^{NDE}$ × OR$^{NIE}$ −1] × 100% for the binary outcome (assuming the outcome of early menopause <45 years is relatively rare) [29] or calculated as ($\beta^{NIE}/\beta^{TE}$) × 100% for the continuous outcome.

Given that women who were excluded from the analysis due to incomplete data were more likely to be less educated, be stressed, be a current smoker, and have a history of IPV, we performed a sensitivity analysis using inverse probability weighting to account for this bias [30]. Logistic regression model was used to calculate propensity scores as the predicted probability of having data observed (i.e. not being missing). We performed a complete-case analysis but weighted the complete cases by the inverse of their probability of being a complete case. Statistical analyses were performed using SAS 9.4 (SAS Institute, Inc., Cary, North Carolina). The paramed program in STATA 14 (StataCorp LP, College Station, Texas) was used to perform the mediation analyses and estimate total, natural direct and natural indirect effects [28]. A 2-sided $p < 0.05$ was considered statistically significant.

## Results

This study included 6138 women experiencing natural menopause. Compared with these women, those who were excluded due to incomplete data were more likely to have a lower level of education, have income difficulties, have a history of IPV, be stressed, be a current smoker and have an early ANM (Additional file 1: Table S1). For women included in the study, the mean ANM was 50.9 years (median 51.0 years, interquartile range: 49.0–54.0), with 7% of the women having early menopause (<45 years).

At baseline (when aged 45–50 years), almost one in six women (15%) reported that they had experienced IPV (Table 1). After adjusting for other factors, women with a history of IPV were more likely to live in rural/remote areas, to have lower education levels, to have income difficulties, to be single or separated/divorced, to have four or more children, and to be obese than women without IPV. Women who had suffered IPV were more

than twice as likely to report being stressed (OR 2.03, 95% CI 1.72–2.40) or be current smokers, with a markedly higher likelihood of being a heavy smoker (20 or more cigarettes per day) (OR 2.77, 2.19–3.51). This was also evident in the higher prevalence of heavy smokers (17%) among women with a history of IPV, compared with other women (7%).

Some similarities were evident in the characteristics of women and their time of ANM (Additional file 2: Table S2). Specifically, the risk factors for women associated with early ANM (before age 45 years) after adjusting for other factors and compared with ANM from 50 to 51 years (Table 2), included lower education levels, having income difficulties, and being a current smoker. The risk of early ANM also increased with the number of cigarettes smoked, such that heavy smokers were three times as likely (RRR 2.98, 95% CI 2.11–4.20) as having early ANM compared with those who had never smoked. Women who reported having an early menarche (at age 11 years or earlier) had an increased risk of having early ANM.

In terms of the relationship between IPV and the timing of menopause (Table 3), women who had a history of IPV were at 54% increased risk (RRR 1.54, 95% CI 1.17–2.01) of early ANM compared to the reference group (women without IPV and ANM at 50–51 years). This increased risk was attenuated (RRR 1.36, 1.03–1.80) after adjustment for education level, income difficulties, age at menarche, parity, BMI, and stress (Model 6). With further adjustment for smoking status (Model 7), the risk of early menopause was further attenuated and no longer significant (RRR 1.20, 0.90–1.59). IPV was still associated with an earlier ANM (effect size: −0.39 years, 95% CI -0.69 to −0.08) in the fully adjusted model that used continuous ANM as the outcome. In the sensitivity analysis which used inverse probability weighting to account for the bias caused by the complete-case analysis, we observed similar results that the risk of early menopause was attenuated from 1.37 (1.06–1.76) to 1.19 (0.92–1.55) after adjusting for smoking status.

The results of the multivariable mediation analysis are presented in Table 4. More than one-third (36.7%) of the association of IPV with increased risk of early menopause (ANM <45 years vs. ≥45 years) (OR 1.49, 95% CI 1.16–1.90) was mediated through the number of cigarettes smoked per day (five categories), after adjusting for education level, income difficulties, and age at menarche. The experience of IPV was also associated with having earlier ANM (−0.60 years, 95% CI -0.89 to −0.30) after full adjustment. As above, the number of cigarettes smoked per day accounted for 37.0% of the effect associated between IPV and the timing of ANM. For both early ANM and the timing of ANM, a similar proportion was mediated through smoking when smoking status was dichotomised as current and non-current smoking.

The role of smoking in the relationship between intimate partner violence and age at natural...

99

**Table 1** Baseline characteristics of women according to their history of intimate partner violence ($n = 6138$)

| | History of intimate partner violence (IPV) | | | |
|---|---|---|---|---|
| | No ($n = 5206$, 84.8%) | Yes ($n = 932$, 15.2%) | Crude OR (95% CI) | Adjusted[a] OR (95% CI) |
| Area of residence | | | | |
| Urban | 1913 (36.7) | 307 (32.9) | Reference | Reference |
| Rural/remote | 3293 (63.3) | 625 (67.1) | 1.18 (1.02–1.37) | 1.25 (1.06–1.47) |
| Education level | | | | |
| No formal qualifications | 666 (12.8) | 168 (18.0) | 1.90 (1.48–2.44) | 1.74 (1.32–2.30) |
| Less than high school/high school | 2497 (48.0) | 468 (50.2) | 1.41 (1.14–1.74) | 1.45 (1.15–1.82) |
| Trade/certificate/diploma | 1102 (21.2) | 171 (18.3) | 1.17 (0.91–1.49) | 1.21 (0.93–1.58) |
| University or higher | 941 (18.1) | 125 (13.4) | Reference | Reference |
| Difficulty on income management | | | | |
| Easy/not bad/some difficult | 4685 (90.0) | 701 (75.2) | Reference | Reference |
| Difficult/impossible | 521 (10.0) | 231 (24.8) | 2.96 (2.49–3.53) | 1.66 (1.36–2.02) |
| Marital status | | | | |
| Married/de facto | 4548 (87.5) | 606 (65.1) | Reference | Reference |
| Separated/divorced | 399 (7.7) | 272 (29.2) | 5.12 (4.29–6.10) | 4.29 (3.55–5.20) |
| Widowed | 97 (1.9) | 18 (1.9) | 1.39 (0.84–2.32) | 1.30 (0.76–2.23) |
| Single | 156 (3.0) | 35 (3.8) | 1.68 (1.16–2.45) | 2.27 (1.45–3.57) |
| Age at menarche (years) | | | | |
| ≤ 11 | 883 (17.0) | 184 (19.7) | 1.23 (1.00–1.52) | 1.10 (0.88–1.38) |
| 12 | 1109 (21.3) | 178 (19.1) | 0.95 (0.77–1.17) | 0.92 (0.74–1.15) |
| 13 | 1526 (29.3) | 258 (27.7) | Reference | Reference |
| 14 | 899 (17.3) | 144 (15.5) | 0.95 (0.76–1.18) | 0.94 (0.74–1.19) |
| ≥ 15 | 789 (15.2) | 168 (18.0) | 1.26 (1.02–1.56) | 1.18 (0.94–1.48) |
| Number of children | | | | |
| 0 | 458 (8.8) | 54 (5.8) | 0.74 (0.55–1.00) | 0.61 (0.43–0.86) |
| 1 | 426 (8.2) | 106 (11.4) | 1.56 (1.24–1.97) | 1.31 (1.02–1.69) |
| 2–3 | 3586 (68.9) | 571 (61.3) | Reference | Reference |
| ≥ 4 | 736 (14.1) | 201 (21.6) | 1.72 (1.43–2.05) | 1.55 (1.28–1.89) |
| Body mass index (kg/m$^2$) | | | | |
| Underweight (<18.5) | 90 (1.7) | 16 (1.7) | 1.03 (0.60–1.77) | 0.79 (0.44–1.44) |
| Normal weight (18.5–24.9) | 2802 (53.8) | 482 (51.7) | Reference | Reference |
| Overweight (25–29.9) | 1494 (28.7) | 243 (26.1) | 0.95 (0.80–1.12) | 0.92 (0.77–1.10) |
| Obese (≥30) | 820 (15.8) | 191 (20.5) | 1.35 (1.13–1.63) | 1.24 (1.02–1.53) |
| Median BMI (Q1, Q3) | 24.5 (22.1, 27.7) | 24.6 (22.3, 28.7) | | |
| Perceived stress | | | | |
| No (stress scores <1) | 4245 (81.5) | 581 (62.3) | Reference | Reference |
| Yes (stress scores ≥1) | 961 (18.5) | 351 (37.7) | 2.67 (2.30–3.10) | 2.03 (1.72–2.40) |
| Median stress scores (Q1, Q3) | 0.5 (0.2, 0.8) | 0.7 (0.4, 1.2) | | |
| Smoking status | | | | |
| Never | 3048 (58.5) | 360 (38.6) | Reference | Reference |
| Ex-smoker | 1469 (28.2) | 316 (33.9) | 1.82 (1.55–2.14) | 1.73 (1.45–2.05) |
| Current smoker, <10 cigarettes/day | 146 (2.8) | 50 (5.4) | 2.90 (2.07–4.07) | 2.52 (1.75–3.63) |
| Current smoker, 10–19 cigarettes/day | 178 (3.4) | 47 (5.0) | 2.24 (1.59–3.14) | 1.80 (1.25–2.58) |

**Table 1** Baseline characteristics of women according to their history of intimate partner violence (*n* = 6138) *(Continued)*

|  | History of intimate partner violence (IPV) | | | |
|---|---|---|---|---|
|  | No (*n* = 5206, 84.8%) | Yes (*n* = 932, 15.2%) | Crude OR (95% CI) | Adjusted[a] OR (95% CI) |
| Current smoker, ≥20 cigarettes/day | 365 (7.0) | 159 (17.1) | 3.69 (2.97–4.58) | 2.77 (2.19–3.51) |

Data are presented as n (%), median (interquartile range) or odds ratio (OR) and 95% confidence interval (95% CI) using logistic regression models. Q1, 25th percentile; Q3, 75th percentile
[a]Adjusted model was adjusted for all the covariates listed in the table

**Table 2** Adjusted associations of socioeconomic, reproductive and lifestyle factors with age at natural menopause (*n* = 6138)

|  | Age at natural menopause (ANM) (years) | | | | |
|---|---|---|---|---|---|
|  | <45 RRR (95% CI) | 45–49 RRR (95% CI) | 50–51 RRR (95% CI) | 52–53 RRR (95% CI) | ≥54 RRR (95% CI) |
| Education level |  |  |  |  |  |
| No formal qualifications | 1.72 (1.11–2.65) | 1.36 (1.03–1.81) | Reference | 0.95 (0.71–1.26) | 0.71 (0.54–0.92) |
| Less than high school/high school | 1.54 (1.08–2.20) | 0.96 (0.77–1.20) | Reference | 0.84 (0.67–1.04) | 0.71 (0.58–0.86) |
| Trade/certificate/diploma | 1.34 (0.90–2.01) | 0.95 (0.74–1.23) | Reference | 0.88 (0.69–1.13) | 0.76 (0.60–0.95) |
| University or higher | Reference | Reference | Reference | Reference | Reference |
| Difficulty on income management |  |  |  |  |  |
| Easy/not bad/some difficult | Reference | Reference | Reference | Reference | Reference |
| Difficult/impossible | 1.47 (1.08–2.02) | 1.14 (0.89–1.45) | Reference | 0.91 (0.71–1.18) | 1.10 (0.88–1.38) |
| Age at menarche (years) |  |  |  |  |  |
| ≤ 11 | 1.54 (1.10–2.16) | 1.30 (1.03–1.64) | Reference | 1.09 (0.86–1.37) | 1.00 (0.80–1.24) |
| 12 | 1.49 (1.10–2.03) | 0.95 (0.76–1.18) | Reference | 0.88 (0.71–1.09) | 0.92 (0.76–1.13) |
| 13 | Reference | Reference | Reference | Reference | Reference |
| 14 | 1.14 (0.80–1.62) | 1.13 (0.90–1.43) | Reference | 0.94 (0.74–1.18) | 1.09 (0.88–1.35) |
| ≥ 15 | 1.34 (0.94–1.91) | 1.09 (0.86–1.39) | Reference | 0.98 (0.77–1.25) | 1.18 (0.95–1.46) |
| Number of children |  |  |  |  |  |
| 0 | 1.28 (0.87–1.89) | 1.32 (1.00–1.73) | Reference | 1.00 (0.76–1.34) | 0.83 (0.63–1.08) |
| 1 | 1.04 (0.71–1.52) | 1.16 (0.89–1.51) | Reference | 0.86 (0.65–1.14) | 0.86 (0.66–1.11) |
| 2–3 | Reference | Reference | Reference | Reference | Reference |
| ≥ 4 | 0.99 (0.73–1.35) | 0.97 (0.78–1.20) | Reference | 1.04 (0.84–1.29) | 0.94 (0.77–1.15) |
| Body mass index (kg/m²) |  |  |  |  |  |
| Underweight (<18.5) | 1.27 (0.57–2.83) | 1.36 (0.77–2.40) | Reference | 1.18 (0.65–2.14) | 0.92 (0.51–1.65) |
| Normal weight (18.5–24.9) | Reference | Reference | Reference | Reference | Reference |
| Overweight (25–29.9) | 1.10 (0.85–1.42) | 1.06 (0.89–1.27) | Reference | 1.12 (0.94–1.34) | 1.34 (1.14–1.58) |
| Obese (≥30) | 1.03 (0.75–1.41) | 1.08 (0.87–1.34) | Reference | 1.10 (0.88–1.37) | 1.26 (1.03–1.55) |
| Perceived stress |  |  |  |  |  |
| No (stress scores <1) | Reference | Reference | Reference | Reference | Reference |
| Yes (stress scores ≥1) | 1.15 (0.88–1.50) | 1.12 (0.93–1.36) | Reference | 0.94 (0.77–1.14) | 1.00 (0.83–1.19) |
| Smoking status |  |  |  |  |  |
| Never | Reference | Reference | Reference | Reference | Reference |
| Ex-smoker | 1.21 (0.93–1.57) | 0.88 (0.74–1.05) | Reference | 0.90 (0.76–1.07) | 0.93 (0.80–1.09) |
| Current smoker, <10 cigarettes/day | 1.69 (0.98–2.92) | 0.84 (0.54–1.30) | Reference | 0.86 (0.56–1.32) | 0.73 (0.49–1.10) |
| Current smoker, 10–19 cigarettes/day | 2.00 (1.22–3.27) | 1.13 (0.77–1.67) | Reference | 0.80 (0.53–1.23) | 0.69 (0.46–1.03) |
| Current smoker, ≥20 cigarettes/day | 2.98 (2.11–4.20) | 1.71 (1.30–2.25) | Reference | 0.82 (0.59–1.12) | 0.81 (0.61–1.09) |

Data are presented as relative risk ratio (RRR) and 95% confidence interval (CI) using multinomial logistic regression models, and all RRRs (95% CI) were adjusted for the covariates listed in the table

**Table 3** Multivariable adjusted association between intimate partner violence and age at natural menopause ($n = 6138$)

| Intimate partner violence | Age at natural menopause (ANM) (years) | | | | | |
| --- | --- | --- | --- | --- | --- | --- |
| | <45 RRR (95% CI) | 45–49 RRR (95% CI) | 50–51 RRR (95% CI) | 52–53 RRR (95% CI) | ≥54 RRR (95% CI) | Continuous ANM β (95% CI) |
| Unadjusted model | 1.54 (1.17–2.01) | 1.06 (0.86–1.30) | Reference | 0.87 (0.70–1.07) | 0.83 (0.68–1.01) | −0.72 (−1.01 to −0.42) |
| Model 1: + education level | 1.49 (1.14–1.95) | 1.04 (0.84–1.28) | Reference | 0.87 (0.70–1.08) | 0.84 (0.69–1.02) | −0.66 (−0.95 to −0.36) |
| Model 2: Model 1 + income difficulties | 1.39 (1.06–1.83) | 1.01 (0.82–1.24) | Reference | 0.88 (0.71–1.09) | 0.82 (0.67–1.00) | −0.60 (−0.89 to −0.30) |
| Model 3: Model 2 + menarche | 1.38 (1.05–1.82) | 1.00 (0.81–1.23) | Reference | 0.87 (0.70–1.09) | 0.82 (0.67–1.00) | −0.60 (−0.89 to −0.30) |
| Model 4: Model 3 + parity | 1.39 (1.05–1.83) | 1.00 (0.81–1.24) | Reference | 0.87 (0.70–1.09) | 0.82 (0.67–1.00) | −0.62 (−0.92 to −0.32) |
| Model 5: Model 4 + BMI | 1.39 (1.05–1.83) | 1.00 (0.81–1.24) | Reference | 0.87 (0.70–1.09) | 0.82 (0.67–1.00) | −0.62 (−0.92 to −0.33) |
| Model 6: Model 5 + stress status | 1.36 (1.03–1.80) | 0.98 (0.80–1.22) | Reference | 0.88 (0.71–1.10) | 0.82 (0.67–1.00) | −0.60 (−0.90 to −0.29) |
| Model 7: Model 6 + smoking status | 1.20 (0.90–1.59) | 0.95 (0.76–1.17) | Reference | 0.91 (0.73–1.13) | 0.84 (0.68–1.03) | −0.39 (−0.69 to −0.08) |

Multinominal logistic regression models were used to estimate relative risk ratio (RRR) and 95% confidence intervals (CI) for the categorical ANM. Linear regression models were used to estimate β (95% CI) for the continuous ANM

## Discussion

Using data from a large population-based cohort, this study underscores that women with a history of IPV in midlife are at increased risk of obesity and are more likely to report having four or more children, being stressed and be current smokers, especially heavy smoking (20 or more cigarettes per day). To our knowledge, this is the first study to show that IPV is also associated with increased risk of early ANM (before age 45 years) after adjusting for other risk factors. This relationship was attenuated, however, after accounting for smoking, which is an established risk factor for early ANM. Findings from the mediation analyses using a counterfactual framework confirmed that a considerable part of the link between IPV and earlier ANM was mediated via current smoking status. Specifically, the number of cigarettes

smoked per day explained more than one third (36.7%) of the overall relationship of IPV with early ANM after adjusting for education level, income difficulties, and age at menarche. These findings are consistent with those from previous studies that have shown the strong links between IPV and higher rates of cigarette smoking [8–10] and between smoking and earlier ANM [18].

The association between IPV and tobacco use is well known and has repeatedly been reported in the literature [8–10]. While causality has not been demonstrated, the direct link approach such as that used in the current analysis is justified. A systematic review of IPV and tobacco use literature found the only factor that influenced the association between IPV and tobacco was pregnancy [31], a factor that is not relevant to the current analysis. The review authors propose that nicotine acts to both

**Table 4** Natural direct and indirect effects of intimate partner violence on the age at natural menopause and the proportion mediated through smoking ($n = 6138$)[a]

| | OR^NDE (95% CI) | OR^NIE (95% CI) | OR^TE (95% CI) | Proportion mediated by smoking (%) |
| --- | --- | --- | --- | --- |
| **Early menopause (ANM <45 vs. ≥45 years)** | | | | |
| Mediator: smoking | | | | |
| Smoking status (5 categories) | 1.31 (1.02–1.68) | 1.14 (1.09–1.18) | 1.49 (1.16–1.90) | 36.7 |
| Current vs. non-current smoking (2 categories) | 1.34 (1.04–1.72) | 1.13 (1.08–1.18) | 1.51 (1.18–1.93) | 33.7 |
| | β^NDE (95% CI) | β^NIE (95% CI) | β^TE (95% CI) | Proportion mediated by smoking (%) |
| **Continuous ANM** | | | | |
| Mediator: smoking | | | | |
| Smoking status (5 categories) | −0.38 (−0.68 to −0.08) | −0.22 (−0.28 to −0.16) | −0.60 (−0.89 to −0.30) | 37.0 |
| Current vs. non-current smoking (2 categories) | −0.41 (−0.71 to −0.11) | −0.18 (−0.23 to −0.12) | −0.59 (−0.94 to −0.24) | 29.8 |

*ANM* age at natural menopause, *NDE* natural direct effect, *NIR* natural indirect effect, *TE* total effect

[a]All estimates were adjusted for education level, income difficulties, and age at menarche. The mediation analysis was performed by fitting a logistic regression model for the binary outcome (ANM <45 vs. ≥45 years) and a linear regression model for the continuous ANM and fitting a linear or logistic regression model for the ordinal or binary mediator. The proportion mediated was calculated as [(OR^NDE (OR^NIE − 1)] / [OR^NDE × OR^NIE −1] × 100% for the binary outcome or (β^NIE/β^TE) × 100% for the continuous outcome

alleviate symptoms of depression that are caused by IPV and the symptoms of anxiety that accompany living with a violent partner [31]. More research is needed to allow for the development of effective smoking cessation interventions for women who have experienced IPV. It is possible that smoking cessation programs designed for those experiencing mental health disorders might be more effective than standard smoking cessation programs, given the much lower quit rates found among those with mental health problems [32]. It should be noted that while certain characteristics seem to cluster together (for example, cigarrette smoking, low education level, income difficulties, being stressed and being exposed to violence), cigarette smoking, by far, has been shown to be consistently linked with age at menopause. We also found that around 5% of the association between IPV and risk of early menopause was mediated through stress (without considering smoking status), but no significant joint effect between smoking status and stress status was observed (data not shown). Therefore, health promotion effort should be placed on smoking cessation programs.

IPV has been linked with sexually transmitted and reproductive disorders (e.g. cervical cancer, vaginal discharge) [2, 6, 7] but this is the first study to demonstrate a clear relationship with early reproductive ageing, which in turn has a known impact on cardiovascular disease [16]. Links have previously been shown between IPV and cardiovascular disease and metabolic syndrome disorder, with a strong focus on health behaviours (e.g. smoking, abdominal obesity) and mental distress as mechanisms that connect IPV with cardiovascular risk [33]. The current study adds to knowledge in this regard by highlighting the importance of reproductive ageing. Future research will need to take into account the multiple social and biological pathways through which IPV acts to influence health and well-being. Early life experience of violence may also affect ovarian function and reproductive ageing via stress response dysregulation [34, 35]. One cohort study found that women who experienced childhood or adolescent violence had more extreme levels of ovarian hormones during perimenopause, suggesting that early experience of violence may lead to neuroendocrine disruption, thereby affecting ovarian function [35]. However, this study found conflicting findings that early life violence was associated with delayed (rather than early) onset of perimenopause (measured by menstrual changes) [34]. Our previous cross-sectional analysis using baseline data found that IPV was associated with surgical menopause but not with postmenopause and perimenopause after adjustment for demographic and health behaviour variables [7]. A number of reasons may explain the conflicting results including different outcomes (hormones and menstrual cycle/status), different forms of violence (physical,

emotional, sexual), and different analytical approaches. Hence, more studies are needed to prove the link between the experience of all forms of violence and reproductive health.

The strengths of our study included large sample size and nationally representative study population, which improves the generalizability of our findings to other middle-aged women. Our study was strengthened by its prospective nature, particularly with respect to longitudinal data on the timing of menopause. This meant that reverse causation could be ruled out for the relationships observed between IPV at baseline and ANM. The extensive survey data collected from the women has also allowed adjustment for a wide range of confounders, including known risk factors for IPV and earlier ANM. However, there were some limitations that should be acknowledged. First, all the data were self-reported, which may have led to some under-reporting of IPV. It was also the case that women who were excluded from the analyses due to incomplete data were more likely to have a history of IPV, be a current smoker, and have an early ANM compared to those who were included. If this potential underestimation of the prevalence of IPV, current smoking, and early menopause were included, it seems likely that the observed associations would be strengthened. Second, since the study is limited to Australian women, these findings should be replicated in other populations. Further research is also needed to investigate potential mechanisms for the relationship between IPV and ANM that is not explained by smoking and other risk factors in this study.

## Conclusions

Women who had a prior history of IPV were at increased risk of early menopause (<45 years), with this relationship substantially mediated through smoking. Our findings suggest that as part of addressing the issue of IPV and its subsequent consequences for women, smoking cessation interventions tailored for women who have lived with IPV will partly mitigate the links with earlier menopause, which is an established risk factor for a range of adverse health outcomes in later life in addition to the effects of smoking.

**Abbreviations**
ALSWH: Australian Longitudinal Study on Women's Health; ANM: Age at natural menopause; BMI: Body mass index; CI: Confidence interval; IPV: Intimate partner violence; NDR: Natural direct effect; NIR: Natural indirect effect; OR: Odds ratio; RRR: Relative risk ratio; TE: Total effect; WHO: World Health Organization

**Acknowledgements**
The research on which this paper is based was conducted as part of the Australian Longitudinal Study on Women's Health, the University of Newcastle,

and the University of Queensland. We are grateful to the Australian Government Department of Health for funding and to the women who provided the survey data.

## Funding
The Australian Longitudinal Study on Women's Health is funded by the Australian Government Department of Health. GDM is supported by the Australian National Health and Medical Research Council Principal Research Fellowship (APP1121844).

## Authors' contributions
GDM conceptualized the study and drafted the manuscript; HFC performed the statistical analysis and contributed to interpretation of results; YAG performed the literature review; DL provided critical revision of the manuscript for important intellectual content. All authors read and approved the final manuscript.

## Competing interests
The authors declare that they have no competing interests.

## Author details
[1]School of Public Health, The University of Queensland, Herston Road, Herston, Brisbane, QLD 4006, Australia. [2]Research Centre for Generational Health and Ageing, The University of Newcastle, Callaghan, NSW, Australia.

## References
1. Basile KC, Black MC, Breiding MJ, Chen J, Merrick MT, Smith SG, et al. National intimate partner and sexual violence survey. Atlanta: Centers for Disease Control and Prevention; 2011.
2. World Health Organization. Global and regional estimates of violence against women: prevalence and health effects of intimate partner violence and non-partner sexual violence. Geneva: WHO Press; 2013.
3. World Health Organization: Violence against women: Intimate partner and sexual violence against women (Fact Sheet No. 239). 2016. http://www.who.int/mediacentre/factsheets/fs239/en/. Accessed 8 Aug 2017.
4. Garcia-Moreno C, Jansen HA, Ellsberg M, Heise L, Watts CH, WHO Multi-country Study on Women's Health and Domestic Violence against Women Study Team. Prevalence of intimate partner violence: findings from the WHO multi-country study on women's health and domestic violence. Lancet. 2006;368:1260–9.
5. Moore M. Reproductive health and intimate partner violence. Fam Plan Perspect. 1999;31:302–6.
6. World Health Organization. Women and health: today's evidence tomorrow's agenda. Geneva: WHO Press; 2009.
7. Loxton D, Schofield M, Hussain R, Mishra G. History of domestic violence and physical health in midlife. Violence Against Women. 2006;12:715–31.
8. Cheng D, Salimi S, Terplan M, Chisolm MS. Intimate partner violence and maternal cigarette smoking before and during pregnancy. Obstet Gynecol. 2015;125:356–62.
9. Yoshihama M, Horrocks J, Bybee D. Intimate partner violence and initiation of smoking and drinking: a population-based study of women in Yokohama, Japan. Soc Sci Med. 2010;71:1199–207.
10. Jun HJ, Rich-Edwards JW, Boynton-Jarrett R, Wright RJ. Intimate partner violence and cigarette smoking: association between smoking risk and psychological abuse with and without co-occurrence of physical and sexual abuse. Am J Public Health. 2008;98:527–35.
11. Begg S, Vos T, Barker B, Stevenson C, Stanley L, Lopez AD. The burden of disease and injury in Australia 2003. Canberra: Australian Institute of Health and Welfare; 2007.
12. García-Moreno C, Zimmerman C, Morris-Gehring A, Heise L, Amin A, Abrahams N, et al. Addressing violence against women: a call to action. Lancet. 2015;385:1685 95.
13. Schei B, Guthrie J, Dennerstein L, Alford S. Intimate partner violence and health outcomes in mid-life women: a population-based cohort study. Arch Womens Ment Health. 2006;9:317–24.
14. Loxton D, Dolja-Gore X, Anderson AE, Townsend N. Intimate partner violence adversely impacts health over 16 years and across generations: a longitudinal cohort study. PLoS One. 2017;12:e0178138.
15. Vos T, Astbury J, Piers L, Magnus A, Heenan M, Stanley L, et al. Measuring the impact of intimate partner violence on the health of women in Victoria, Australia. Bull World Health Organ. 2006;84:739–44.
16. Mishra GD, Cooper R, Kuh D. A life course approach to reproductive health: theory and methods. Maturitas. 2010;65:92–7.
17. Lisabeth LD, Beiser AS, Brown DL, Murabito JM, Kelly-Hayes M, Wolf PA. Age at natural menopause and risk of ischemic stroke: the Framingham heart study. Stroke. 2009;40:1044–9.
18. Schoenaker DA, Jackson CA, Rowlands JV, Mishra GD. Socioeconomic position, lifestyle factors and age at natural menopause: a systematic review and meta-analyses of studies across six continents. Int J Epidemiol. 2014;43: 1542–62.
19. Dobson AJ, Hockey R, Brown WJ, Byles JE, Loxton DJ, McLaughlin D, et al. Cohort profile update: Australian longitudinal study on Women's health. Int J Epidemiol. 2015;44:1547a–f.
20. Lee C, Dobson AJ, Brown WJ, Bryson L, Byles J, Warner-Smith P, et al. Cohort profile: the Australian longitudinal study on Women's health. Int J Epidemiol. 2005;34:987–91.
21. Mishra GD, Pandeya N, Dobson AJ, Chung HF, Anderson D, Kuh D, et al. Early menarche, nulliparity and the risk for premature and early natural menopause. Hum Reprod. 2017;32:679–86.
22. Bell S, Lee C. Development of the perceived stress questionnaire for young women. Psychol Health Med. 2002;7:189–201.
23. Bell S, Lee C. Perceived stress revisited: the Women's health Australia project young cohort. Psychol Health Med. 2003;8:343–53.
24. Gee RE, Mitra N, Wan F, Chavkin DE, Long JA. Power over parity: intimate partner violence and issues of fertility control. Am J Obstet Gynecol. 2009;201:148. e141-7
25. Bosch J, Weaver TL, Arnold LD, Clark EM. The impact of intimate partner violence on women's physical health: findings from the Missouri behavioral risk factor surveillance system. J Interpers Violence. 2017;32:3402–19.
26. Robins JM, Greenland S. Identifiability and exchangeability for direct and indirect effects. Epidemiology. 1992;3:143–55.
27. Pearl J. Direct and Indirect Effects. Proceedings of the Seventeenth conference on Uncertainty in Artificial Intelligence. Seattle, WA; 2001: 411–20.
28. Valeri L, Vanderweele TJ. Mediation analysis allowing for exposure-mediator interactions and causal interpretation: theoretical assumptions and implementation with SAS and SPSS macros. Psychol Methods. 2013;18:137–50.
29. Vanderweele TJ, Vansteelandt S. Odds ratios for mediation analysis for a dichotomous outcome. Am J Epidemiol. 2010;172:1339–48.
30. Seaman SR, White IR. Review of inverse probability weighting for dealing with missing data. Stat Methods Med Res. 2013;22:278–95.
31. Crane CA, Hawes SW, Weinberger AH. Intimate partner violence victimization and cigarette smoking: a meta-analytic review. Trauma Violence Abuse. 2013;14:305–15.
32. Cook BL, Wayne GF, Kafali EN, Liu Z, Shu C, Flores M. Trends in smoking among adults with mental illness and association between mental health treatment and smoking cessation. JAMA. 2014;311:172–82.
33. Stene LE, Jacobsen GW, Dyb G, Tverdal A, Schei B. Intimate partner violence and cardiovascular risk in women: a population-based cohort study. J Women's Health (Larchmt). 2013;22:250–8.
34. Allsworth JE, Zierler S, Lapane KL, Krieger N, Hogan JW, Harlow BL. Longitudinal study of the inception of perimenopause in relation to lifetime history of sexual or physical violence. J Epidemiol Community Health. 2004; 58:938–43.
35. Allsworth JE, Zierler S, Krieger N, Harlow BL. Ovarian function in late reproductive years in relation to lifetime experiences of abuse. Epidemiology. 2001;12:676–81.

# 11

# Perceived stress across the midlife: longitudinal changes among a diverse sample of women, the Study of Women's health Across the Nation (SWAN)

Elizabeth Hedgeman[1]*[iD], Rebecca E. Hasson[2], Carrie A. Karvonen-Gutierrez[1], William H. Herman[3] and Siobán D. Harlow[1]

## Abstract

**Background:** In women, midlife is a period of social and physiological change. Ostensibly stressful, cross-sectional studies suggest women experience decreasing stress perceptions and increasing positive outlook during this life stage. The aim of this paper was to describe the longitudinal changes in perceived stress as women transitioned through the midlife.

**Methods:** Premenopausal women (n = 3044) ages 42–52 years at baseline, were recruited from seven sites in the Study of Women's Health Across the Nation, and followed approximately annually over 13 visits with assessment of perceived stress and change in menopausal status. Longitudinal regression models were used to assess the effects of age, menopausal status and baseline sociodemographic variables on the trajectory of perceived stress over time.

**Results:** At baseline, mean age was 46.4 ± 2.7 years; participants were white (47%), black (29%), Hispanic (7%), Japanese (9%), or Chinese (8%). Hispanic women, women with lesser educational attainment, and women reporting financial hardship were each more likely to report high perceived stress levels at baseline (all $p < 0.0001$). After adjustment for baseline sociodemographic factors, perceived stress decreased over time for most women ($p < 0.0001$), but increased for both Hispanic and white participants at the New Jersey site ($p < 0.0001$). Changing menopausal status was not a significant predictor of perceived stress.

**Conclusions:** Self-reported stress decreased for most women as they transitioned across the midlife; changing menopausal status did not play a significant role after adjustment for age and sociodemographic factors. Future studies should explore the stress experience for women by racial / ethnic identity and demographics.

**Keywords:** Women's health, Stress, Minority health/disparities/SES, Aging, Menopausal transition, Epidemiology

## Background

The midlife, bounded by young adulthood and old age, has heretofore received only limited scientific attention. Modern social scientists place the beginning of midlife at 35 or 40 years of age, to highlight the period when most adults have finished schooling, entered the workforce, and embarked into marriage with childbearing and rearing [1] – a period of "life past the initial putting together [2]." Clinically this life phase coincides with the age at which chronic conditions begin to appear, an age that can vary by cultural and sociodemographic identity [3]. When asked themselves, adults cite midlife as beginning anywhere from 35 to 45 and ending around 55–60 years of age [2, 4, 5].

For modern women 40¯65 years of age, these middle years are marked by the potential for profound social and physiological changes [6]. Households are changing, with children leaving and "boomerang" children returning [7, 8]. Aging parents may require more care as their health and functioning decline. Workplace stress may

* Correspondence: ehedgeman@gmail.com; hedgeman@umich.edu
[1]Department of Epidemiology, School of Public Health, University of Michigan, 6610B SPH I, 1415 Washington Heights, Ann Arbor, MI 48109-2029, USA
Full list of author information is available at the end of the article

increase with the attainment of seniority, additional job strain, and concomitantly increasing time demands [9, 10]. The menopausal transition – a period beginning in the early forties, marking reproductive senescence, changing estrogen levels, and ultimate cessation of the menstrual cycle – can bring vasomotor and genitourinary symptoms, disrupted sleep cycles and mood changes [2, 11–14]. Though the 'midlife crisis' has been largely debunked [15], the midlife years appear to be a period ripe for stress. Previous work has demonstrated that positive affect – a measure of positive mood and outlook – was significantly lower in midlife women (ages 35–64 years in 1995–1996) as compared to younger and older women, with relationship stress and occupational stress found to be strong drivers of the observed dissatisfaction [16, 17].

And yet, perhaps contrary to expectation, research suggests that perceived stress – a self-reported, subjective measure of individual control and coping – decreases, and quality of life increases, through midlife in some populations. Among nearly 14,000 women ages 40–55 years, contacted in 1994 for the Study of Women's Health Across the Nation (SWAN) cross-sectional screening study, increased age was positively associated with quality of life for white and black women, though not for Chinese, Hispanic or Japanese women [18]. Similar cross-sectional results from the first wave of the Midlife Development in the United States (MIDUS; 1995–1996) study suggest that overall quality of life reaches a nadir in the late 30s to early 40s, only to increase through the remaining midlife and beyond [19]. Cross-sectional studies from both the United States (1983) and United Kingdom (circa 2006) suggest that levels of perceived stress decrease over the entire lifespan for all race / ethnicities [20, 21]. Corresponding with these cross-sectional findings of lower stress perception with age, the longitudinal Melbourne Women's Midlife Health Project of Australian-born midlife women (ages 45–55 in 1991) found that negative moods – feelings of tension, confusion, helplessness, loneliness, insignificance – decreased significantly over the 11 years of follow-up [22]. However, missing from this literature is a longitudinal assessment of perceived stress, particularly across the midlife.

The aim of this study was to describe the longitudinal reports of perceived stress as women transitioned through the midlife in the SWAN cohort. Specific hypotheses, based on the findings from prior research, were that perceived stress (i) would decrease over time for some, but not all women, due to differing racial / ethnic experiences of aging, and (ii) would increase as women progressed through perimenopause, but generally decrease with age. Socioeconomic factors were included in models as modifying factors expected to influence perceived stress. Secondary data were obtained

from this large, sociodemographically diverse cohort of women, with individual perceived stress assessed at multiple points over 15 years and 13 visits. Potential differences in the experience of perceived stress by race / ethnicity, adjusted for socioeconomic status, and whether stress profiles were influenced by stage of the menopausal transition, considered a key biological hallmark of this lifestage, were assessed for longitudinal differences over time.

## Methods
### Study population
A full description of the Study of Women's Health Across the Nation (SWAN) longitudinal cohort and methodology has been published in detail elsewhere [23]. Briefly, SWAN was instituted in 1996 as an observational cohort study of women, their lifestyles, and their health through the menopausal transition with longitudinal follow-up to determine outcomes over time. Eligibility was based on age (42–52 years), self-reported race / ethnicity, and reproductive status (not pregnant or lactating; at least one menstrual cycle in previous three months; uterus and at least one ovary intact; not taking exogenous hormones affecting ovarian function at time of enrollment). Study sites – located in Boston, Massachusetts (MA); Chicago, Illinois (IL); Southeast Michigan (MI); Los Angeles, California (CA); Newark, New Jersey (NJ); Pittsburgh, Pennsylvania (PA); and Oakland, CA – invited recruitment from white, black, Hispanic, Chinese and Japanese communities. All sites recruited white participants, four sites recruited black participants (MA, MI, IL, PA) and one site each recruited Chinese (Oakland, CA), Japanese (Los Angeles, CA) or Hispanic (NJ) participants. At baseline, the full study included 3302 women. Women were followed approximately annually for 13 visits with study participation at 74.5% by visit 13.

For this analysis, women were excluded if they had fewer than two perceived stress scores ($n = 253$) or experienced a pregnancy ($n = 5$) over follow-up. The final analytical sample included 3044 women. Data from the NJ site were truncated at visit five due to an interruption in site operations, affecting 108 white and all 212 Hispanic women.

### Variables
Age, self-reported race / ethnicity, educational attainment (less than high school, high school degree [or equivalent], college degree, post-college training) and smoking status (current smoker yes or no) were ascertained by questionnaire at baseline for all participants. Baseline financial hardship was estimated by self-report to the question: "How hard is it for you to pay for the very basics like food, housing, medical care, and heating". Available responses

were 'Very Hard', 'Somewhat Hard' and 'Not very hard at all'. Baseline physical measures including height (centimeters), weight (kilograms) and lightly-clothed waist circumference (in centimeters) were assessed by trained staff during the clinic visit. Body mass index (BMI) was calculated as weight (kg) divided by height (cm) squared.

Perceived stress was self-reported at each visit using the four-item Perceived Stress Scale questionnaire (PSS4) developed and validated by Cohen et al. [20, 24]. PSS4 questions included:

1. In the past two weeks, how often have you felt you were unable to control the important things in your life?
2. In the past two weeks, how often have you felt confident about your ability to handle your personal problems?
3. In the past two weeks, how often have you felt that things were going your way?
4. In the past two weeks, how often have you felt difficulties were piling up so high that you could not overcome them?

Participants indicated the frequency they experienced each of the four stressful situations using a 5-point Likert scale (1 = never, 2 = almost never, 3 = sometimes, 4 = fairly often, 5 = very often). For scoring total perceived stress, responses to negative questions were summed with the reverse of the responses to positive questions, yielding a composite score ranging from 4 to 20. Larger PSS4 scores indicated increased time experiencing stressful situations in the prior two weeks. Perceived stress questions were asked at baseline (year 0) and each follow-up visit, for a total of 13 possible measurements. The mean number of available perceived stress scores per woman was 10.2 (median: 12, range: 2–13); 15.6% had five or fewer perceived stress scores.

Menopausal status was assessed at each visit based on participant's report of menstrual irregularity [25] or complete cessation of cycles, plus self-reported information on hysterectomy and / or oophorectomy and current hormone use. Menopausal status was coded as premenopausal (menses has occurred in previous 3 months with no change in predictability over past 12 months), early perimenopausal (menses has occurred in previous 3 months, but with less predictability), late perimenopausal (menses has occurred in previous 12 months, but without menses in previous 3 months) or postmenopausal (no menses in past 12 months and / or both ovaries removed). Unknown menopausal status due to hormone use or hysterectomy was collapsed into a single 'unknown' category.

## Statistical analysis

Baseline descriptive information was compared for all participants and by baseline reported perceived stress level (categorized as low [≤ 25th percentile], moderate, high [≥ 75 percentile]). Women without a baseline PSS score ($n = 86$) were not included in analyses focused on stress at baseline, but were included in the longitudinal models of perceived stress. Logistic regression, adjusting for age, was used to assess the association of sociodemographic variables with high (versus low + moderate) perceived stress at baseline. To assess for potential bias due to selective loss of participants reporting higher baseline perceived stress, linear regression, adjusting for age, was used to test the difference in baseline perceived stress by loss to follow-up status over the 13 visits.

To guide modeling, change in mean perceived stress was first explored graphically by age, stratified by selected sociodemographic variables expected to contribute to perceived stress (race / ethnicity, educational attainment, baseline financial hardship, site of recruitment). For graphing crude means, age was truncated at 65 years (55 years for Hispanic women) to prevent leverage in slope estimation due to cohort attrition and the smaller numbers of women at the upper tail of the age distribution.

A linear mixed model was examined to understand the contribution of sociodemographic variables and menopausal status to change in perceived stress over time. Variables of interest were first reviewed individually for their effects on perceived stress. Model building was performed sequentially, using a forward stepwise approach, with statistical significance of added variables assessed by variable significance and model fit tested by Likelihood Ratio with alpha set to 0.05. Appropriateness of random effects in models were tested using restricted maximum likelihood and mixed effects were tested using maximum likelihood. An unstructured variance-covariate matrix was assumed. All models incorporated race / ethnicity and age, centered at 42 years, as a time-varying variable and included a random slope for age. Potential interactions of longitudinal age with sociodemographic variables were evaluated to assess differences in slope. Additional interactions with race / ethnicity and socio-economic variables were assessed in separate models, but small cell sizes resulted in model instability.

Final models were assessed for appropriate specification by review of the errors from the random effects (age) as well as the conditional errors for the fixed effects. All errors were assessed for normality graphically. All graphing and statistics were performed using SAS version 9.4 (SAS Institute, Cary, NC).

## Results

### Baseline characteristics

At baseline, the 3044 women eligible for this analysis were a mean age of 46.4 years (range: 42.0–53.0 years) with a racial / ethnic distribution of 47.4% white, 28.7% black, 8.9% Japanese, 8.0% Chinese and 7.0% Hispanic (Table 1). The majority of the cohort (> 90%) had obtained at least a high school degree while 44.1% had attained a college degree or higher. Financial difficulty was reported by nearly 40% of women, with 8.7% reporting that it was 'very hard' to pay for the basics of living. Among the 2958 women reporting perceived stress at baseline, mean perceived stress score was 8.5 (median: 8.0, range: 4–19). Characteristics of 86 women without a baseline perceived stress score are available in Additional file 1: Table S1.

At baseline, Hispanic women were significantly more likely to report high perceived stress as compared to any other race / ethnicity (all comparisons $p < 0.0001$), while Chinese women were significantly less likely to report high stress ($p < 0.0001$ for white, black and Hispanic women, $p = 0.0185$ for Japanese women) (Table 1). Women reporting higher levels of financial hardship were more likely to report high perceived stress than

**Table 1** Population characteristics by baseline perceived stress score

| | N | Overall (n = 3044) | Category of Baseline Perceived Stress[a][b] | | |
| | | | Low (n = 844) | Moderate (n = 1352) | High (n = 762) |
| --- | --- | --- | --- | --- | --- |
| Perceived Stress[c] | 2958 | 8.5 ± 2.9 | 5.1 ± 0.8 | 8.5 ± 1.1 | 12.4 ± 1.5 |
| Age[c] | 3044 | 46.4 ± 2.7 | 46.3 ± 2.7 | 46.4 ± 2.7 | 46.2 ± 2.7 |
| Race / Ethnicity (%) | | | | | |
| White | 1443 | – | 29.1 | 48.1 | 22.8 |
| Black | 874 | – | 32.3 | 39.0 | 28.7 |
| Hispanic | 212 | – | 18.0 | 31.0 | 51.0 |
| Japanese | 272 | – | 22.7 | 54.6 | 22.7 |
| Chinese | 243 | – | 26.3 | 59.4 | 14.3 |
| Education (%) | | | | | |
| Less than High School | 191 | – | 15.4 | 35.1 | 49.5 |
| High School | 1496 | – | 26.6 | 44.0 | 29.3 |
| College Degree | 627 | – | 30.0 | 48.5 | 21.5 |
| Post-College | 705 | – | 34.5 | 49.9 | 15.6 |
| Difficulty paying for Basics (%) | | | | | |
| Very Hard | 263 | – | 10.0 | 38.6 | 51.4 |
| Somewhat Hard | 899 | – | 17.4 | 44.2 | 38.5 |
| Not hard | 1865 | – | 36.5 | 47.3 | 16.2 |
| Site of Recruitment (%) | | | | | |
| PA | 439 | – | 29.9 | 42.8 | 27.3 |
| MI | 503 | – | 30.7 | 40.0 | 29.3 |
| MA | 424 | – | 25.1 | 51.6 | 23.4 |
| IL | 433 | – | 34.4 | 41.8 | 23.8 |
| Oakland, CA | 442 | – | 27.1 | 54.9 | 18.1 |
| Los Angeles, CA | 483 | – | 30.4 | 50.7 | 18.9 |
| NJ | 320 | – | 18.7 | 36.0 | 45.3 |
| Smoking Status (%) | | | | | |
| Non-Smoker | 2522 | – | 29.0 | 47.6 | 23.4 |
| Smoker | 498 | – | 26.6 | 36.5 | 36.9 |
| BMI (kg/m$^2$)[c] | 3009 | 28.2 ± 7.2 | 27.9 ± 6.8 | 27.9 ± 7.1 | 29.3 ± 7.8 |
| Waist Circumference (cm)[c] | 3012 | 86.1 ± 16.1 | 85.4 ± 15.6 | 85.6 ± 15.7 | 88.7 ± 17.2 |

[a]Categorical variable *rows* sum to 100%. Numbers may not sum to 100 due to rounding
[b]Note that 86 women had missing baseline PSS4 scores
[c]Mean ± SD

women reporting some or no financial hardship ($p$ = 0.0003 and < 0.0001, respectively); and women without a high school diploma were significantly more likely to report high perceived stress than women with a high school diploma, college or other advanced degree (all $p$ < 0.0001). Likewise, women who were current smokers were more likely to report high levels of perceived stress as compared to women who were not ($p$ < 0.0001), and women with increased BMI or waist circumference were also more likely to report high perceived stress ($p$ < 0.0001 for each).

### Perceived stress and increasing age

Mean cohort age increased to 62.0 years at the 13th follow-up visit while unadjusted mean perceived stress scores declined by − 0.06 ± 0.00 points with each increased year of age. No difference was seen in baseline perceived stress between women retained and those who died or were lost to follow-up (8.4 ± 2.9 vs 8.5 ± 3.0, respectively, $p$ = 0.38). Trajectories for change in perceived stress with age are displayed in Fig. 1a-d, by race / ethnicity, educational attainment, financial hardship, and site of recruitment. Corresponding with the baseline results, women with less educational attainment, women reporting increased financial hardship and women recruited from NJ had higher mean reported levels of perceived stress than their counterparts. In addition, mean perceived stress was observed to decline with age across all sociodemographic categories with the exception of Hispanic women.

Unadjusted regressions for each variable and the final multivariable regression model evaluating the effects of age, menopausal status, race / ethnicity, educational attainment, baseline financial hardship and site of recruitment on longitudinal change in perceived stress are displayed in Table 2. In the final multivariate regression model, women reporting financial hardship and with lesser attained education reported significantly higher levels of perceived stress at baseline as compared to women reporting no financial hardship or training beyond a college degree. Only Japanese race / ethnicity remained as a statistically significant predictor of higher perceived stress after adjustment for financial hardship and educational attainment. Interactions between financial strain and age suggested that moderate and severe baseline financial hardship were associated with a steeper decline in perceived stress over time as compared to no financial hardship. Though mean reported perceived stress decreased over time for most women, for white and Hispanic women located in NJ, perceived stress increased (0.07 ± 0.03 points with each increased year of age) over the five available visits for this site. For interpretation purposes, within this cohort a 42-year-old white woman living near Pittsburgh, with a high school

diploma and no reported baseline financial hardship (the 'reference category') had a perceived stress score of 7.93, that decreased by 0.10 points over each increasing year of age. In comparison, a Japanese woman of the same age, living near Los Angeles, with a high school education and no baseline financial hardship, reported a perceived stress of 8.17 that decreased by 0.01 points each year, and a Hispanic woman of the same age, living near New Jersey, without a high school education and no baseline financial hardship had a mean perceived stress score of 8.05 that increased by 0.11 points each year.

When menopausal status was added to the final adjusted model with longitudinal age, model fit increased significantly (Likelihood Ratio $p$ < 0.00001). Results suggested that progression through each stage of the menopausal transition (from pre-menopause onward) was associated with a further decrease in perceived stress, however the menopausal status variable did not reach statistical significance ($p$ = 0.5203; data not shown) and thus was omitted from the final model.

### Discussion

This study is one of the first to describe longitudinal change in perceived stress levels in a multi-ethnic sample of midlife women in the United States. Mean levels of self-reported stress, as measured annually by Cohen's Perceived Stress Scale, decreased for most women as they transitioned across the midlife. Compared to similar black, white and Chinese women within SWAN, mean levels of perceived stress decreased in a more attenuated fashion for Japanese women, but increased over time for white and Hispanic women living in New Jersey. In addition, women with lower educational attainment, and in particular, baseline financial hardship, consistently reported higher levels of perceived stress, though this difference diminished with time. After adjustment for other sociodemographic variables, race / ethnicity was a significant predictor of increased perceived stress for only Japanese women. Changing menopausal status did not play a significant role in change in perceived stress after adjustment for age and sociodemographic factors.

Cross-sectional studies performed both in the United States and the United Kingdom have suggested that perceived stress decreases with age. A 1983 population-based survey of adults in the United States reported a mean PSS4 of 4.9 ± 3.0 for adults ages 18–29 years, 4.4 ± 2.9 for adults ages 45–54 years and 4.0 ± 3.0 for adults ages 65 years and older using a 0–15 scale (corresponding to mean PSS4 scores of 8.9, 8.4 and 8.0, respectively, on the 4–20 scale used here) [20]. Reported perceived stress was higher among women compared to men, Hispanics and blacks as compared to whites, and increased with lower annual income and educational attainment. Similarly, a more recent cross-sectional review

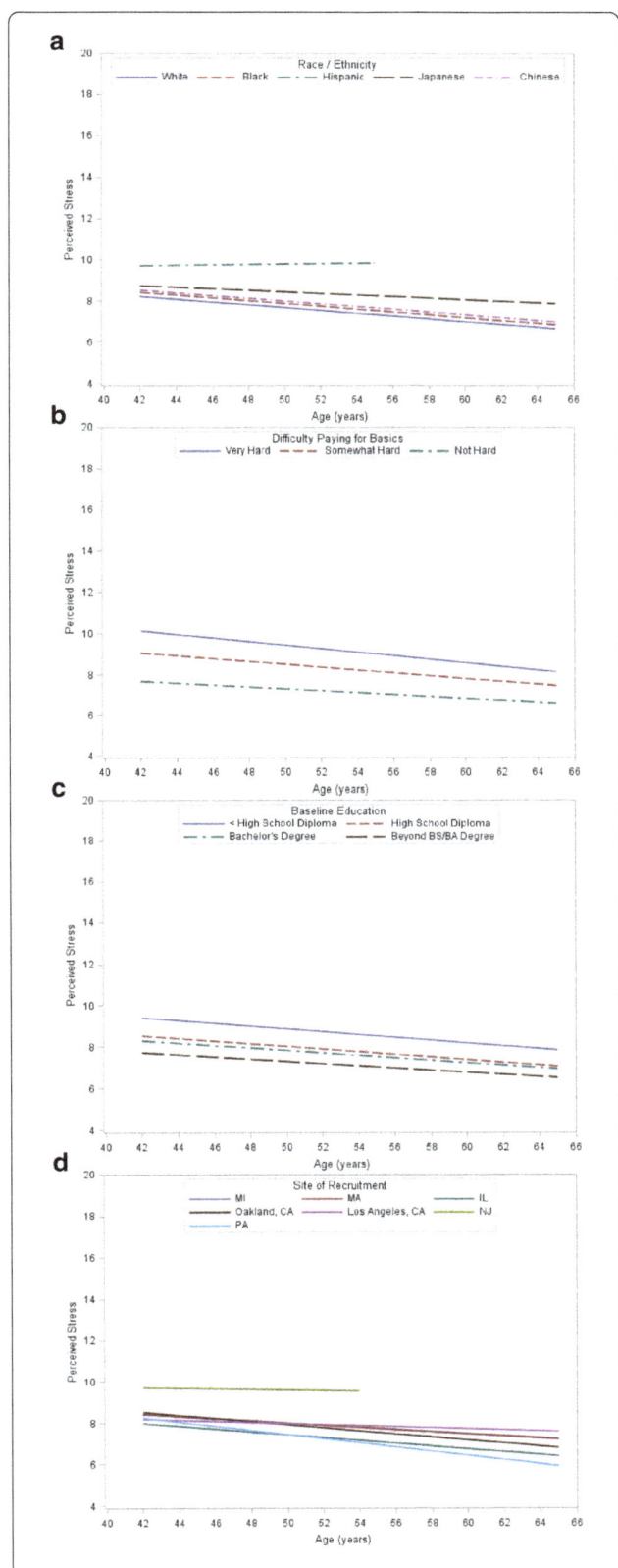

**Fig. 1** Change in perceived stress over age; age is truncated at 65 years (55 years for Hispanic women) to prevent leverage due to cohort attrition and small numbers. Note the data truncation due to New Jersey site limitation. **a** Race / ethnicity includes all eligible women. **b** Baseline difficulty paying for the basics; New Jersey participants omitted. **c** Baseline education; New Jersey participants omitted. **d** Site of recruitment includes all eligible women

of reported perceived stress from individuals ages 16–85 years living in the United Kingdom indicated that younger age, female sex, reduced social support and black, Asian (Indian, Pakistani, Bangladeshi, other) or mixed (as compared to white) race were associated with higher PSS4 scores [21].

While the unadjusted results indicated that women of non-white ethnicity or with lower socioeconomic means tended to report higher perceived stress, supporting the findings from the above referenced studies, the *adjusted* analyses presented here indicated that black women and Hispanic women reported lower perceived stress at baseline as compared to similar white, Japanese and Chinese women in SWAN. Although these differences did not reach statistical significance, our findings are in contrast to studies of SWAN participants that indicate that black women (in particular) and Chinese women report higher levels of perceived discrimination and unfair treatment than their peers, and that these reports are tied to increased biological stress reactivity and decreased mental and physical health [26–28]. This paradox – lower perceived stress reports among subgroups showing higher biological response to stressors – may be explained by a tendency for women with lower social standing to internalize and normalize stressors that are experienced frequently [29–31]. For example, Lee and Bierman found that, in older adults experiencing discrimination, decreased social status was associated with fewer outward expressions of anger, but more suppressed or internalized experiences of anger; the authors theorized that anger suppression was a coping mechanism and a method to de-escalate potentially dangerous situations [30]. These finding with the SWAN cohort are intriguing and warrant further investigation.

In further comparison to the cross-sectional studies, the work presented here indicates that there are variations in the rate of change of perceived stress in some subgroups of women and, moreover, that not all individuals experience decreases over time. The faster rate of decrease in perceived stress scores for women initially in the higher categories of baseline financial hardship may be due to alleviation of the stressor as women age into retirement [32] or may reflect acute baseline financial stressors associated with only temporary increases in perceived stress. Conversely, the results may reflect selective cohort loss over time among women reporting

**Table 2** Unadjusted and fully adjusted random effects model explaining perceived stress over increasing age

| | Unadjusted Parameters | | Fully Adjusted Model* | |
| --- | --- | --- | --- | --- |
| | β (95% CI) | P (Type 3) | β (95% CI) | P (Type 3) |
| Intercept | – | – | 7.93 (7.65, 8.20) | – |
| Age | −0.06 (−0.07, −0.06) | < 0.0001 | −0.10 (−0.12, −0.08) | < 0.0001 |
| Race / Ethnicity | | < 0.0001 | | < 0.0001 |
| White | REF | | REF | |
| Black | 0.16 (−0.02, 0.35) | | −0.06 (−0.26, 0.14) | |
| Hispanic | 2.06 (1.73, 2.39) | | −0.33 (−0.86, 0.20) | |
| Japanese | 0.71 (0.43, 0.99) | | 0.84 (0.47, 1.21) | |
| Chinese | 0.31 (0.01, 0.61) | | 0.28 (−0.11, 0.67) | |
| Difficulty paying for Basics (%) | | < 0.0001 | | < 0.0001 |
| Not hard | REF | | REF | |
| Somewhat Hard | 1.26 (1.09, 1.43) | | 1.28 (1.06, 1.51) | |
| Very Hard | 2.20 (1.92, 2.48) | | 2.37 (2.00, 2.74) | |
| Education | | < 0.0001 | | 0.0016 |
| Less than High School | 1.37 (1.03, 1.71) | | 0.34 (−0.02, 0.69) | |
| High School | REF | | REF | |
| College Degree | −0.23 (−0.43, −0.02) | | −0.02 (−0.22, 0.18) | |
| Post-College Degree | −0.79 (−0.99, −0.60) | | −0.32 (−0.52, −0.12) | |
| Site of Recruitment | | < 0.0001 | | 0.0487 |
| PA | REF | | REF | |
| MI | 0.67 (0.40, 0.95) | | −0.20 (−0.54, 0.15) | |
| MA | 0.59 (0.3, 0.87) | | 0.01 (−0.34, 0.37) | |
| IL | 0.02 (−0.27, 0.31) | | −0.04 (−0.40, 0.32) | |
| Oakland, CA | 0.44 (0.15, 0.72) | | 0.03 (−0.39, 0.44) | |
| Los Angeles, CA | 0.61 (0.33, 0.89) | | −0.59 (−0.99, −0.18) | |
| NJ | 2.21 (1.89, 2.53) | | 0.11 (−0.47, 0.70) | |
| Menopausal Status | | < 0.0001 | – | – |
| Pre | REF | | – | – |
| Early peri | −0.20 (−0.29, −0.10) | | – | – |
| Late peri | −0.30 (−0.42, −0.17) | | – | – |
| Post | −0.67 (−0.76, −0.58) | | – | – |
| Unknown | −0.33 (−0.47, −0.20) | | – | – |
| Age * Difficulty paying for Basics Interaction | – | – | | < 0.0001 |
| Age*Not hard | – | – | REF | |
| Age*Somewhat Hard | – | – | −0.02 (−0.04, −0.01) | |
| Age*Very Hard | – | – | −0.05 (−0.08, −0.02) | |
| Age * Site Interaction | – | – | | |
| Age*PA | – | – | REF | < 0.0001 |
| Age*MI | – | – | 0.08 (0.05, 0.10) | |
| Age*MA | – | – | 0.06 (0.03, 0.08) | |
| Age*IL | – | – | 0.02 (−0.00, 0.05) | |
| Age*Oakland, CA | – | – | 0.04 (0.02, 0.07) | |
| Age*Los Angeles, CA | – | – | 0.09 (0.06, 0.11) | |
| Age*NJ | – | – | 0.21 (0.16, 0.26) | |

*The multivariate model includes all variables listed; menopausal status was not statistically significant (*p* > 0.05) in the final model higher financial hardship, although mean baseline perceived stress scores did not vary by attrition status. Curiously, while our results indicate that perceived stress decreased for all women to some varying degree as they aged across the midlife, Hispanic and white women living in or near Newark, NJ reported increasing perceived stress over the course of their five visits from baseline. Due to the interruption of activities at the NJ site, it is impossible to determine whether the observed perceived stress trajectory would have continued to increase or reverse course over the remaining 8 visits. Notably, the fifth follow-up occurred primarily in 2001/2002, and results may have been influenced by the World Trade Center bombing in September 2001 [33]. Moreover, as Hispanic women were recruited only from this site, it is impossible to disentangle the site effect from the experience of being a midlife Hispanic woman in the United States.

Our results found no increase in perceived stress associated with changing menopausal status after adjustment for aging and sociodemographic characteristics. These findings are in contrast to existing cross-sectional work and some longitudinal work suggesting that the menopausal transition is associated with higher stress and depression. Freeman et al. found that higher perceived stress was independently associated with higher menopausal symptom severity including: hot flushes, poor sleep quality, depression and general aches and stiffness [34]. Though these findings are intriguing, they excluded assessment of general socioeconomic status – obscuring the role of general life stressors during the experience of menopause [35]. More recently, when adjusting for study visit, Falconi et al. found that early and late perimenopause were significantly associated with increases in perceived stress [36], but they did not adjust for age or sociodemographic indicators. Prior publications have indicated that women who proceed through menopause at an earlier age are socioeconomically disadvantaged [37–39] and already prone to increased life stress [40]. Woods et al., in longitudinal analyses from the Seattle Midlife Women's Study, which included predominately white women but adjusted for age, found that factors such as employment and health status, but also pre-existing mood disturbances, were the only significant predictors of perceived stress over a decade, and not the menopausal transition itself [41]. Our findings are consistent with Woods et al. as we found that the role of socioeconomic factors such as educational attainment, employment and financial hardship were stronger predictors of perceived stress over midlife than the menopausal transition itself in this larger, more diverse sample of midlife women. These findings may suggest that women experience the menopausal transition as a series of acute stressors (e.g., hot flashes, sleep disturbances) that

can be attenuated by chronic, socioeconomic-based life stressors, however further work would be necessary to substantiate this theory.

Explanations for the observed decreases in perceived stress with age are suggestive yet incomplete. Research suggests that older adults show more maturity and regulation of emotion [42, 43], leading to increased feelings of optimism and fewer symptoms of psychological distress than younger adults [44, 45], however the cross-sectional nature of most extant studies can not rule out a cohort effect based on era of birth. Beyond changes in the appraisal and regulation of stress, changing life roles with age, such as retirement or the relinquishment of parenting, may lead to the occurrence of fewer stressful events even as individual health may be declining [46]. Focus groups performed with women in the United States suggest that the midlife is a time of reduced child-rearing responsibilities leading to role restructuring, more control over one's time, and an increased sense of personal power and freedom [47–50] – concepts embedded in Cohen's Perceived Stress Scale. Finally, recent longitudinal work performed by Lachman et al. for the Midlife in the United States (MIDUS) study shows that life satisfaction significantly increases across the midlife decades (4th to 5th, 5th to 6th decades) [5], again corresponding with the decreases in perceived stress seen in this work.

Despite the decreasing perception of stress with age, individuals who report relatively greater stress at the start of the midlife continue to report higher stress levels as they age, an important finding given that more highly stressed individuals are at greater health risk than their less-stressed peers. Arnold et al. found that high or moderate baseline perceived stress increased mortality risk for adults hospitalized with acute myocardial infarction (high/moderate vs. low PSS4 score: aHR = 1.42 [95% CI = 1.15–1.76]) [51]. Investigators for the REGARDS study found that, for individuals with household incomes < \$35,000/ yr., baseline PSS4 score was associated with all-cause mortality risk (high vs. no stress: aOR = 1.55 [95%CI: 1.31–1.82]), and marginally associated with incident coronary heart disease (high vs. no stress: aOR = 1.29 [95%CI: 0.99–1.69]) [52]. Similarly, Aggarwal et al. identified increased baseline perceived stress, as measured by a modified 'PSS6' score, to be predictive of future cerebral infarct in older adults (high vs. low PSS6 score: aOR = 1.94, 95% CI = 1.11–3.40) [53]. As individuals in lower socioeconomic and sociocultural strata are more at risk of adverse health outcomes such as diabetes, stroke and myocardial infarct [54–59], it is plausible that individual perception and internal assimilation of stress is one of many factors directly influencing health [60]. Future work will assess whether the women of SWAN who report higher perceived stress, and lower socioeconomic means, are more at risk of adverse outcomes.

The primary limitation of this study was our limited ability to understand perceived stress among women reporting the highest levels over time. Hispanic women, women reporting extreme financial hardship at baseline, and those with the least education, each comprised less than 10% of the study sample, limiting power and preventing analyses to disentangle potential interactions among these subgroups. Similarly, the disruption of operations at the NJ site, a site situated to recruit Hispanic women and women of lower socioeconomic means, prevented a complete review of change in reported perceived stress over time at that site. Only baseline financial hardship was assessed in these models as it was not measured at every follow-up visit. Fluctuating hardship levels may explain additional variability over time. It is also worth noting that we are ascribing self-reports of perceived stress over a two-week period to women's perceptions over the course of a year, ruling out a detailed assessment of stress that women may feel on a day-to-day basis. This broader view of stress, in addition to our exploration of menopausal *stages* versus menopausal *symptoms*, may have precluded the assessment of the impact of stressors that fluctuate on a daily basis, such as from vasomotor symptoms. Finally, we have chosen to review and model mean change over time, which may obscure subtle differences in trajectories of stress that are non-linear; a subject worth further exploration. Nonetheless, the analyses presented, incorporating the diverse cohort from the SWAN longitudinal study, provide important information about stress over the midlife and menopausal transition.

## Conclusion

In conclusion, this study found that the perception of stress decreased over time for the majority of this diverse set of midlife women in the United States. Perceived stress increased for the Hispanic and white women recruited from New Jersey, and was consistently greater among women with lesser education attainment and women experiencing financial difficulty. Concomitant with the increased reporting of stress, those with higher stress were more likely to smoke and have higher BMIs at baseline. While we are limited to observing the change in stress over the thirteen years of study – and solely within women – our results add credence to the original surveys performed by Cohen et al. [20, 24], and provide further evidence that decreases in stress are truly age-related and not related to era of birth. Future work is necessary to further explore the stress experience for women in the United States, especially as it varies by racial / ethnic identity, but also to assess longitudinal trajectories of stress that are non-linear or unchanging over time, change with changing life roles, and to tie the observed perceived stress differences with adverse mental and clinical outcomes.

## Acknowledgements
We thank all the women who participated in SWAN and the study personnel at each site.
Clinical Centers: University of Michigan, Ann Arbor – Siobán Harlow, PI 2011 – present, MaryFran Sowers, PI 1994-2011; Massachusetts General Hospital, Boston, MA – Joel Finkelstein, PI 1999 – present; Robert Neer, PI 1994 – 1999; Rush University, Rush University Medical Center, Chicago, IL – Howard Kravitz, PI 2009 – present; Lynda Powell, PI 1994 – 2009; University of California, Davis/Kaiser – Ellen Gold, PI; University of California, Los Angeles – Gail Greendale, PI; Albert Einstein College of Medicine, Bronx, NY – Carol Derby, PI 2011 – present, Rachel Wildman, PI 2010 – 2011; Nanette Santoro, PI 2004 – 2010; University of Medicine and Dentistry – New Jersey Medical School, Newark – Gerson Weiss, PI 1994 – 2004; and the University of Pittsburgh, Pittsburgh, PA – Karen Matthews, PI.
NIH Program Office: National Institute on Aging, Bethesda, MD – Chhanda Dutta 2016- present; Winifred Rossi 2012–2016; Sherry Sherman 1994 – 2012; Marcia Ory 1994 – 2001; National Institute of Nursing Research, Bethesda, MD – Program Officers.
Central Laboratory: University of Michigan, Ann Arbor – Daniel McConnell (Central Ligand Assay Satellite Services).
SWAN Repository: University of Michigan, Ann Arbor – Siobán Harlow 2013 - Present; Dan McConnell 2011 - 2013; MaryFran Sowers 2000 - 2011.
Coordinating Center: University of Pittsburgh, Pittsburgh, PA – Maria Mori Brooks, PI 2012 - present; Kim Sutton-Tyrrell, PI 2001 – 2012; New England Research Institutes, Watertown, MA - Sonja McKinlay, PI 1995 – 2001.
Steering Committee: Susan Johnson, Current Chair; Chris Gallagher, Former Chair.

## Funding
The Study of Women's Health Across the Nation (SWAN) has grant support from the National Institutes of Health (NIH), DHHS, through the National Institute on Aging (NIA), the National Institute of Nursing Research (NINR) and the NIH Office of Research on Women's Health (ORWH) (Grants U01NR004061; U01AG012505, U01AG012535, U01AG012531, U01AG012539, U01AG012546, U01AG012553, U01AG012554, U01AG012495). The content of this article is solely the responsibility of the authors and does not necessarily represent the official views of the NIA, NINR, ORWH or the NIH. SDH gratefully acknowledge use of the services and facilities of the Population Studies Center at the University of Michigan, funded by NICHD Center Grant R24 HD041028.
The National Institute of Aging and National Institute of Nursing Research program officers participated in the design of the SWAN study. They were not involved in the data analysis, interpretation of data or writing of this manuscript.

## Authors' contributions
EH conducted the literature review and data analyses, and had primary responsibility for the drafting the manuscript. SDH and CKG made substantial contributions to the design and oversaw the data analyses. All authors contributed to the critical review and revision of the manuscript for intellectual content. All authors read and approved the final manuscript.

## Competing interests
The authors declare that they have no competing interests.

## Author details
[1]Department of Epidemiology, School of Public Health, University of Michigan, 6610B SPH I, 1415 Washington Heights, Ann Arbor, MI 48109-2029, USA. [2]School of Kinesiology, School of Public Health, University of Michigan, Ann Arbor, USA. [3]Department of Internal Medicine, School of Public Health, University of Michigan, Ann Arbor, USA.

## References
1. Lachman ME. Development in Midlife. Annu Rev Psychol. 2004;55:305–31.
2. Woods NF, Mitchell ES. Women's images of midlife: observations from the Seattle midlife women's health study. Health Care Women Int. 1997;18:439–53.
3. Ward BW, Schiller JS, Goodman RA. Multiple chronic conditions among US adults: a 2012 update. Prev Chronic Dis. 2014;11 https://doi.org/10.5888/pcd11.130389.
4. Brim OG, Ryff CD, Kessler RC, editors. How healthy are we?: a national study of well-being at midlife. Chicago: University of Chicago Press; 2004.
5. Lachman ME, Teshale S, Agrigoroaei S. Midlife as a pivotal period in the life course: balancing growth and decline at the crossroads of youth and old age. Int J Behav Dev. 2015;39:20–31.

6. Williams K, Kurina LM. The social structure, stress, and women's health. Clin Obstet Gynecol. 2002;45:1099–118.

7. Jacobsen L, Mather M, Dupuis G. Household change in the United States. Popul Bull. 2012;67 http://www.prb.org/Publications/Reports/2012/us-household-change.aspx. Accessed 23 Oct 2016

8. Fry R. For first time in modern era, living with parents edges out other living arrangements for 18- to 34-year-olds. Washington, D.C.: Pew Research Center; 2016. http://www.pewsocialtrends.org/2016/05/24/for-first-time-in-modern-era-living-with-parents-edges-out-other-living-arrangements-for-18-to-34-year-olds/. Accessed 27 Sep 2016

9. Amick BC, Kawachi I, Coakley EH, Lerner D, Levine S, Colditz GA. Relationship of job strain and iso-strain to health status in a cohort of women in the United States. Scand J Work Environ Health. 1998;24:54–61.

10. Lundberg U, Frankenhaeuser M. Stress and workload of men and women in high-ranking positions. J Occup Health Psychol. 1999;4:142–51.

11. Woods NF, Mitchell ES. Symptoms during the perimenopause: prevalence, severity, trajectory, and significance in women's lives. Am J Med. 2005; 118(Suppl 12B):14–24.

12. Davis SR, Castelo-Branco C, Chedraui P, Lumsden MA, Nappi RE, Shah D, et al. Understanding weight gain at menopause. Climacteric J Int Menopause Soc. 2012;15:419–29.

13. Hall JE. Endocrinology of the menopause. Endocrinol Metab Clin N Am. 2015;44:485–96.

14. Santoro N, Epperson CN, Mathews SB. Menopausal symptoms and their management. Endocrinol Metab Clin N Am. 2015;44:497–515.

15. Freund AM, Ritter JO. Midlife crisis: a debate. Gerontology. 2009;55:582–91.

16. Mroczek DK, Kolarz CM. The effect of age on positive and negative affect: a developmental perspective on happiness. J Pers Soc Psychol. 1998;75:1333–49.

17. Mroczek D. Positive and negative affect at midlife. In: Brim OG, Ryff CD, Kessler RC, editors. How healthy are we?: a national study of well-being at midlife. Chicago, IL: University of Chicago Press; 2004. p. 205–26.

18. Avis NE, Assmann SF, Kravitz HM, Ganz PA, Ory M. Quality of life in diverse groups of midlife women: assessing the influence of menopause, health status and psychosocial and demographic factors. Qual Life Res Int J Qual Life Asp Treat Care Rehabil. 2004;13:933–46.

19. Fleeson W. The quality of American life at the end of the century. In: Brim O, Ryff C, Kessler R, editors. How healthy are we?: a National Study of well-being at midlife. Chicago, IL: University of Chicago Press; 2004. p. 252–72.

20. Cohen S. Perceived stress in a probability sample of the United States. In: The social psychology of health. Newbury Park, Calif: sage publications; 1988. p. 31–67.

21. Warttig SL, Forshaw MJ, South J, White AK. New, normative, English-sample data for the short form perceived stress scale (PSS-4). J Health Psychol. 2013;18:1617–28.

22. Dennerstein L, Guthrie JR, Clark M, Lehert P, Henderson VW. A population-based study of depressed mood in middle-aged. Australian-born women Menopause N Y N. 2004;11:563–8.

23. Sowers M, Crawford SL, Sternfeld B, Morganstein D, Gold E, Greendale G, et al. SWAN: a multicenter, multiethnic, community-based cohort study of women and the menopausal transition. In: Lobo RA, Kelsey JL, Marcus R, editors. Menopause: biology and pathobiology. San Diego, CA: Academic Press; 2000. p. 175–88.

24. Cohen S, Kamarck T, Mermelstein R. A global measure of perceived stress. J Health Soc Behav. 1983;24:385–96.

25. Brambilla DJ, McKinlay SM, Johannes CB. Defining the perimenopause for application in epidemiologic investigations. Am J Epidemiol. 1994;140:1091–5.

26. Guyll M, Matthews KA, Bromberger JT. Discrimination and unfair treatment: relationship to cardiovascular reactivity among African American and European American women. Health Psychol Off J Div Health Psychol Am Psychol Assoc. 2001;20:315–25.

27. Brown J, Matthews KA, Bromberger JT, Chang Y. The relation between perceived unfair treatment and blood pressure in a racially/ethnically diverse sample of women. Am J Epidemiol. 2006;164:257–62.

28. Pascoe EA, Smart Richman L. Perceived discrimination and health: a meta-analytic review. Psychol Bull. 2009;135:531–54.

29. Thomas SA, González-Prendes AA. Powerlessness, anger, and stress in African American women: implications for physical and emotional health. Health Care Women Int. 2009;30:93–113.

30. Lee Y, Bierman A. A longitudinal assessment of perceived discrimination and maladaptive expressions of anger among older adults: does subjective social power buffer the association? J Gerontol. Series B, Psychol Sci Soc Sci. 2016.

31. Krieger N. Discrimination and health inequities. Int J Health Serv Plan Adm Eval. 2014;44:643–710.

32. van der Heide I, van Rijn RM, Robroek SJ, Burdorf A, Proper KI. Is retirement good for your health? A systematic review of longitudinal studies. BMC Public Health. 2013;13 https://doi.org/10.1186/1471-2458-13-1180.

33. Silver RC, Holman EA, McIntosh DN, Poulin M, Gil-Rivas V. Nationwide longitudinal study of psychological responses to September 11. JAMA. 2002;288:1235–44.

34. Freeman EW, Sammel MD, Lin H, Gracia CR, Pien GW, Nelson DB, et al. Symptoms associated with menopausal transition and reproductive hormones in midlife women. Obstet Gynecol. 2007;110(2 Pt 1):230–40.

35. Nosek M, Kennedy HP, Beyene Y, Taylor D, Gilliss C, Lee K. The effects of perceived stress and attitudes toward menopause and aging on symptoms of menopause. J Midwifery Womens Health. 2010;55:328–34.

36. Falconi AM, Gold EB, Janssen I. The longitudinal relation of stress during the menopausal transition to fibrinogen concentrations: results from the study of Women's health across the nation. Menopause N Y N. 2016;23:518–27.

37. Stanford JL, Hartge P, Brinton LA, Hoover RN, Brookmeyer R. Factors influencing the age at natural menopause. J Chronic Dis. 1987;40:995–1002.

38. Gold EB. Factors associated with age at natural menopause in a multiethnic sample of midlife women. Am J Epidemiol. 2001;153:865⁻74.

39. Gold EB, Crawford SL, Avis NE, Crandall CJ, Matthews KA, Waetjen LE, et al. Factors related to age at natural menopause: longitudinal analyses from SWAN. Am J Epidemiol. 2013;178:70–83.

40. Bromberger JT, Matthews KA, Kuller LH, Wing RR, Meilahn EN, Plantinga P. Prospective study of the determinants of age at menopause. Am J Epidemiol. 1997;145:124–33.

41. Woods NF, Mitchell ES, Percival DB, Smith-DiJulio K. Is the menopausal transition stressful? Observations of perceived stress from the Seattle midlife Women's health study. Menopause N Y N. 2009;16:90–7.

42. Boeninger DK, Shiraishi RW, Aldwin CM, Spiro A. Why do older men report low stress ratings? Findings from the veterans affairs normative aging study. Int J Aging Hum Dev. 2009;68:149–70.

43. Brummer L, Stopa L, Bucks R. The influence of age on emotion regulation strategies and psychological distress. Behav Cogn Psychother. 2014;42:668–81.

44. Lawton MP, Kleban MH, Rajagopal D, Dean J. Dimensions of affective experience in three age groups. Psychol Aging. 1992;7:171–84.

45. Chang E. Optimism–pessimism and stress appraisal: testing a cognitive interactive model of psychological adjustment in adults. Cogn Ther Res. 2002;26:675–90.

46. Aldwin CM, Sutton KJ, Chiara G, Spiro A. Age differences in stress, coping, and appraisal: findings from the normative aging study. J Gerontol B Psychol Sci Soc Sci. 1996;51:P179–88.

47. Berg JA, Taylor DL. Symptom responses of midlife Filipina Americans. Menopause N Y N. 1999;6:115–21.

48. Sampselle CM, Harris V, Harlow SD, Sowers M. Midlife development and menopause in African American and Caucasian women. Health Care Women Int. 2002;23:351–63.

49. Kagawa-Singer M, Wu K, Kawanishi Y, Greendale GA, Kim S, Adler SR, et al. Comparison of the menopause and midlife transition between Japanese American and European American women. Med Anthropol Q. 2002;16:64–91.

50. Villarruel AM, Harlow SD, Lopez M, Sowers M. El cambio de Vida: conceptualizations of menopause and midlife among urban Latina women. Res Theory Nurs Pract. 2002;16:91–102.

51. Arnold SV, Smolderen KG, Buchanan DM, Li Y, Spertus JA. Perceived stress in myocardial infarction: long-term mortality and health status outcomes. J Am Coll Cardiol. 2012;60:1756–63.

52. Redmond N, Richman J, Gamboa CM, Albert MA, Sims M, Durant RW, et al. Perceived stress is associated with incident coronary heart disease and all-cause mortality in low- but not high-income participants in the reasons for geographic and racial differences in stroke study. J Am Heart Assoc. 2013;2: e000447.

53. Aggarwal NT, Clark CJ, Beck TL, Mendes de Leon CF, DeCarli C, Evans DA, et al. Perceived stress is associated with subclinical cerebrovascular disease in older adults. Am J Geriatr Psychiatry Off J Am Assoc Geriatr Psychiatry. 2014; 22:53–62.

54. Salomaa V, Niemela M, Miettinen H, Ketonen M, Immonen-Raiha P, Koskinen S, et al. Relationship of socioeconomic status to the incidence and prehospital, 28-day, and 1-year mortality rates of acute coronary events in the FINMONICA myocardial infarction register study. Circulation. 2000;101:1913–8.

56.  Krishnan S, Cozier YC, Rosenberg L, Palmer JR. Socioeconomic status and
     incidence of type 2 diabetes: results from the black Women's health study.
     Am J Epidemiol. 2010;171:564–70.
57.  Addo J, Ayerbe L, Mohan KM, Crichton S, Sheldenkar A, Chen R, et al.
     Socioeconomic status and stroke: an updated review. Stroke. 2012;43:
     1186–91.
58.  Hasson RE, Adam TC, Pearson J, Davis JN, Spruijt-Metz D, Goran MI. Sociocultural
     and socioeconomic influences on type 2 diabetes risk in overweight/obese
     African-American and Latino-American children and adolescents. J Obes. 2013;
     2013:1–9.
59.  Schneiderman N, Llabre M, Cowie CC, Barnhart J, Carnethon M, Gallo LC, et al.
     Prevalence of diabetes among Hispanics/Latinos from diverse backgrounds:
     the Hispanic community health study/study of Latinos (HCHS/SOL). Diabetes
     Care. 2014;37:2233–9.
60.  Marshall IJ, Wang Y, Crichton S, McKevitt C, Rudd AG, Wolfe CDA. The effects of
     socioeconomic status on stroke risk and outcomes. Lancet Neurol. 2015;14:
     1206–18.

# 12

# Bone mineral density in midlife long-term users of hormonal contraception in South Africa: relationship with obesity and menopausal status

Mags E. Beksinska[1]*[iD], Immo Kleinschmidt[2] and Jenni A. Smit[1]

## Abstract

**Background:** In South Africa, hormonal contraception is widely used in women over the age of 40 years. One of these methods and the most commonly used is depot-medroxyprogesterone acetate (DMPA) which has been found to have a negative effect on bone mass. Limited information is available on the effect of norethisterone enanthate (NET-EN) on bone mass, and combined oral contraceptives (COCs) have not been found to be associated with loss of bone mass. The aim of this study was to investigate bone mineral density (BMD) in pre and perimenopausal women (40–49 years) in relation to use of DMPA, NET-EN and COCs for at least 12 months preceding recruitment into the study and review associations with body mass index (BMI) and menopausal status.

**Methods:** One hundred and twenty seven users of DMPA, 102 NET-EN users and 106 COC users were compared to 161 nonuser controls. Menopausal status was assessed, BMI and forearm BMD was measured at the distal radius using dual X-ray absorptiometry. Comparison analysis was conducted at baseline and 2.5 years.

**Results:** There was no significant difference in BMD between the four contraceptive user groups ($p = 0.26$) with and without adjustment for age at baseline or at 2.5 years ($p = 0.52$). The BMD was found to be significantly associated with BMI ($p = < 0.0001$) with an increase of one unit of BMI translating to an increase of 0.0044 g/cm$^2$ in radius BMD. Follicle stimulating hormone (FSH) level $\geq$ 25.8 mIU/mL was associated with a decrease of 0.017 g/cm$^2$ in radius BMD relative to women with FSH < 25.8 mIU/mL. Significant interaction between FSH and BMI in their effect on BMD was observed ($p = .006$).

**Conclusion:** This study found no evidence that long-term use of DMPA, NET-EN and COCs affects forearm BMD in this population at baseline or after 2.5 years of follow-up. This study also reports the complex relationship and significant interaction between FSH and BMI in their effect on BMD. BMD research in older women needs to ensure that women are assessed for menopausal status and BMI.

**Keywords:** Depot-medroxyprogesterone acetate, Norethisterone enanthate, Combined oral contraceptives, Bone mineral density, Menopause, Follicle stimulating hormone, Body mass index

* Correspondence: mbeksinska@matchresearch.co.za
[1]MatCH Research Unit [Maternal, Adolescent and Child Health Research Unit],
Department of Obstetrics and Gynaecology, Faculty of Health Sciences,
University of the Witwatersrand, 40 Dr AB Xuma Street,11th floor, Suite
1108-9,Commercial City, Durban 4001, South Africa
Full list of author information is available at the end of the article

## Background

In South Africa hormonal contraceptive use is high as reported in the last South African Demographic and Health Survey [1]. Of the two available hormonal injections, older women (> 40 years) almost exclusively use depot medroxyprogesterone acetate (DMPA) (81%) compared to norethisterone enanthate (NET-EN) (19%) [1]. These highly effective methods of contraception may be the method of choice for many women over 40 who have completed childbearing and are concerned about avoiding pregnancy. Hormonal injectables are not generally recommended in perimenopausal women where use of these methods is viewed as "contraceptive overkill" [2]. Most studies have found that current users of DMPA have lower BMD compared to nonusers [3–7]. However, a recent Cochrane review concludes that existing information cannot confirm whether steroidal contraceptives influence future fracture risk [8].

Specifically there is limited information on the effect of hormonal contraception on BMD in women in their midlife (> 40 years of age) [9–12]. As few studies have included women in this age group. Results of these studies have been mixed with some finding no differences in BMD between older DMPA users and nonusers or normal population means [9–11], while one study found a negative effect of DMPA on BMD compared to nonusers [12].

Studies investigating combined oral contraceptive (COC) use in perimenopausal users have not found a negative impact on BMD compared to nonusers of COCs [3]. Two cross-sectional studies have looked at BMD in NET-EN users. In one of these studies [13], current NET-EN users aged 40–44 had lower ultrasound measures in the calcaneus compared to nonusers, while the second study found no difference in forearm BMD between current users and controls [10].

Other potential factors that may play a role in BMD in midlife include menopausal status [14] and obesity [15]. However, evidence suggesting that being overweight / obese may be protective of BMD, is conflicting [16]. This study aimed to investigate BMD in pre and perimenopausal users (40 to 49 years) of DMPA, NET-EN, COC and nonusers of contraception in a 4–5 year follow-up study and review associations with BMI and menopausal status.

## Methods

A cohort of women aged 40 to 49 years old using DMPA, NET-EN, or COCs, and nonusers of hormonal contraception were recruited from a large family planning clinic in Durban, South Africa. For inclusion as a hormonal contraceptive user, women had to have used either DMPA, NET-EN or COCs for at least 1 year. For inclusion in the nonuser control group women should not have used any form of hormonal contraception in the past year. Women who were postmenopausal were

excluded from the study at screening using menstrual history (no bleeding for 2 years or more) and follicle-stimulating hormone (FSH) levels from blood samples. An FSH level of ≥25.8 m International Units per milliliter (mIU/mL) was considered to be in the menopausal range (King Edward VIII Hospital Durban; Chemical Pathology Laboratory criteria using Roche Elecsys FSH expected values). Women with an FSH ≥25.8 m (mIU/mL) who reported irregular bleeding within the last 2 years were classified as perimenopausal and were eligible for this study.

On recruitment, a questionnaire was administered to elicit information on lifetime contraceptive history, fertility history, menopausal symptoms and regularity of the menstrual cycle. The examination included height, weight, blood pressure and waist and hip measurement. Forearm BMD was measured by dual energy x-ray absorptiometry (DXA model DTX-200). Osteometer MediTech A/S Co, Rodovre, Denmark). BMD was measured in grams/centimetre$^2$ (g/cm$^2$) in the distal forearm (radius). The DXA equipment was standardized daily using a phantom as prescribed by the manufacturers instructions. Accuracy to the standard during the recruitment period was 0.53%. and in vivo precision was 0.94%. Study participants were followed-up at six-monthly intervals for a total of four to 5 years depending on time of recruitment. BMD was measured at each 6-monthly follow-up visit. Final comparison analysis was conducted at 2.5 years as the majority of women (87%) had stopped using a method of contraception by end of study. The study was conducted between 2000 and 2008.

The characteristics of women in the study were quantified as means ± standard deviations (SD), medians, or percentages. FSH levels were divided into two categories according to laboratory cut-off levels for premenopausal (< 25.8 mIU/mL) and perimenopausal/menopausal (≥25.8 mIU/mL). Differences in BMD between contraceptive groups, and the associations between BMD and selected characteristics of the study participants by contraceptive group were assessed using one-way analysis of variance and multiple variable linear regression.

The study aimed to be able to detect a half standard deviation difference in BMD between users and non-users of injectable contraceptives. This would be of biological significance as this difference would translate into a large difference in the risk of fracture in the older woman. Information on the mean and standard deviation of cross sectional measurements of forearm bone mass made in white, European, premenopausal, women as was reported by Nordin [17], was used to estimate sample size. The sample size required for each category assuming a two-tailed statistical test with a probability value (alpha) of 0.05 and with a power (beta) of 0.80 was 63 subjects. Loss to follow up was estimated at 8–10% per year. Sample size was adjusted to 100 per user group to ensure that a statistically significant difference could be detected. Data were analysed using the statistical package STATA (V.12 College station, TX, USA).

Ethical approval was granted by the University of the Witwatersrand, Human Subjects Research Committee (ref M981001), and by the Scientific and Ethical Review Group of the World Health Organization.

## Results

In total, 496 women were recruited. Baseline demographic and reproductive characteristics are summarised in Table 1. The mean age was approximately 43 years in the three hormonal contraceptive user groups with the nonusers on average 2 years older. Almost all women were African except for the COC group which included a higher proportion of Indian and Coloured women. Most women took no regular exercise and the mean BMI of the women in each user group fell into the upper end of obese class 1 (30–34.99 kg/m$^2$) group [18]. Women in the contraceptive groups had used their method for approximately four of the previous 5 years prior to recruitment, with all having used the method without a break for the last 12 consecutive months. Only 19.7% of women in the DMPA group and 33.0% of the

NET-EN group reported a regular menstrual cycle (between 21 and 35 days), compared with 90.0% of the COC group and 93% of the non-users.

In total, 48.5% of women in the non-user group were classified as perimenopausal (reported at least one vasomotor symptom in the last 3 months and had an FSH in the perimenopausal/menopausal range). This was a higher proportion than in the other 3 groups (40.2% DMPA, 31.4% NET-EN, 30.1% COCs); however, after adjusting for age, there was no evidence of a difference between the 4 groups in terms of menopausal status (DMPA $p = 0.48$; NET-EN $p = 0.93$; COC $p = 0.29$).

There was no significant difference in BMD at baseline between the four contraceptive user groups at the radius ($p = .26$), with and without adjustment for age (Table 2). Although a small decrease in BMD was noted per year over the age range – 0.0017 g/cm$^2$ (95% CI -0.0041-0.0008) this was not statistically significant ($p = .18$). Length of use of method in the last 5 years and total lifetime use was not associated with difference in BMD.

Body mass index, FSH level (equal to and above 25.8 mIU/mL versus below 25.8 mIU/mL) and interaction of BMD with FSH level were all significantly associated with BMD in a multiple regression model ($r^2 = 0.2$). According to this model, for women of median BMI of

**Table 1** Baseline characteristics of subjects in the 40–49 year age range by contraceptive method use

| Characteristics | DMPA ($n = 127$) | NET-EN ($n = 102$) | COC ($n = 106$) | Non-user Controls ($n = 161$) | P-value |
|---|---|---|---|---|---|
| Mean age, years (SD) | 43.6 (2.7) | 43.0 (2.2) | 43.7 (2.5) | 45.4 (2.5) | < 0.001 |
| Ethnicity % | | | | | |
| African | 98.4 | 95.2 | 67.0 | 94.4 | 0.007 |
| Coloured | 1.6 | 1.0 | 7.5 | 2.5 | |
| Indian | 0 | 3.8 | 25.5 | 3.1 | |
| Exercise | | | | | |
| No regular exercise (%) | 96.9 | 96.0 | 94.3 | 93 | 0.48 |
| Dieted in last 6 months (%) | 0 | 0 | 4.7 | < 1 | 0.003 |
| Current smoker (%) | 4.7 | 5.6 | 5.7 | 9.9 | 0.23 |
| Parity (median) | 4 | 3 | 3 | 3 | 0.04 |
| Ever lactated % | 88.2 | 91.3 | 87.7 | 83.2 | 0.34 |
| Mean age at menarche, years(SD) | 15.2± 1.7 | 15.5 ± 1.7 | 14.8 ± 1.7 | 14.8 ± 1.6 | 0.014 |
| Lactation (yrs) median | 3.5 | 3.2 | 3.0 | 3.2 | 0.06 |
| FSH | | | | | |
| < 25.8 mIU/mL, % | 72 | 94 | 90 | 68 | < 0.0001 |
| ≥ 25.8 mIU/mL, % | 28 | 6 | 10 | 32 | |
| Use of group method* | | | | | |
| Median use last 5 yrs. (months) | 53 | 45 | 52 | NA | |
| Median lifetime use (months) | 84 | 49 | 89 | NA | |
| Median age at first use | 36 | 37 | 36 | NA | |
| Radius BMD g/cm$^2$ | 0.514 | 0.514 | 0.500 | 0.518 | 0.26 |

*Only group method shown i.e. group to which women using that method at the time of recruitment were allocated

**Table 2** Factors potentially associated with Radius BMD (unadjusted) at baseline

| Factors | Radius BMD g/cm$^2$ 95% CI | P value |
|---|---|---|
| Contraceptive group | | 0.26 |
| DMPA | 0.514 (0.501–0.527) | |
| NET-EN | 0.514 (0.499–0.528) | |
| COC | 0.500 (0.486–0.514) | |
| Nonuser | 0.518 (0.506–0.529) | |
| Ethinicity | | |
| African | 0.516 (0.509–0.523) | |
| Indian | 0.491 (0.451–0.531) | 0.007 |
| Coloured | 0.479 (0.456–0.503) | |
| Age, per year | −0.0017 (−0.0041–0.0008) | 0.188 |
| BMI, change per kg/m$^2$ | 0.0044 (0.0036–0.0052) | < 0.001 |
| FSH | | 0.029 |
| < 25.8 mIU/mL, % | 0.516 (0.508)-0.524) | |
| ≥ 25.8 mIU/mL, % | 0.498 (0.483–0.512) | |

33.9 units, mean radius BMD varied from 0.514 g/cm$^2$ [95% CI 0.507–0.521] with FSH < 25.8 mIU/mL, to 0.501 g/cm$^2$ [95% CI 0.488–0.513] for women with FSH ≥ 25.8 mIU/mL, ($p = 0.066$). The effect of FSH on BMD was significantly modified by BMI, and vice-versa ($p = .006$). For women with FSH < 25.8 mIU/mL, BMD increased by 0.0038 [95%CI 0.0028–0.0047] (g/cm$^2$) per unit increase in BMI, whereas for women with FSH ≥ 25.8 mIU/mL, BMD increased by 0.0067 g/cm$^2$ [95% CI 0.0048–0.0086] for each unit increase in BMI (Table 3).

Follicle-stimulating hormone level was found to be significantly different between user groups ($p = < 0.0001$). However, after adjusting for age, the difference between the 4 groups was no longer significant ($p = 0.13$). An increase of 1 year in age increased FSH level by 3 mIU/mL ($p < 0.001$).

Although differences were noted between the contraceptive groups, most were not associated with BMD except for BMI, ethnic group and FSH level. A statistically significant difference in BMD was found between the Indian and African women ($p = .014$); however after

adjusting for BMI the difference in BMD was no longer significant.

During follow-up all nonusers of hormonal contraception remained as nonusers, however many women in the user groups continued participation in the study but ceased using a contraceptive method. At baseline 32% of women recruited were nonusers of contraception, this increased to 71% after 3 years of follow-up and by end of the follow-up period the majority of women (87%) had ceased using a method of contraception. Due to small numbers of hormonal contraceptive users from 3 years of follow-up, comparison of user groups was conducted at the 2.5 year visit. At this follow up visit 278 women continued with the same method they were using at baseline. Women were excluded from the analysis if they stopped or changed their method. No difference was found in BMD between the groups at the 2.5 year visit (Table 4).

## Discussion

This longitudinal study found no difference in forearm BMD between pre and perimenopausal users and nonusers of hormonal contraception at baseline or after 2.5 years of follow-up. This is in agreement with other studies of COC users in the perimenopause, where no change in BMD occurred [3]. The populations investigated in previous studies looking at the effect of DMPA and NET-EN on BMD have included women using the method in their 40s but there is limited information in this age group specifically. The age ranges of women in some studies have included users up to the age of 52, however the numbers have been small. In one cross-sectional study older DMPA users were disaggregated in the data [11] and no differences were found in BMD in women aged between 40 and 49 and a slightly older group of 50–52 compared to a normal population mean in the lumber spine and femoral neck. Tang et al., conducted a 3-year prospective study of perimenopusal women (mean age 43 years) who had used DMPA for 5 years or more [12]. At baseline significantly lower BMD in the spine, femoral neck, trochanter and ward's triangle were reported compared to never users. At the three-year follow up, women had a mean age of 46 years

**Table 3** Results of multiple regression model with BMI and FSH level

| Factors | Radius BMD units 95% CI | P value |
|---|---|---|
| Effect of [a]FSH (for women of median BMI = 33.9 kg/m$^2$) | | |
| < 25.8 mIU/mL | 0.514 (0.507–0.521) | < 0.066 |
| ≥ 25.8 mIU/mL | 0.501 (0.488–0.513) | |
| Effect of BMI, unit BMD per unit change in BMI For | | < 0.001 |
| FSH < 25.8 mIU/mL For | 0.0038 (0.0028–0.0047) | |
| FSH ≥ 25.8 mIU/mL | 0.0067 (0.0048–0.0086) | |

[a]Significant interaction between FSH level and BMI ($p = 0.006$)

**Table 4** Mean Radius BMD at 2.5 years by contraceptive group[a]

|  | N | Radius BMD g/cm$^2$ (SD) | P value |
|---|---|---|---|
| Contraceptive group |  |  | 0.522 |
| DMPA | 63 | 0.511 (.071) |  |
| NET-EN | 38 | 0.501 (.081) |  |
| COC | 48 | 0.500 (.082) |  |
| Nonuser | 129 | 0.504 (.075) |  |

[a]Only women continuing with the same method from baseline were included in this analysis

with a mean length of DMPA use of 10.1 years. At this follow up it was projected that the loss from baseline would be linear, however only small losses were noted of less than 1% in all sites aside from the trochanter where a small increase was noted [12]. The authors of the Tang study concluded that rate of BMD loss may be faster in the first 5 years of DMPA use with a levelling off thereafter. Our DMPA user sample was of similar age and reported length of DMPA use to the Tang study. It may be that users in our study had reached a steady state and further bone loss had not occurred. A further longitudinal study [9] followed up women who had been longterm users of either DMPA or the IUD until menopause. This study found no difference in BMD between these two groups at each of the three forearm sites at one-year follow-up post-menopause.

The absence of differences between the groups in BMD at baseline and follow up in our study is in agreement with some studies of BMD in hormonal contraceptive users in the midlife [3]. Although most studies adjust for BMI as it is a known to be associated with BMD [15], it may also be important to review the overall weight of the sample population to assess the proportion that may be obese. The majority of women in our study were classified in the upper range of obese class 1 which may have conferred some protective effect on their BMD. In 2013, South Africa had an obesity rate of 42% for women and 13.5% for men, the highest overweight and obesity rate in sub-Saharan Africa [19].

Another possible reason for the lack of difference in BMD between the groups may be related to the sensitivity of the measurement using forearm BMD. Forearm DXA has been shown to give good precision [20] and accuracy [21] with the added advantages of equipment that is portable and considerably less cost to purchase and maintain compared to DXA equipment measuring central sites. In a large European osteoporosis cohort, a logistic regression analysis for identification of group (HRT or control), the prediction was best for whole body (82.6%) and spine (80.9%), followed by total hip (78.5%) and lastly, forearm (74.7%). The authors concluded that for clinical diagnosis axial DXA is recommended [22].

The study recruited from a public sector urban family planning clinic in a South African city. There was no locally available public health facility with DXA equipment to measure central body sites due to the high cost of the equipment, maintenance and staff to undertake scans. The Forearm DXA scanner was purchased through the study funding which was only able to cover the cost of a forearm DXA scanner.

Many women may continue to use hormonal injectables into their late forties and beyond menopause as menopausal symptoms such as amenorrhea may be masked by use of progestogen-only hormonal contraceptives which also cause amenorrhea [2]. DMPA has been shown to relieve vasomotor symptoms in perimenopausal women [23, 24]. and DMPA and NET-EN are known to suppress the midcycle surge of folliclestimulating hormone (FSH) and luteinising hormone (LH), thereby reducing raised FSH levels, although the tonic release of these gonadotrophins continues at luteal phase levels [25]. Data from South Africa presents some evidence that a raised FSH level, although initially supressed, will return to its raised level within the three monthly DMPA and two-monthly NET-EN cycles of use and could be potentially used to assist as a menopausal indicator without interrupting method use in this group of contraceptive users [26]. Detection of menopause or perimenopause does therefore present some challenges in this group of injectable contraceptive users, whose BMD may be compromised by any risk associated with hormonal contraception use.

## Conclusions

This study adds to evidence on the effect of hormonal contraception on BMD in the midlife. This study also reports the complex relationship and significant interaction between FSH and BMI in their effect on BMD. BMD research in older women needs to ensure that women are assessed for menopausal status and BMI.

**Acknowledgements**
Not applicable.

**Funding**
Funding for the study was provided by the World Health Organization. The funding body had some input into the design of the study and final approval of the protocol and had some minimal input into the interpretation.

**Authors' contributions**
MB developed the protocol and data collection instruments, assisted in the analysis of the data under the supervision of IK and interpreted the results and led the manuscript writing. IK analysed and interpreted the data. JS interpreted the data and was a major contributor in writing the manuscript. All authors read and approved the final manuscript.

**Competing interests**
The authors declare that they have no competing interests (MB IK JS).

**Author details**
[1]MatCH Research Unit [Maternal, Adolescent and Child Health Research Unit], Department of Obstetrics and Gynaecology, Faculty of Health Sciences, University of the Witwatersrand, 40 Dr AB Xuma Street,11th floor, Suite 1108-9,Commercial City, Durban 4001, South Africa. [2]London School of Hygiene and Tropical Medicine, Keppel Street, London WC1E, England.

**References**
1. Department of Health South Africa, Medical Research Council and Measure DHS. South African demographic and health survey 1998, full report. Pretoria (South Africa) Department of Health; 2002.
2. Guillebaud, J. 2001. Contraception: your questions answered. Edinburgh : Churchill Livingstone: 1993. 280
3. Curtis KM, Martins SL. Progestogen-only contraception and bone mineral density: a systematic review. Contraception. 2006;73:470–87.
4. Wanichsetakul P, Kamudhamas A, Watanaruagkovit P, Siripakam Y, Visutakul P. Bone mineral density at various anatomic bone sites in women receiving combined oral contraceptives and depot-medroxyprogesterone acetate for contraception. Contraception. 2002;65:407–10.
5. Petitti DB, Piaggio G, Mehta S, Cravioto MC, Meirik O. Steroid hormone contraception and bone mineral density: a cross-sectional study in an international population. Obstet Gynecol. 2000;95:736–43.
6. Scholes D, Lacroix AZ, Ott SM, Ichikawa LE, Barlow WE. Bone mineral density in women using depot medroxyprogesterone acetate for contraception. Obstet Gynecol. 1999;93:233–8.
7. Cundy T, Farquhar CM, Cornish J, Reid IR. Short-term effects of high dose oral Medroxyprogesterone acetate on bone density in premenopausal women. J Clin Endocrinol Meta. 1996;81:1014–7.
8. Lopez LM, Grimes DA, Schulz KF, Curtis KM, Chen M. Steroidal contraceptives: effect on bone fractures in women. Cochrane Database Syst Rev. 2014;6:CD006033. https://doi.org/10.1002/14651858.CD006033.pub5.
9. Sanches L, Marchi NM, Castro S, et al. Forearm bone mineral density in postmenopausal former users of depot medroxyprogesterone acetate. Contraception. 2008;78:365–9.
10. Beksinska M, Smit J, Kleinschmidt I, Farley T, Mbatha F. Bone mineral density in women aged 40-49 years using depot-medroxyprogesterone acetate, norethisterone enanthate or combined oral contraceptives for contraception. Contraception. 2005;71:170–5.
11. Globade B, Ellis S, Murphy B, Randall S, Kirkman R. Bone density amongst long term users of medroxyprogesterone acetate. Br J Obstet Gynaecol. 1998;105:790–4.
12. Tang OS, Tang G, Yip PSF, Li B. Further evaluation of long-term depot-medroxyprogesterone acetate use and bone mineral density; a longitudinal cohort study. Contraception. 2000;62(4):161.
13. Rosenberg L, Zhang Y, Constant D, Cooper D, Kalla AA, Micklesfield L, et al. Bone status after cessation of use of injectable progestin contraceptives. Contraception. 2007;76:425–31.
14. Salamat MR, Salamat AH, Janghorbani M. Association between obesity and bone mineral density by gender and menopausal status. Endincrinol Metab. 2016;31(4):547–58. https://doi.org/10.3803/EnM.2016.31.4.547.
15. Cummings SR, Black DM, Nevitt MC, Browner W, Cauley J, Ensrud K, et al. Bone mineral density at various sites for prediction of hip fractures. The study of osteoporotic fractures research group. Lancet. 1993;31:72–5.
16. Migliaccio S, Greco EA, Fornari R, Donini DM, Lenzi A. Is obesity in women protective of osteoporosis? Diab Metab Syndrome Obes Targets Ther. 2011;4:273–82.
17. Nordin BE. The definition and diagnosis of osteoporosis. Calcif Tissue Int. 1987;40:57–8.
18. World Health Organisation Global data on body mass. BMI Classification. http://apps.who.int/bmi/index.jsp. Accessed 11 Mar 2018.
19. Ng M, Fleming T, Robinson M, Thomson B, Graetz N, Margono C, Mullany EC, Biryukov S, et al. Global, regional, and national prevalence of overweight and obesity in children and adults during 1980–2013: a systematic analysis for the Global Burden of Disease Study 2013. Lancet. 2014;384(9945):766–81.
20. Davis JW, Ross PD, Wasnich RD, MacLean CJ, Vogel JM. Long-term precision of bone loss rate measurements among postmenopausal women. Calcif Tissue Int. 1991;48:311–8.
21. Stock JL, Coderre JA, Mallette LE. Effects of a short course of estrogen on mineral metabolism in postmenopausal women. J Clin Endocrinol Metab. 1985;61:595–600.
22. Abrahamsen BL, Stilgren LS, Hermann AP, Tofteng CL, Barenholdt O, Vestergaard P, et al. Discordance between changes in bone mineral density measured at different skeletal sites in perimenopausal women—implications for assessment of bone loss and response to therapy: the Danish osteoporosis prevention study. J Bone Miner Res. 2001;16:1212–9.
23. Bullock JL, Massey FM, Gambrell RD Jr. Use of medroxyprogesterone acetate to prevent menopausal symptoms. Obstet Gynecol. 1975;46:165–8.
24. Morrison JC, Martin DC, Blair RA, Anderson GD, Kincheloe BW, Bates GW, et al. The use of medroxyprogesterone acetate for the relief of climacteric symptoms. Am J Obstet Gynecol. 1980;138:99–104.
25. Franchimont P, Cession G, Ayalon D, Musters A, Legros JJ. Suppressive action of norethisterone enanthate and depo medroxyprogesterone acetate on gonadotropin levels. Obstet Gynecol. 1970;36:93–100.
26. Beksinska ME, Smit JA, Kleinschmidt I, Rees HV, Farley TM, Guidozzi F. Detection of raised FSH levels among older women using depo medroxyprogesterone acetate and norethisterone enanthate. Contraception. 2003;68:339–43.

# 13

# Work outcomes in midlife women: the impact of menopause, work stress and working environment

Claire Hardy[1], Eleanor Thorne[1], Amanda Griffiths[2] and Myra S. Hunter[1]*

**Abstract**

**Background:** There is growing research interest in the question of whether menopause impacts upon mid-aged women's work outcomes, but the evidence to date is inconclusive. This paper examines whether: (i) menopausal status, and experience of hot flushes and night sweats (HFNS), and whether (ii) work stress and work environment, are associated with work outcomes (absenteeism, job performance, turnover intention, and intention to leave the labor force).

**Methods:** An online survey (sociodemographic, menopause, health, well-being and aspects of work) was completed by 216 (pre-, peri- and postmenopausal) women aged 45–60 years.

**Results:** Work outcomes were not associated with menopausal status but were significantly associated with job stress and aspects of the work environment, such as demand, control and support. HFNS presence, frequency and problem-rating were not significantly associated with work outcomes. HF problem rating at work was significantly associated with intention to leave the labor force, after controlling for age (F(2,101), 6.742, $p = .002$).

**Conclusions:** The main predictors of work outcomes in this sample of mid-aged women were aspects of the working environment (particularly role clarity and work stress). Menopausal status was not associated with work outcomes but having problematic hot flushes at work was associated with intention to stop working. These results challenge assumptions about the menopause transition by providing evidence that the menopause does not impact on women's self-reported work performance and absence. However, support for women with problematic HFNS at work may be beneficial, as might addressing working environment issues for mid-aged women.

**Keywords:** Menopausal status, Absenteeism, Job performance, Turnover intention, Intention to leave the labor force, Job stress, Working environment

## Background

The increasing age of the working population in most European countries means that more women will be working during their menopausal transition than ever before [1]. The menopause - the last menstrual cycle - generally occurs on average between the ages of 50 and 51 in western cultures [2]. The perimenopause or menopause transition is the time from the onset of menstrual cycle changes until one year after the final menstrual period [3]. Although highly variable between women, the menopausal transition can last on average two to four years, but can last up to ten years [4, 5].

It has been estimated that between 20 and 40% of menopausal women experience hot flushes and night sweats (HFNS), also referred to as vasomotor symptoms, which can impact negatively on quality of life, including personal and work life [6]. Women tend to report that these symptoms are more difficult to manage in the work place, due to embarrassment and concern about the reactions of others [7–9]. Menopausal status and HFNS are often kept hidden [10] and not disclosed to managers at work [11]; consequently menopause taboos are not challenged and women may not obtain practical support that could be helpful. This has led to various

* Correspondence: myra.hunter@kcl.ac.uk
[1]Department Psychology (at Guy's), Institute of Psychiatry, Psychology and Neuroscience, Kings College London, 5th Floor Bermondsey Wing, Guy's Campus, London SE1 9RT, UK
Full list of author information is available at the end of the article

guidance and recommendations that menopause at work warrants attention and support for women. For example, the UK Faculty of Occupational Medicine of the Royal College of Physicians has published guidance on how employers can best support menopausal women in the workplace [12].

Recent research on this topic has focused on two main areas: (i) that menopause can have negative effects at work and (ii) that certain working environments negatively impact on experience of menopausal symptoms. A recent systematic review by Jack and colleagues [13] explored menopause at work and found a number of studies suggesting that women with problematic menopausal symptoms may experience impairments on a range of work outcomes. For example, in an Australian survey of approximately 1000 women aged 40–70 years, HFNS frequency was significantly associated with reduced job satisfaction, work engagement, organizational commitment, and a higher intention to quit their job [14]. In the US, a significant relationship was found between night sweat severity and impaired worker productivity on a large sample of over 3000 mid-aged women [15]. Overall, however, the systematic review concluded that evidence was still inconclusive in terms of the impact of menopause on work outcomes. It is important to note that almost without exception, evidence relating to performance at work is based on self-perceived measures.

Since the review's publication, a further cross-sectional study of 1274 female workers aged 40–65 years in Australia found that having HFNS were associated with a greater likelihood of poor self-rated work ability [16]. In another recent study Hickey and colleagues [17] examined relationships between work outcomes and stage of menopause, in a study of over 1000 women in Australia. Self-reported work engagement, job satisfaction, organizational commitment, or work limitations did not differ with menopausal status. Postmenopausal women were less likely to report intention to leave their employing organization (turnover intention) than pre- or peri-menopausal women. However, the study did not control for the potential impact of age on these variables, which the authors noted may have been important to consider.

Finally, a recent report published in 2017 systematically reviewed the economic evidence of possible impact of menopause upon work outcomes, i.e. whether the menopause transition is a problem for UK working women and, in turn, workplaces and the wider labor market [18]. Both positive and negative effects were found for women transitioning whilst in employment, and some evidence suggested that menopausal women were unable to seek employment, were reducing their working hours, leaving or losing their job whilst in

transitions, and identifying negative impact on their career. However, they, like Jack and colleagues [13], stated that evidence for the menopause having an economic impact remains inconclusive. It is also important to note that evidence relating to women's performance is based on self-perceived performance not objective measures.

A key aspect of the workplace is job or work stress. Work-related stress is one of the main reasons reported for sickness absence in many developed countries; for example in the UK work stress has been the focus of much research over the last several decades [19]. Job stress is generally understood as a result of an employee's cognitive appraisal that their working environment may be imposing greater demands (stressors) on them than they can cope with. The relationships between these cognitive appraisals and psychosocial environmental stressors has been largely influenced by Lazarus's transactional model [20], which posits that stress results when person/environment transactions lead the individual to perceive a discrepancy between the demands of a situation and his/her resources or ability to cope with those demands. Stress has been examined in many populations and occupations, yet, mid-aged women have been largely overlooked.

Researchers have attempted to identify aspects of the work environment that might result in job stress and work outcomes. For example, early work was influenced by role stress theory [21] and the Person-Environment fit theory [22]. These theories proposed that the employee's role was key and that if the employee did not fit the working environment appropriately then stress would occur. More recently this field has been more heavily influenced by Karasek's jobs demands-control model [23] and the spin-off job demands-resources (JDR) model [24]. Within these theories, if an employee has insufficient control or resources or lack of support to be able to meet the demands of their job, then stress would occur. The JDR model [24] refers to control as a resource, specifically, but also suggests that other resources are available in the employee's physical, psychological, social, or organizational domains.

In the context of female employees at midlife, there is a need for more research exploring job stress in menopausal women as well as the possible impact of menopausal status on work outcomes. This paper attempts to contribute by addressing the following research questions: (i) are menopausal status and the experience of menopausal symptoms – hot flushes and night sweats – associated with key work outcomes, including absenteeism, job performance, turnover intention (leaving the current employing organization), intention to leave the labor force, and (ii) what is the association of job stress and the working environment on these work outcomes?

## Method

An electronic survey was sent via email to female members of a trade union and professional association for family court and probation staff in England, Wales and Northern Ireland in June 2016. The workforce had undergone organizational change during the past three years and was considered a suitable population to explore job stress. Self-report data was collected on demographic and health-related questions, including age, ethnicity, educational level, general health, work-related variables included: employment status (full-time, part-time), working hours, flexible working, manual working, and managerial/supervisory responsibilities.

Job stress was measured using a single-item asking women how stressful they find their jobs (1 = not stressful to 4 = extremely stressful, [25]). The working environment was measured using the Health and Safety Executive's Management Standards Indicator Tool (MSIT) which includes 35 items to measure six aspects of work which if badly managed are known to be associated with the experience of stress; demands, control, support (manager and peer), relationships, role and change [26]. Responses are given using a 5-point Likert-scale (1 = never to 5 = always) and were all shown to have acceptable levels of reliability ($\alpha$ = .68–.87).

Menopausal status was determined according to menstrual criteria: regular periods (regular for them), changes in menstrual periods but had menstruated in the last 6 months, or had not menstruated for a least 1 year. Participants were grouped as pre, peri-, and postmenopausal, respectively; perimenopause or menopause transition being the time from the onset of menstrual cycle changes until one year after the final menstrual period [3]. HFNS were assessed using the Hot Flush Rating Scale [7] including the presence of HFNS, HFNS frequency in the past week, HFNS problem rating (3 ten point scales items assessing interference, distress and problem ratings of HFNS $\alpha$ = .87), and an additional single item 10 point scale assessing HFNS problem rating specifically when at work.

Dependent variables were: number of days affected by work absence in the last 4 weeks (summed total number of full days, arriving to work late, and leaving early), a self-rated job performance item (a single item, 1 = poor-5 = excellent, [27, 28]), turnover intention was measured using an existing 4-item measure, with 5-point Likert scales, to assess the employee's intention to leave the organization ($\alpha$ = 0.78) [29]), and intention to leave the work force was measured using a single-item (1 = no, 2 = sometimes, 3 = yes).

Univariate regression analyses were conducted to determine any significant associations between sociodemographic variables and the outcomes. Only age was significantly related to intention to leave the labor force

only ($r$ = .36, $p$ = .000) and was controlled for in the main analyses. ANOVA was used to determine if there were menopausal group differences in the outcome variable absence; Kruskal-Wallis H Tests were used to determine if there were differences in perceived job performance and turnover intentions between the menopausal groups, and ANCOVAs were conducted to determine whether there were group differences in the outcome intention to stop working, controlling for age. Mann-Whitney U tests were used to determine whether there was an association between HFNS presence and the work outcomes. Bivariate linear regression analyses were conducted to determine whether experience of HFNS was associated with the outcome variables, and multiple regression analyses were used to determine the relative associations between significant univariate variables with the outcomes variable.

Ethical approval was given by King's College London, Ethical Review Committee (reference number: HR-15/16–2492) and all participants gave their consent to participate and publish the results.

## Results
### Sample characteristics

Two hundred and sixteen women aged 40–65 years were included in this study. Table 1 shows the characteristics of the sample. Women were on average 53 years, white (88.7%), mostly educated to at least degree or professional qualification level (85.6%) and were generally healthy. Over half exercised a minimum of 2 times per week (55.1%). The sample's mean BMI score (29.30) is considered at the upper end of being overweight.

Fifty-eight per cent of the women were postmenopausal, with the remainder divided roughly equally between peri- or pre-menopausal. 62% were experiencing HFNS, on average, 19 times in the past week. Apart from one participant, none were taking HRT. A small proportion of women were taking non-prescribed medication for the menopause (7.7%) and fewer were taking prescribed medication (4.8%).

The majority of women worked full-time, for an average of 36 h per week in non-manual jobs (97.7%), within a public sector organization. Most of the women in the sample had degree level education and were employed in non-manual work. The majority (81.5%) were experiencing moderate to severe levels of job stress with only 2.3% reporting no job stress.

Women had been affected by absence, on average, for 4 days in the last 4 weeks. Specifically, they took an average of 2.37 (sd = 5.59) full days, arrived late to work 1.26 (sd = 3.56) times in the past 4 weeks, and left work early 1.13 (sd = 2.90) times in the past 4 weeks.

Self-rated work performance was generally perceived as high with three-quarters (74.9%) rating their performance

**Table 1** Sample characteristics

| Characteristic | | Mean (SD) or N (%) |
|---|---|---|
| Age (n = 216) | Mean (sd) | 52.51 (5.75) |
| Ethnicity (n = 212) | White | 188 (88.7%) |
| | Black | 19 (9.0%) |
| | Asian | 5 (2.4%) |
| Menopausal status (n = 216) | Pre (regular periods) | 48 (22.2%) |
| | Peri (irregular periods for last 6 months) | 42 (19.4%) |
| | Post (no period for 12 months) | 126 (58.3%) |
| HFNS frequency in past week (n = 102) | Mean (sd) | 19.45 (17.90) |
| | | range: 0–89 |
| HFNS problem rating (n = 104) | Mean (sd) | 4.77 (2.11) |
| HFNS Problem rating at work (n = 104) | Mean (sd) | 5.03 (2.71) |
| General health (n = 216) | Mean (sd) | 2.81 (1.07) |
| BMI (n = 199) | Mean (sd) | 29.30 (7.39) |
| Education level (n = 215) | 'O' Grade/ 'O' Level/ Standard Grade | 17 (7.9%) |
| | Higher/ 'A' Level/ National Grade | 14 (6.5%) |
| | Degree or professional qualification | 106 (49.3%) |
| | Post-graduate qualification | 78 (36.3%) |
| Relationship status (n = 214) | Single/Divorced/ Separated/Widowed | 63 (29.4%) |
| | Married/With partner | 151 (70.6%) |
| Work full-time (n = 212) | | 155 (73.1%) |
| Working hours (n = 211) | Mean (SD) | 36.44 (9.68) |
| Flexible working (n = 212) | | 148 (69.8%) |
| Non-manual job (n = 215) | | 210 (97.7%) |
| Managerial/supervisory responsibilities (n = 212) | | 59 (27.8%) |
| Sector (n = 216) | Public | 131 (60.6%) |
| | Private | 85 (39.4%) |
| How stressful do you find your job? (n = 216) | Not stressful | 5 (2.3%) |
| | Mildly stressful | 35 (16.2%) |
| | Moderately stressful | 95 (44%) |
| | Extremely stressful | 81 (37.5%) |

as very good/excellent compared to others in a similar role. Approximately half of the women (52.3%) indicated that they have considered leaving the labor force altogether.

## Menopause and work outcomes

Table 2 shows the scores for the menopausal status groups on the key work outcomes.

No significant differences were found between menopausal status and any work outcome, i.e. number of days affected by absence (total number of days taken off, arrived late, left early), job performance, turnover intention. Intention to leave the labor force was significantly different between the menopausal groups, $H = 19.300$, $p = .001$, with post-menopausal women showing a significantly higher intention than pre- or peri-menopausal women. However, this difference became non-significant after controlling for age.

### Job stress and work environment

Relationships between job stress and work environment were considered as possible predictors of work outcomes. To improve normality of the job stress variable, responses were recoded to combine the lower two response options and create a 3-point scale (i.e. low, moderate, high stress) for use in the following analyses. Higher perceived job stress was significantly associated with lower self-rated job performance, $F(1, 209) = 22.317$, $p = .0001$, higher turnover intention, $F(1, 214) = 37.016$, p = .0001, and higher intention to leave the labor force controlling for age, $F(2, 213) = 23.012$, $p = .0001$. Job stress was not associated with number of days affected by absence.

Regarding the working environment, higher self-rated job performance was associated with lower demands, $F(1, 209) = 11.59$, $p = .001$, clearer job role, $F(1, 209) = 30.53$, $p = .0001$, and having more control at work, $F(1, 209) = 7.771$, $p = .006$.

Higher turnover intention was associated with higher demands at work, $F(1, 214) = 18.575$, $p = .000$, lower role clarity, $F(1, 214) = 41.683$, $p = .0001$, low control, $F(1, 214) = 21.611$, $p = .000$, better relationships, $F(1, 214) = 4.019$, $p = .046$, lower manager support, $F(1, 214) = 23.99$, $p = .000$, lower peer support, $F(1, 214) = 10.155$, $p = .002$, and poor change management, $F(1, 214) = 24.467$, $p = .0001$.

Higher intention to leave the labor force, controlling for age, was associated with higher demands, $F(2, 213) = 20.307$, $p = .0001$, poor role clarity, $F(2, 213) = 5.826$, $p = .017$, lower control, $F(2, 213) = 16.199$, $p = .022$, lower peer support, $F(2, 213) = 19.766$, $p = .014$, and poorer change management, $F(2, 213) = 19.639$, $p = .015$.

Absence (more days/part days off work) in the last four weeks were associated with lower perceived levels of control, $F(1, 214) = 5.826$, $p = .017$, and better relationships, $F(1, 214) = 9.256$, $p = .003$.

### The role of HFNS

A subsample (n = 168) of peri and post-menopausal women provided data relating to HFNS, and relationships between HFNS and work outcomes were examined. Neither the presence of vasomotor symptoms (HFNS) nor

**Table 2** Total sample and pre, peri, and postmenopausal status groups on work outcomes

| | Number | Pre-menopause M (SD) | Number | Peri-menopause M (SD) | Number | Post-menopause M (SD) | Number | Total M (SD) |
|---|---|---|---|---|---|---|---|---|
| Absence (Number of days affected by absence in last 4 weeks) | 48 | 5.49 (6.59) | 42 | 4.60 (6.13) | 126 | 3.89 (6.20) | 216 | 4.38 (6.28) |
| Job performance | 47 | 3.00 (0.75) | 39 | 2.87 (0.73) | 125 | 2.86 (0.75) | 211 | 2.89 (0.75) |
| Turnover intention | 48 | 3.19 (0.99) | 42 | 3.11 (0.99) | 126 | 3.18 (1.04) | 211 | 3.17 (1.02) |
| Intention to leave the labor force | 48 | 0.48 (0.80) | 42 | 0.64 (0.88) | 126 | 1.07 (0.87) | 216 | 0.84 (0.89) |

HFNS frequency or Problem-rating were associated with work outcomes. However, reporting more problematic hot flushes *at work* was significantly associated with intention to stop working, $F(2, 101) = 6.742$, $p = .002$. Specifically, higher problem ratings were associated with a greater intention to leave ($B = .082$).

### Relationships between age, job stress, working environment, HFNS, and work outcomes

Significant variables in univariate analyses were entered into stepwise linear regression analyses to determine the strongest predictors of each work outcome (see Table 3). Overall, the number of days affected by work absence was predicted by (better) relationships at work and (lower) control at work, but together these variables only accounted for a small (6%) amount of the variance. Job performance was best predicted by the working environment subscales, (higher) job role and (lower) job stress, which accounted for 16.1% of the variance. Intention to leave the employing organization was best predicted by (poorer) role clarity, (higher) job stress, and (poorer) managerial support, which accounted for 24.9% of the

variance. Intention to stop working was best predicted by (older) age, (poorer) role clarity, and (higher) problematic hot flushes at work, which account for 22.5% of the variance.

### Discussion

This study contributes to the evidence regarding the potential impact of menopausal experience, and of work stress and work environment on work outcomes. The sample was highly educated and generally healthy, but reported moderate and severe levels of work stress and fairly high levels of work absence (2.37 full days absence in past 4 weeks), compared with a national average for annual sickness absence in the UK of 4.3 days [30]. There was not a particularly strong intention to leave their employing organization, but approximately half of the women had considered leaving the labor force altogether. Despite this, their subjective ratings of their own work performance were relatively high. The organization had recently undergone substantial change, which is known to be associated with a high report of stress. The results also suggest that performance

**Table 3** Predictors of work outcomes: step-wise linear regression analyses

| Work outcome | Variable | Regression statistics |
|---|---|---|
| Number of days affected by absence ($n = 216$) | Relationships | $B = 2.667$, 95% CI = .746–4.587, $p = .007$ |
| | Control | $B = -1.498$, 95% CI = −2.957–.040, $p = .044$ |
| | | $R^2 = .060$ |
| Job performance ($n = 211$) | Role | $B = .324$, 95% CI = .189–.459, $p = .0001$ |
| | Job stress | $B = .-206$, 95% CI = −.346–.066, $p = .004$ |
| | | $R^2 = .161$ |
| Turnover intention ($n = 216$) | Role | $B = -.342$, 95% CI = −.529–.156, $p = .0001$ |
| | Job stress | $B = .344$, 95% CI = .164–.524, $p = .0001$ |
| | Managerial support | $B = -.184$, 95% CI = −.317–.051, $p = .0001$ |
| | | $R^2 = 249$ |
| Intention to leave the labor force ($n = 104$) | Age | $B = .072$, 95% CI = .037–.107, $p = .0001$ |
| | Role | $B = -.264$, 95% CI = −.475–.054, $p = .014$ |
| | HF Problem rating at work | $B = .065$, 95% CI = .006–124, $p = .031$ |
| | | $R^2 = .225$ |

remained high despite considerable work stress, absence and intention to leave the labor force. There is some evidence from qualitative data that women might work harder in order that their performance is not affected [11].

We found that there were no differences between pre, peri, and post-menopausal women with respect to work absence, job performance, turnover intention, and intention to leave the labor force. Neither were dimensions of HFNS reporting (prevalence, frequency and problem-rating) associated with work outcomes. However, having problematic hot flushes, specifically at work, was associated with a higher intention to leave the labor force. These results suggest that any impact of menopause or menopausal symptoms on work outcomes is likely to be minimal and quite specific. Interestingly, it is the problematic nature of HFNS, not their frequency that had an impact on the work outcomes studied here. This supports previous findings that it is how bothersome or problematic that HFNS are that is associated with quality of life, rather than their frequency [6].

Overall, our results support those of Hickey and colleagues [17] who found few differences between reproductive status on a range of work outcomes. Women rated their work performance positively in both studies. Hickey and colleagues found one significant association - that postmenopausal women had a lower intention to leave the labor force than pre- and peri-menopausal women. However, age was not controlled for in this study. In contrast we found that post-menopausal women reported a higher intention to leave the labor force than pre- or peri-menopausal women. However, this difference became non-significant after controlling for age.

The impact of work stress and the work environment was also examined and found to be significantly associated with key work outcomes. Successive Health and Safety Executive Labour Force Surveys on self-reported work-related illness have revealed that mid-life women (aged 45–54) are the group reporting most work-related stress [19]. We did not find an association between work stress and menopausal status. However, levels of work stress were relatively high across these stages. The results are similar to those reported by professionals in a similar occupational field (i.e. the police, [25]). In the UK, public service industries show the highest levels of stress and it is the main reason for absence from work [19].

Work stress and the working environment appeared to play a greater role in the work outcomes than menopausal status or experience. Specifically, job stress was associated with job performance, and turnover intention, although not significantly for days affected by absence. The working environment appeared to be more strongly

associated with absence, especially having better relationships at work and less control over work. Job role clarity was also a key influence on these work outcomes, especially for intention to leave the employing organization and labor force. Managerial support was associated with turnover intention but none of the other outcomes. Intention to leave the labor force was additionally influenced by age and problematic hot flushes at work, which was the only outcome to be associated with the menopausal experience.

With regards to the menopause transition, there is guidance [1, 12] that encourages managers to be informed about the menopause and to foster a culture where women feel empowered to speak up about any difficulties. Increased flexibility, attention to workplace temperatures and access to information and advice are also recommended [11]. In a recent study of how mid-aged women wanted to be treated in the workplace [31] most women mentioned that employers/managers should not consider the menopause in an overly negative light, for example, as an 'affliction' or a 'condition' affecting all older female employees. They believed that employers/managers should be aware that the menopause is a normal process and one that is highly variable between women.

It is also important to mention other symptoms that may be associated with the menopause that we did not examine. These include tiredness, poor concentration and memory, and low confidence, and sleep disturbance [9, 11, 15]. Hickey et al. [17] found that sleep problems were most commonly reported by peri-menopausal women, while for postmenopausal women it was joint and muscular discomfort. Only hot flushes and vaginal dryness were significantly more frequent in peri- and post, compared to premenopausal women. Whitely and colleagues [9] concluded, from a study examining the effects of menopausal symptoms on work impairment, that whilst women with menopausal symptoms reported significantly higher work impairment, there was no specific symptom that significantly predicted work productivity losses.

In this context and in the light of the current findings and those of Hickey et al. [17], we suggest that specific symptoms or physical changes, such as HFNS, are considered since menopausal status does not appear to be associated with most work outcomes. This is likely to reduce general stereotyping of 'menopausal women' and address women's concerns about being perceived as 'not good at their jobs' because they are going through the menopause. In addition, work outcomes, such as performance and work intentions, appear to differ markedly in their relationship to HFNS, so future studies might usefully include a broad range of work outcomes. It is also important to report positive findings, for example in the current study work performance was highly rated in this sample of working mid-aged women.

Attempts to retain women in the labor force might focus on providing support to those women who are having problematic HFNS specifically at work, as well as modifying aspects of the work environment that can exacerbate experience and women's ability to cope with symptoms [1, 11, 12]. Information and advice on managing symptoms using a cognitive behavioural approach is available [32, 33], including a self-help approach for working women with problematic symptoms [28], and may be offered as needed. The results also suggest that steps need to be taken to help employees to have clarity of roles, feel supported, and have more control over their work.

Future research might investigate changes at work and their impact on menopause experience: for example, providing information and training about the menopause to all staff. Such enquiries might compare different delivery methods (face to face, paper or online). Research might explore attempts to improve workplace culture regarding health-related issues for women. The effectiveness of risk assessment and risk management initiatives could be explored, where key factors affecting women are identified and interventions designed to reduce them.

Some limitations should also be noted. The overall sample size was relatively small and also derived from one job sector (i.e. the probation service) that had undergone organizational change in the past 3 years. This may influence the generalizability of the findings, and further research exploring a range of different job sectors is recommended.

The women appeared to be experiencing relatively high levels of stress, but we did not explore non-work sources of stress, which are commonly reported during midlife, such as caring roles and family responsibilities [34].

## Conclusion

This study presents evidence that menopausal status does not appear to be associated with work outcomes (absence, performance, turnover intention and intention to leave the labor force) and most women maintained high levels of self-rated performance at work despite menopause and high levels of work stress. The results therefore challenge the assumptions that the menopause has a negative impact on work performance and levels of absence from work. The findings suggest implications for possible changes to workplace practices and policy that may benefit those mid-aged women experiencing difficulties during mid-life and/or the menopause. In particular, providing support for women with problematic HFNS at work, as well as addressing working environment issues. Investigations examining the impact of such workplace changes and tailored interventions are needed.

## Acknowledgements
We would like to thank Sarah Friday and colleagues for their feedback and input to the study.

## Funding
This research was funded by the charity Wellbeing of Women RG1701.

## Authors' contributions
CH and MSH designed the study, drafted the manuscript; ET contributed to data collection and the statistical analysis; AG contributed to the final draft; all authors read and approved the manuscript.

## Competing interests
The authors declare that they have no competing interests.

## Author details
[1]Department Psychology (at Guy's), Institute of Psychiatry, Psychology and Neuroscience, Kings College London, 5th Floor Bermondsey Wing, Guy's Campus, London SE1 9RT, UK. [2]Division of Psychiatry & Applied Psychology, School of Medicine, University of Nottingham, Nottingham, UK.

## References
1. Griffiths A, Ceausu I, Depypere H, Lambrinoudaki I, Mueck A, Pérez-López FR, van der Schouw YT, Senturk LM, Simoncini T, Stevenson JC, Stute P. EMAS recommendations for conditions in the workplace for menopausal women. Maturitas. 2016;85:79–81.
2. Freeman EW, Sammel MD, Lin H, Gracia CR. Anti-mullerian hormone as a predictor of time to menopause in late reproductive age women. J Clin Endocrinol. 2012;97(5):1673–80.
3. Harlow SD, Gass M, Hall JE, Lobo R, Maki P, Rebar RW, Sherman S, Sluss PM, De Villiers TJ. STRAW+ 10 Collaborative Group. Executive summary of the Stages of Reproductive Aging Workshop+ 10: addressing the unfinished agenda of staging reproductive aging. J Clin Endocrinol Metab. 2012 Apr 1;97(4):1159–68.
4. Hunter MS, Gentry-Maharaj A, Ryan A, Burnell M, Lanceley A, Fraser L, Jacobs I, Menon U. Prevalence, frequency and problem rating of hot flushes persist in older postmenopausal women: impact of age, body mass index, hysterectomy, hormone therapy use, lifestyle and mood in a cross-sectional cohort study of 10 418 British women aged 54–65. BJOG: An International Journal of Obstetrics & Gynaecology. 2012;119(1):40–50.
5. Avis NE, Crawford SL, Greendale G, Bromberger JT, Everson-Rose SA, Gold EB, Hess R, Joffe H, Kravitz HM, Tepper PG, Thurston RC. Duration of menopausal vasomotor symptoms over the menopause transition. JAMA Intern Med. 2015;175(4):531–9.
6. Ayers B, Hunter MS. Health-related quality of life of women with menopausal hot flushes and night sweats. Climacteric. 2013;16(2):235–9.
7. Hunter MS, Liao K. A psychological analysis of menopausal hot flushes. Br J Clin Psychol. 1995;34(4):589–99.
8. Smith MJ, Mann E, Mirza A, Hunter MS. Men and women's perceptions of hot flushes within social situations: are menopausal women's negative beliefs valid? Maturitas. 2011;69(1):57–62.
9. Woods NF, Mitchell ES. Symptoms during the perimenopause: prevalence, severity, trajectory, and significance in women's lives. Am J Med. 2005;118(12):14–24.
10. Sergeant J, Rizq R. 'Its all part of the big CHANGE': a grounded theory study of women's identity during menopause. J Psychosom Obstet Gynecol. 2017;6:1–6.
11. Griffiths A, MacLennan SJ, Hassard J. Menopause and work: an electronic survey of employees' attitudes in the UK. Maturitas. 2013;76(2):155–9.
12. Faculty of Occupational Medicine. http://www.fom.ac.uk/health-at-work-2/information-for-employers/dealing-with-health-problems-in-the-workplace/advice-on-the-menopause. Accessed 12th September 2017.

13. Jack G, Riach K, Bariola E, Pitts M, Schapper J, Sarrel P. Menopause in the workplace: what employers should be doing. Maturitas. 2016;85:88–95.

14. Jack G, Bariola E, Riach K, Schnapper J, Work PM. Women and the menopause: an Australian exploratory study. Climacteric. 2014;17(Suppl 2):34.

15. Whiteley J, DiBonaventura MD, Wagner JS, Alvir J, Shah S. The impact of menopausal symptoms on quality of life, productivity, and economic outcomes. J Women's Health. 2013;22(11):983–90.

16. Gartoulla P, Worsley R, Bell RJ, Davis SR. Moderate to severe vasomotor and sexual symptoms remain problematic for women aged 60 to 65 years. Menopause. 2015;22(7):694–701.

17. Hickey M, Riach K, Kachouie R, Jack G. No sweat: managing menopausal symptoms at work. J Psychosom Obstet Gynecol. 2017;22:1–8.

18. Brewis J, Beck V, Davies A, Matheson J. The effects of menopause transition on women's economic participation in the UK. Research Report. 2017. https://www.gov.uk/government/publications/menopause-transition-effects-on-womens-economic-participation

19. Health and Safety Executive. http://www.hse.gov.uk/statistics/causdis/stress/stress.pdf. Accessed 12th September.

20. Lazarus RS. Psychological stress and the coping process. New York: McGraw-Hill.

21. Kahn RL, Wolfe DM, Quinn RP, Snoek JD. Rosenthal RA. Organizational stress: Studies in role conflict and ambiguity; 1964.

22. Harrison RV. The person-environment fit model and the study of job stress', Human Stress and Cognition in Organizations: An Integrated Perspective, ed. by TA Beehr and RS Bhagat.1985.

23. Karasek Jr RA. Job demands, job decision latitude, and mental strain: implications for job redesign. Adm Sci Q. 1979:285–308.

24. Demerouti E, Bakker AB, Nachreiner F, Schaufeli WB. The job demands-resources model of burnout. J Appl Psychol. 2001;86(3):499.

25. Houdmont J, Kerr R, Randall R. Organisational psychosocial hazard exposures in UK policing: management standards Indicator tool reference values. Policing: An Int J Police Strateg & Manage. 2012;35(1):182–97.

26. Health and Safety Executive (HSE). Management Standards Indicator Tool. http://www.hse.gov.uk/stress/standards/pdfs/indicatortool.pdf. Accessed 12th September 2017.

27. Hunter MS, Hardy C, Norton S, Griffiths A. Study protocol of a multicenter randomized controlled trial of self-help cognitive behavior therapy for working women with menopausal symptoms (MENOS@work). Maturitas. 92:186–92.

28. Hardy C, Griffiths A, Norton S, Hunter MS. Self-help cognitive behavior therapy for working women with problematic hot flushes and night sweats (MENOS@ Work): a multicenter randomized controlled trial. Menopause. 2018;25,(5) on line DOI: https://doi.org/10.1097/GME.0000000000001048.

29. Shore LM, Martin HJ. Job satisfaction and organizational commitment in relation to work performance and turnover intentions. Human relations. 1989;42(7):625–38.

30. Office of National Statistics (ONS). Table A05: Labour market by age group: Women by economic activity and age (seasonally adjusted). https://www.ons.gov.uk/employmentandlabourmarket/peopleinwork/employmentandemployeetypes/datasets/employmentunemploymentandeconomicinactivitybyagegroupseasonallyadjusteda05sa. Accessed 12th September 2017.

31. Hardy C, Griffiths A, Hunter MS. What do working menopausal women want? A qualitative investigation into women's perspectives on employer and line manager support. Maturitas. 2017;101:37–41.

32. Women's Health Concern. https://www.womens-health-concern.org/help-and-advice/factsheets/cognitive-behaviour-therapy-cbt-menopausal-symptoms. Accessed 12th September 2017.

33. Hunter MS, Smith M. Managing hot flushes and night sweats: a cognitive behavioural self-help guide to the menopause: Routledge; 2014.

34. Woods NF, Mitchell ES, Percival DB, Smith-DiJulio K. Is the menopausal transition stressful? Observations of perceived stress from the Seattle midlife Women's health study. Menopause. 2009;16:90–7.

# 14

# Stress and the menopausal transition in Campeche, Mexico

Lynnette Leidy Sievert[1*] (iD), Laura Huicochea-Gómez[2], Diana Cahuich-Campos[2], Dana-Lynn Ko'omoa-Lange[3] and Daniel E. Brown[4]

## Abstract

**Background:** Stress has been implicated as a factor in the presence and severity of symptoms during the menopausal transition. Our primary aim was to test the hypothesis that stress-sensitive biological measures and self-reported stress would be positively associated with a greater likelihood and intensity of hot flashes. Our secondary aim was to examine measures of stress in relation to the most often reported symptoms in Campeche, Mexico. We also hypothesized ethnic differences (Maya versus non-Maya) in relation to measures of stress and symptom reports.

**Methods:** Participants aged 40–60 ($n = 305$) were drawn from multiple sites across the city of San Francisco de Campeche to achieve a generally representative sample. Measures included C-reactive protein (CRP), an indicator of inflammation; Epstein-Barr virus antibodies (EBV-Ab), an indicator of immune function; the Perceived Stress Scale (PSS); a symptom checklist; anthropometric measures; and a questionnaire that elicited symptoms, ethnicity (based on language, birthplace, and last names of the woman, her parents, and her grandparents) and ten dimensions of socioeconomic status (SES). The relationships between symptoms and stress-sensitive biological and self-reported measures were examined in bivariate analyses, and with logistic and linear regressions.

**Results:** The twelve most common symptoms reported, in descending order of frequency, were tiredness, muscle and joint pain, nervous tension, problems concentrating, feeling depressed, difficulty sleeping, headaches, feeling of ants crawling on the skin, loss of interest in sex, urinary stress incontinence, hot flashes, and night sweats. PSS scores were significantly associated with the likelihood of seven symptoms (yes/no), and with the intensity of ten symptoms after controlling for ethnicity, SES, education, cohabitation status, parity, smoking, body mass index, and menopausal status. The stress-sensitive biological measures of immune function (EBV-Ab and CRP) were not significantly associated with midlife symptoms. The PSS was associated with more symptoms among the Maya (e.g., feeling nervous/tense and having difficulty concentrating) than non-Maya.

**Conclusion:** PSS scores were associated with the intensity, but not the likelihood, of hot flashes. Other symptoms were also associated with self-reported stress but not with physiological measures. Maya/non-Maya differences may indicate that either symptoms or stress were experienced and/or reported in culture-specific ways.

**Keywords:** Menopause, Stress, Hot flashes, Night sweats, Fatigue, Sleep difficulties, Depression

* Correspondence: leidy@anthro.umass.edu
[1]Department of Anthropology, Machmer Hall, 240 Hicks Way, UMass Amherst, Amherst, MA 01003-9278, USA
Full list of author information is available at the end of the article

## Background

The menopausal transition is often characterized by hot flashes and night sweats [1], fatigue and body aches [2], difficulty sleeping [3], and transient depression [4]. Some symptoms can be attributed to the changing hormone levels associated with the loss of ovarian follicles, including fluctuating estradiol and increases in follicle stimulating hormones [5, 6]. However, some symptoms may be better explained by combining physiological information with the social changes that coincide with this time of life. For example, a woman's children are likely to be adolescents with their own challenges, husbands may be undergoing transition in social status such as retirement or struggling with health issues, and parents may be in need of substantial levels of care [7, 8].

During the menopausal transition, stress may be a contributor to trouble sleeping, depression [9, 10], and/or symptoms that may have a psychosomatic component [11]. For example, in cross-cultural work among women aged 45–55, Sievert et al. [12] found that *job* change was associated with an increased likelihood of nervous tension, difficulty concentrating, headaches, and fatigue in the U.S., but not in Spain. In Spain, but not the U.S., *household* change was associated with depressed mood and difficulty concentrating. These differences show that stress is variable and context dependent. It appears that job change may be experienced as more stressful in the U.S., whereas household change may be more stressful in Spain.

Specific to hot flashes, stress has been identified as a determinant in some [13–17], but not all [12, 18, 19] studies of factors associated with hot flashes. In a laboratory setting, where symptomatic women were exposed to a variety of stressors, there were 57% more self-reported hot flashes during stress periods compared to non-stress periods [20]. In the Study of Women's Health Across the Nation (SWAN), after adjusting for ethnicity, lifestyle, and other confounding variables, self-reported perceived stress was significantly associated with self-reported vasomotor symptoms (adjusted odds ratio 1.4, 95% confidence interval 1.2–1.6) [15], and significantly related to a longer persistence of self-reported hot flashes into the postmenopausal period [13]. In a 13-year longitudinal study in Philadelphia, women who reported moderate or severe hot flashes during the study period had a higher baseline Perceived Stress Scale (PSS) score (21.9) compared to women with mild hot flashes (19.5) or no hot flashes (18.2, $p < 0.01$). Stress was not significantly associated with the duration of self-reported hot flushes in a multivariable model [14].

Cortisol is a stress-sensitive biological measure [21] that has been examined in relation to hot flashes. Two early laboratory studies showed an increase in cortisol levels during and after monitored hot flashes [22, 23]. In the Seattle Women's Health Study, women with increased urinary cortisol had significantly greater self-reported hot flash and cold sweat symptom severity compared to women without increased cortisol [24]. In Modena, Italy, women with self-reported severe hot flashes had significantly higher levels of 24-h urinary cortisol compared to women with none to moderate vasomotor symptoms [25]. Hot flash report has also been associated with higher salivary cortisol levels in the early afternoon [26]. In a small study where women with hot flashes were measured by an ambulatory monitor, objectively measured hot flashes were associated with significantly higher salivary cortisol levels at 15, 30, and 45 min post-waking compared to women without biometrically measured hot flashes [27].

Not all studies have shown a consistently positive relationship between hot flashes and cortisol levels. For example, hot flash report has not been associated with the cortisol awakening response or diurnal variation in cortisol levels [26, 28, 29]. One study found greater self-reported hot flash severity associated with a flatter diurnal slope in salivary cortisol [30].

Self-reported hot flashes and other symptoms have been shown to vary across ethnicity within the same country [31–33]. Self-reported stress has also been shown to vary with ethnicity. For example, Brown [34, 35] compared levels of stress across two Filipino-American ethnic groups to show that individuals from Visayan backgrounds self-reported significantly higher levels of stress compared to individuals of Ilocano descent. At the same time, there was no difference in the 24-h excretion rates of norepinephrine and epinephrine between the two groups. Brown also found that Filipino American women (mostly Ilocanos) were significantly more likely to record being anxious in a diary compared to European American women, but European Americans had higher elevations in ambulatory blood pressure when they did report anxiety [36]. Ethnic differences were also found in response to doing household chores: Filipino American women were more likely to report being anxious during chores than European Americans, but the European American women had higher diastolic BP while doing chores than the Filipino Americans [36]. Ethnic differences in the report of stress may reflect psychosocial differences [37], or culturally-based reporting biases [38]. For these reasons, the study reported here examined self-reported stress and symptom frequencies between Maya and non-Maya women.

Previous studies of menopause among Maya women in the Yucatán Peninsula of Mexico found an early mean recalled age at natural menopause of 44 years, compared to 52.5 years in the U.S. [39–41]. An in-depth ethnographic study documented an absence of self-reported hot flashes among rural Maya women [42]. According to

Beyene, Maya women explained menopause as something that occurred when a woman used up her menstrual blood ([43], page 119). These women perceived menopause to be "a life stage free of taboos and restrictions, offering increased freedom of movement" (p.120). Other investigators recorded higher levels of hot flash frequencies among urban (49%) and rural (41%) Maya women in the Yucatán peninsula [44].

This study administered the PSS, as used in the SWAN and Philadelphia studies, to measure self-reported stress. To our knowledge, this will be the first study to examine hot flashes and other symptoms at midlife in relation to Epstein-Barr virus antibodies (EBV-Ab) [45, 46]. Both C-reactive protein (CRP) and EBV-Ab have been positively associated with high stress levels [47, 48]. CRP is an acute-phase protein that is commonly used as a measure of general inflammation. Because chronic stress is associated with elevated inflammation levels [49], this protein has been used as a marker of both acute and chronic stress [50, 51]. With regard to EBV-Ab, most people are chronically infected with EBV. When an individual is stressed, down-regulation of the immune system allows the virus to replicate, and antibodies to the virus increase in the blood stream. Accordingly, an elevated EBV-Ab level has been used as a biological marker of stress [47, 52].

The primary aim of this study was to test the hypothesis that two biological measures potentially sensitive to stress and a self-reported measure of stress would be associated with a higher likelihood and intensity of hot flashes after controlling for potential confounders. Our secondary aim was to examine the stress-sensitive measures and self-reported stress in relation to the most commonly reported symptoms in Campeche, Mexico. Based on the results of other cross-cultural studies [12, 36] detailed above, we paid particular attention to ethnic differences in nervous tension, difficulties concentrating, headaches, fatigue, and depressed mood, as well as hot flashes and trouble sleeping. We hypothesized that all stress measures would be associated with the frequency and intensity of each of the 12 most-reported symptoms in bivariate analyses, and after controlling for potential confounders. We also hypothesized ethnic differences (Maya vs. non-Maya) in relation to measures of stress and symptom reports [38]. Other variables that could affect both stress measures and symptoms were collected, including age, menopausal status, level of education, socioeconomic status (SES), body mass index (BMI), ethnicity, marital status and cohabitation with husband or partner, parity, and smoking habits.

## Methods
### Sample
The study took place in San Francisco de Campeche, a city of approximately 250,000 people [53] located on the western coast of the Yucatan peninsula. Nearly 12% of the city's population speaks Maya [53]. Women aged 40–60 years were drawn from businesses, schools, the city market, and by presentations given in homes. The use of several recruitment methods assured a diverse, although not random, sample of the city's population. These participants make up the urban component of a larger study of menopause in the state of Campeche [54]. In the city, a total of 305 women participated in interviews and anthropometric measures, with a sub-sample of 162 participants providing finger stick blood samples. Of those 162 women, 109 provided sufficient blood for the assay of both CRP and EBV-Ab levels.

The study was approved by the Institutional Review Board of the University of Massachusetts Amherst; the Human Subjects Committee of the University of Hawaii at Hilo; and the Committee for Ethics in Research of the Secretary of Health in the State of Campeche, Mexico. All participants signed a letter of consent after lengthy explanation in Spanish.

### Measures
All participants answered questions related to their age, education, parity, and smoking status. An SES index was created from 10 dimensions related to housing construction, household composition, and infrastructure, such as, access to drinking water and type of cooking fuel. Within the city of Campeche, the range in SES index was from 22 to 39. With regard to marital status, 96% of married women ($n = 160$) and 73% of women with a partner ($n = 26$; *union libre*) lived with their partner and, therefore, the variable of interest used in the analyses here was whether or not a woman cohabited with a husband or partner.

Maya/non-Maya ethnicity was assessed on the basis of each woman's two last names, whether she could speak or understand Maya, and place of birth. The same information was collected with regard to her parents and grandparents. Women were categorized as Maya, not Maya, or not able to be clearly defined on the basis of this information from all three generations. There were 40 participants for whom an ethnic was unclear because of missing information (e.g., not everyone knew the language spoken by their grandparents).

Menopausal status was defined by STRAW+ 10 stages: (1) regular menstruation, (2) changes in the number of days or quantity of blood, (3) more or less frequent menstruation, (4) a change in periods of more than 6 days, (5) 2 months or more have passed without a period, and (6) more than 12 months have passed without a period [55]. Stages 1 and 2 were categorized as pre-menopausal, stages 3 to 5 as peri-menopausal, and stage 6 as postmenopausal.

Stature was measured with a Seca 213 stadiometer to the nearest 0.1 cm. Weight was measured to the nearest 0.1 kg with a digital scale. BMI was computed as $kg/m^2$.

All participants completed the PSS that has been previously used in Mexican populations [56]. The PSS is a well validated 10-item questionnaire that directly queries levels of stress experienced in the past month, and the degree to which one's life is unpredictable, uncontrollable, and overloaded [57, 58].

Participants were asked about the presence or absence of 19 symptoms during the past 2 weeks including hot flashes (*Ha tenido calores o bochornos?*) and night sweats (*En la noche ha tenido sudoraciones?*). This "everyday symptom list" has been used in many studies [59–61], including in Mexico [62]. Symptom intensities were reported as: 0 = *nada*; 1 = *un poco*; 2 = *mucho*; and 3 = *muchisimo*. Twelve symptoms had a frequency of 45% or higher in the city of Campeche. The cut off of 45% was selected in order to include hot flashes and night sweats in the analyses below. The 12 symptom reports were totaled to derive a total number of symptoms reported for each individual. Also, the intensity of the 12 symptoms were totaled to derive a total symptom intensity score for each participant.

Blood was collected by finger stick onto Whatman #903 Protein Saver filter paper sample cards [47], dried for 4 h, and immediately frozen in the Huicochea laboratory at ECOSUR, Campeche. The cards were carried to the United States by LLS, and mailed overnight to the University of Hawaii at Hilo with ice packs. The cards were then transferred to freezer storage at – 30 °C until analysis.

To determine the presence of EBV – Viral Capsid Antigen (VCA) in dried blood spot samples, an EBV-VCA enzyme-linked immunosorbent assay (Diamedix Corporation, Miami Lakes, FL), was modified for sampling dried blood spots. Briefly, a sample of each blood spot was taken by punching a single 6 mm disc using a standard hand held hole puncher. The blood spot samples were incubated in elution buffer overnight, on a platform shaker at low speed. 100 uL of the cut-off calibrator, controls and samples were transferred to the antigen wells. The samples and controls were allowed to incubate at room temperature for 30 min. The contents of the wells were discarded, and the wells were washed three times with wash solution. 100 uL of conjugate was pipetted into each well, and allowed to incubate at room temperature for 30 min. The contents were discarded, and the wells were washed three times in wash solution. Next, 100 uL of the substrate was pipetted into each well, and the wells were incubated at room temperature for 30 min. After incubation with substrate, 100 uL of stop solution was pipetted into each well. The absorbance was determined at 450 nm. All controls and samples were assayed in duplicate [45].

To determine the index value for each participant, the following formula was used:

$$\frac{\text{Absorbance of sample}}{\text{Mean absorbance of cut-off calibrator}} = \text{Index value}$$

Samples with an index value ≥1.10 were determined to be positive for VCA IgG antibody.

CRP enzyme-linked immunosorbent assay (Abcam, Cambridge, MA) was used to quantitatively measure human CRP in blood spots following the methods of McDade et al. [63]. CRP values in blood spots were converted into the equivalent values of CRP in plasma by the following: $(CRP_{bloodspot} * 1.15) – 0.13 = CRP_{Plasma}$ [63]. None of the participants had a $CRP_{Plasma}$ value greater than 10.0 mg/L, an indicator of an active infection which would have led to exclusion from analyses involving CRP and EBV-Ab [64].

### Analyses

PSS scores, EBV-Ab levels, and $CRP_{Plasma}$ levels were appraised for normal distribution. PSS scores were normally distributed and examined in relation to ethnic categories (Maya, not Maya, difficult to categorize) by ANOVA and in relation to each symptom (yes/no) by t-tests. EBV-Ab and $CRP_{Plasma}$ levels were not normally distributed, and therefore were examined in relation to ethnic categories and in relation to each symptom by two-tailed Mann Whitney tests. Spearman correlations were examined between EBV-Ab values, $CRP_{Plasma}$ levels, and PSS scores.

Logistic regressions were performed with each of the 12 symptoms (none vs. any level of symptom experience) as a dependent variable in a separate regression model. Analyses were carried out separately for each of the three stress measures – PSS scores, EBV-Ab values, and $CRP_{Plasma}$ levels; therefore, there were three analyses carried out for each of the 12 symptoms. BMI, SES, education, ethnicity, cohabiting with a husband or partner, parity, smoking, and menopausal status were covariates. Because of the correlation among the covariates SES and education ($r = .465$, $p < 0.001$), and in order to achieve the best set of variables associated with each symptom, backward stepwise regression was carried out with a probability for entry set at 0.05 and probability for removal set to 0.10. Because of the multiple testing, we applied an adjusted p-value of $p \le 0.001$ to determine significance. Logistic regressions were repeated separately for women categorized as Maya and non-Maya.

Linear regressions with backwards elimination were carried out for all participants with intensity of symptom reports (*nada, un poco, mucho, muchisimo*) as dependent variables and PSS scores, EBV-Ab values, $CRP_{Plasma}$ levels,

BMI, SES, education, ethnicity, cohabiting with a husband or partner, parity, smoking, and menopausal status as co-variates. As described above, analyses for each symptom were carried out separately for the three stress variables, and analyses were repeated separately for women categorized as Maya and non-Maya, respectively.

## Results

Table 1 presents some characteristics of the sample by ethnicity. The Maya had a significantly lower SES index than non-Maya, but there were otherwise no significant ethnic differences in the listed characteristics. There were no significant differences in the PSS score between Maya and non-Maya women ($t = 1.3$, ns); Maya women had significantly higher EBV-Ab (two-tailed Mann Whitney test, $p < 0.05$), but there was no significant ethnic difference in $CRP_{Plasma}$ levels. There were no significant ethnic differences in the frequency of symptoms, the total number of reported symptoms, or the total symptom intensity scores (two-tailed t-tests, ns). Figure 1 shows the frequency of reported symptoms for the entire sample.

For all women in the sample, there was a significant correlation between EBV-Ab values and $CRP_{Plasma}$ levels (Spearman $\rho = 0.57$, $p < 0.001$), but PSS scores were not significantly correlated with either EBV-Ab values ($\rho = -0.08$, ns) or $CRP_{Plasma}$ levels ($\rho = -0.02$, ns). Similar correlation results among stress measures were obtained when the ethnic groups were considered separately.

Table 2 presents results for bivariate analyses of the relation between stress measures and reported symptoms (none vs. any level of symptom experience) for all participants. The table gives means and standard deviations of the PSS scores, and medians of the $CRP_{Plasma}$ and EBV-Ab levels. For nine of the 12 symptoms, women who reported the symptom had a significantly higher PSS score compared to women who did not report the symptom ($p \leq 0.001$). Women with hot flashes and headaches had higher PSS scores, with p-values of 0.004 and 0.006, respectively – slightly above the conservative Bonferroni correction of $p \leq 0.001$. EBV-Ab and $CRP_{Plasma}$ values were not significantly higher among women reporting any symptom.

The total number of reported symptoms for each individual was significantly correlated with the PSS score

**Table 1** Participant information. Means ± standard deviations, numbers of participants, or percentages shown

|  | Maya | Non-Maya | Could not classify | All |
|---|---|---|---|---|
| N | 144 | 121 | 40 | 305 |
| Age at interview Mean ± s.d. | 47.9 ± 5.0 | 46.9 ± 5.0 | 47.5 ± 5.0 | 47.5 ± 5.0 |
| BMI (kg/m²) Mean ± s.d. | 31.3 ± 5.2 | 30.3 ± 5.8 | 29.1 ± 5.3 | 30.6 ± 5.5 |
| SES Index[a] Range 22–39. Mean ± s.d. | 32.8 ± 2.4 | 33.4 ± 2.3 | 33.4 ± 2.4 | 33.1 ± 2.4 |
| Education (yrs) Mean ± s.d. | 12.8 ± 4.4 | 13.8 ± 4.0 | 13.3 ± 4.4 | 13.2 ± 4.2 |
| Menopause status (%) |  |  |  |  |
| Pre-menopausal | 40.3 | 47.9 | 42.5 | 43.6 |
| Perimenopausal | 20.8 | 24.0 | 22.5 | 22.3 |
| Post – menopausal | 38.9 | 28.1 | 35.0 | 34.1 |
| % cohabiting with husband or partner | 59.0 | 57.0 | 70.0 | 59.7 |
| Parity Mean ± s.d. | 2.0 ± 1.1 | 2.1 ± 1.2 | 2.0 ± 1.4 | 2.0 ± 1.2 |
| Smoking (%) | 10.4 | 14.9 | 12.5 | 12.5 |
| PSS score Mean ± s.d. n = 305 | 1.55 ± 1.6 | 1.04 ± 0.6 | 1.58 ± 1.7 | 1.35 ± 1.3 |
| EBV-Ab level* Mean ± s.d. n = 162 | 4.59 ± 1.4 | 4.06 ± 1.7 | 3.83 ± 1.6 | 4.30 ± 1.6 |
| $CRP_{plasma}$ level Mean ± s.d. n = 157 | 16.78 ± 5.2 | 17.65 ± 5.9 | 17.95 ± 4.5 | 17.28 ± 5.4 |
| Total symptom score (range 0–12, based on 12 most common symptoms) | 7.4 ± 3.0 | 7.4 ± 2.7 | 6.9 ± 3.1 | 7.3 ± 2.9 |
| Total symptom intensity score (range 0–33, based on 12 most common symptoms) | 10.9 ± 6.4 | 10.4 ± 6.0 | 9.3 ± 5.5 | 10.5 ± 6.0 |

[a]Ethnic difference, Maya versus non-Maya, $p < 0.05$

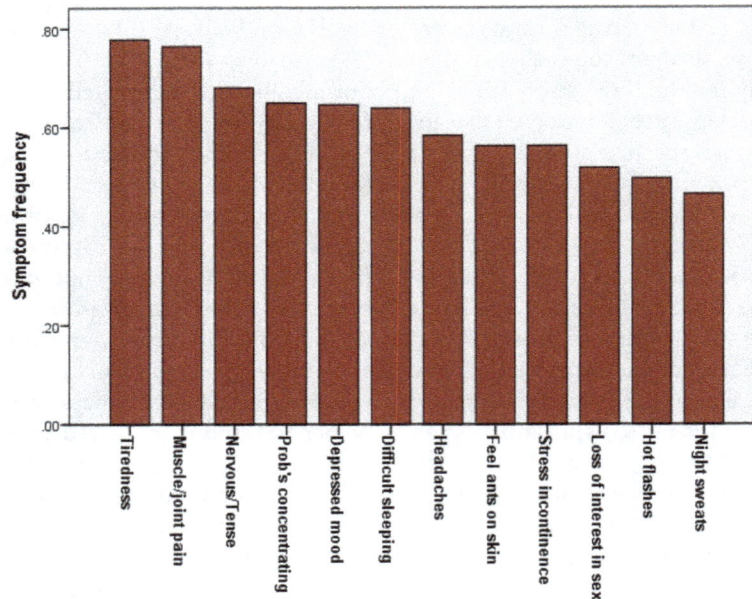

**Fig. 1** Frequency of the 12 most often reported symptoms among Maya and non-Maya women living in the city of Campeche, Mexico (*n* = 305)

(two-tailed Spearman correlations, ρ = 0.42, *p* < 0.001), but not with CRP$_{Plasma}$ (ρ = − 0.02, ns) nor EBV-Ab (ρ = − 0.08, ns) levels. The total symptom intensity score was significantly correlated with the PSS score (ρ = 0.46, *p* < 0.001) and EBV-Ab values (ρ = 0.17, *p* < 0.05).

Table 3 presents the covariates that remained in the models following backwards stepwise logistic regression for each symptom among all participants. PSS score was significantly, positively associated with the report of

tiredness, muscle/joint pain, feeling nervous/tense, problems concentrating, depressed mood, difficulty sleeping, and loss of interest in sex after controlling for BMI, SES, education, ethnicity, cohabiting with a husband or partner, parity, smoking, and menopausal status. Odds Ratios for PSS ranged from 1.10 (95% CI 1.04–1.15) for loss of interest in sex to 1.22 (95% CI 1.13–1.32) tiredness. Hot flashes, night sweats, and the feeling of ants crawling on the skin had *p*-values of 0.007, 0.004,

**Table 2** Bivariate comparisons of stress levels by symptom complaints. Means ± standard deviations for PSS scores or medians for CRP$_{Plasma}$ and EBV-Ab levels shown

| Symptom | PSS score by symptom | | EBV-Ab value by symptom | | CRPPlasma level by symptom | |
|---|---|---|---|---|---|---|
| | No | Yes | No | Yes | No | Yes |
| Tiredness or lack of energy | 13.9 ± 4.2 | 18.2 ± 5.3*** | 0.81 | 1.00* | 5.28 | 5.69 |
| Muscle and joint pain | 15.1 ± 4.6 | 17.9 ± 5.5*** | 1.00 | 0.96 | 5.61 | 5.64 |
| Nervous or tense | 15.3 ± 4.5 | 18.2 ± 5.5*** | 0.93 | 1.00 | 5.28 | 5.68 |
| Problems concentrating | 15.4 ± 4.5 | 18.3 ± 5.6*** | 0.94 | 0.99 | 5.57 | 5.65 |
| Depressed mood or sadness | 15.3 ± 4.3 | 18.4 ± 5.6*** | 0.93 | 1.00 | 4.86 | 5.72* |
| Difficulty sleeping | 15.1 ± 5.0 | 18.6 ± 5.2*** | 0.86 | 1.01 | 5.34 | 5.68 |
| Headaches | 16.3 ± 4.7 | 18.0 ± 5.8** | 0.94 | 1.00 | 5.48 | 5.69 |
| Feeling of ants crawling on skin | 16.0 ± 4.7 | 18.3 ± 5.7*** | 0.82 | 0.94* | 5.33 | 5.48 |
| Urinary stress incontinence with effort or laughter | 16.4 ± 4.9 | 17.9 ± 5.7* | 0.93 | 0.98 | 5.34 | 5.68 |
| Loss of interest in sexual relations | 16.3 ± 5.2 | 18.4 ± 5.4*** | 1.00 | 0.96 | 5.65 | 5.65 |
| Hot flashes | 16.4 ± 5.2 | 18.2 ± 5.4** | 0.94 | 0.98 | 5.59 | 5.67 |
| Night sweats | 16.4 ± 5.0 | 18.5 ± 5.7*** | 0.84 | 1.02 | 5.34 | 5.68 |

Two tailed t-tests or Mann-Whitney tests, *p < 0.05; **p < 0.01; ***p ≤ 0.001

**Table 3** Logistic regression analyses of symptom reports. 95% Confidence Intervals shown for Odds Ratios

| With PSS scores | | | With CRP$_{Plasma}$ | | | With EBV–Ab | | |
|---|---|---|---|---|---|---|---|---|
| Variable | Odds Ratio (95% CI) | Signif. | Variable | Odds Ratio (95% CI) | Signif. | Variable | Odds Ratio (95% CI) | Signif. |
| **Tiredness** | | | | | | | | |
| PSS Score | 1.22 (1.13–1.32) | **<0.001** | [none remained in model] | | | Parity | 1.41 0.94–2.10 | <0.1 |
| Parity | 1.36 (1.02–1.83) | <0.05 | | | | | | |
| **Muscle and Joint Pain** | | | | | | | | |
| PSS Score | 1.11 (1.04–1.18) | **<0.001** | SES | 0.80 0.64–1.01 | <0.1 | [none remained in model] | | |
| Education | 0.95 (0.80–0.95) | <0.01 | | | | | | |
| **Nervous or Tense** | | | | | | | | |
| PSS Score | 1.12 (1.06–1.18) | **<0.001** | Cohabiting (ref) | | | EBV-Ab | 1.76 (1.00–3.12) | = 0.05 |
| Parity | 1.36 (1.06–1.74) | <0.05 | not cohabiting | 0.41 (0.19–1.01) | <0.05 | Cohabiting (ref) | | |
| BMI | 0.96 0.91–1.01 | <0.1 | | | | not cohabiting | 0.39 (0.18–0.85) | <0.05 |
| **Problems concentrating** | | | | | | | | |
| PSS Score | 1.14 (1.08–1.21) | **<0.001** | Menopause Pre- (Ref) | | | Non-smoker (ref) | | |
| | | | Peri- | 3.99 (1.31–12.09) | <0.05 | Smoker | 3.50 (0.97–12.59) | <0.1 |
| | | | Post- | 1.57 (0.65–3.80) | ns | | | |
| | | | BMI | 1.09 (1.00–1.19) | <0.05 | | | |
| **Depressed mood** | | | | | | | | |
| PSS Score | 1.14 (1.07–1.20) | **<0.001** | BMI | 1.10 (1.02–1.18) | <0.05 | BMI | 1.09 (1.01–1.18) | <0.05 |
| BMI | 1.07 (1.02–1.13) | = 0.01 | | | | Education | 0.92 (0.83–1.01) | <0.1 |
| **Difficulty sleeping** | | | | | | | | |
| PSS Score | 1.18 (1.11–1.25) | **<0.001** | Education | 0.85 (0.76–0.96) | = 0.01 | Education | 0.91 (0.81–1.01) | <0.1 |
| Cohabiting (ref) | | | Menopause Pre- (Ref) | | | BMI | 0.94 (0.87–1.01) | <0.1 |
| Not cohabiting | 2.04 (1.12–3.70) | <0.05 | Peri- | 1.21 (0.49–2.98) | ns | | | |
| | | | Post- | 3.56 (1.37–9.25) | <0.05 | | | |
| **Ethnicity** | | | | | | Ethnicity | | |
| Maya (ref) | | | | | | Maya (ref) | | |
| Non-Maya | 0.53 (0.30–0.92) | <0.05 | | | | Non-Maya | 0.34 (0.16–0.74) | <0.01 |

**Table 3** Logistic regression analyses of symptom reports. 95% Confidence Intervals shown for Odds Ratios (Continued)

| With PSS scores | | | With CRP$_{Plasma}$ | | | With EBV–Ab | | |
|---|---|---|---|---|---|---|---|---|
| Variable | Odds Ratio (95% CI) | Signif. | Variable | Odds Ratio (95% CI) | Signif. | Variable | Odds Ratio (95% CI) | Signif. |
| Parity | 1.25 (0.97–1.61) | < 0.1 | | | | | | |
| Headaches | | | | | | | | |
| PSS Score | 1.06 (1.01–1.11) | < 0.05 | CRP$_{Plasma}$ | 1.19 (0.97–1.45) | p< 0.1 | [none remained in model] | | |
| Education | 0.93 (0.87–0.99) | < 0.05 | Ethnicity Maya (ref) | | | | | |
| | | | Non–Maya | 2.24 (1.07–4.67) | < 0.05 | | | |
| Cohabiting (ref) | | | | | | | | |
| Not cohabiting | 0.63 (0.38–1.05) | < 0.1 | | | | | | |
| Feeling of ants crawling on skin | | | | | | | | |
| PSS Score | 1.08 (1.03–1.13) | = 0.002 | CRP$_{Plasma}$ | 1.22 1.00–1.49 | < 0.1 | Education | 0.90 (0.81–1.00) | = 0.05 |
| | | | Menopause Pre- (ref) | | | | | |
| | | | Peri- | 2.89 (1.08–7.76) | < 0.05 | | | |
| | | | Post- | 1.58 (0.69–3.66) | ns | | | |
| Stress Incontinence | | | | | | | | |
| PSS Score | 1.05 (1.00–1.10) | < 0.05 | [none remained in model] | | | [none remained in model] | | |
| Menopause Pre- (ref) | | | | | | | | |
| Peri- | 0.72 (0.38–1.38) | ns | | | | | | |
| Post- | 0.54 (0.30–0.95) | < 0.05 | | | | | | |
| Loss of interest in sex | | | | | | | | |
| PSS Score | 1.10 (1.04–1.15) | **< 0.001** | Cohabiting (ref) | | | Cohabiting (ref) | | |
| Cohabiting (ref) | | | not cohabiting | 0.30 (0.14–0.64) | = 0.002 | not cohabiting | 0.48 (0.23–1.01) | = 0.05 |
| Not cohabiting | 0.26 (0.15–0.43) | **< 0.001** | | | | SES | 0.83 (0.69–0.99) | < 0.05 |
| Ethnicity | | | | | | | | |
| Maya (ref) | | | | | | | | |
| Non-Maya | 0.60 (0.36–1.02) | < 0.1 | | | | | | |
| Hot flashes | | | | | | | | |
| PSS Score | 1.07 (1.02–1.12) | = 0.007 | [none remained in model] | | | Cohabiting (ref) | | |
| | | | | | | not cohabiting | 0.54 (0.26–1.13) | = 0.1 |

**Table 3** Logistic regression analyses of symptom reports. 95% Confidence Intervals shown for Odds Ratios (Continued)

| With PSS scores | | | With CRP$_{Plasma}$ | | | With EBV–Ab | | |
| --- | --- | --- | --- | --- | --- | --- | --- | --- |
| Variable | Odds Ratio (95% CI) | Signif. | Variable | Odds Ratio (95% CI) | Signif. | Variable | Odds Ratio (95% CI) | Signif. |
| Menopause Pre- (ref) | | | | | | Menopause Pre- (ref) | | |
| Peri- | 1.90 (0.99–3.66) | < 0.1 | | | | Peri- | 2.12 (0.94–4.77) | < 0.1 |
| Post- | 1.73 (0.97–3.08) | < 0.1 | | | | Post- | 2.22 (0.91–5.43) | < 0.1 |
| Parity | 1.23 (0.99–1.53) | < 0.1 | | | | | | |
| Night sweats | | | | | | | | |
| PSS Score | 1.07 (1.02–1.13) | = 0.004 | CRP$_{Plasma}$ | 1.26 (1.01–1.57) | < 0.05 | | | |
| Cohabiting (ref) | | | Cohabiting (ref) | | | Cohabiting (ref) | | |
| Not cohabiting | 0.40 (0.23–0.69) | **= 0.001** | not cohabiting | 0.28 (0.12–0.63) | = 0.002 | not cohabiting | 0.24 (0.11–0.53) | **< 0.001** |
| Menopause Pre- (ref) | | | Menopause Pre- (ref) | | | Menopause Pre- (ref) | | |
| Peri- | 2.06 (1.05–4.06) | < 0.05 | Peri- | 2.37 (0.92–6.10) | ns | Peri- | 3.03 (1.27–7.21) | < 0.05 |
| Post- | 2.12 (1.16–3.88) | < 0.05 | Post- | 2.60 (1.05–6.42) | < 0.05 | Post- | 2.02 (0.78–5.22) | ns |

Variables entered into the logistic models: ethnicity, SES, education, cohabitation status, parity, smoking, body mass index, and menopausal status. Significance set to $p <= 0.001$

and 0.002, respectively – slightly above the conservative Bonferroni correction of $p \leq 0.001$. EBV-Ab and $CRP_{Plasma}$ levels were not significantly associated with any of the symptoms.

Along with the PSS score, not cohabiting with a husband or partner significantly decreased report of the loss of interest in sex and the likelihood of night sweats. Along with the PSS score, number of children was positively associated with the risk of tiredness and nervousness, although not at the level of $p \leq 0.001$. Overall, the PSS score was the variable most likely to be associated with symptom frequencies.

When the logistic regressions were carried out separately by ethnicity, for Maya, the PSS score was significantly associated with tiredness, feeling nervous/tense, difficulty concentrating, depressed mood, and night sweats ($p \leq 0.001$); for non-Maya, the PSS score was significantly associated with reported tiredness, depressed mood, and sleep difficulties (not shown). $CRP_{Plasma}$ levels and EBV-Ab values were not significantly associated with any symptom reports for Maya or non-Maya when ethnic groups were examined separately.

As shown in Table 4, the PSS score was significantly associated with the intensity (*nada* = 0 to *muchisimo* = 3) of ten of the 12 reported symptoms, including hot flashes and night sweats ($p \leq 0.001$). $CRP_{Plasma}$ levels and EBV-Ab values were not significantly associated with the intensity of any symptom reports. When regressions were carried out separately by ethnicity, among Maya participants, the PSS score was significantly associated with the intensity of feeling tired, muscle/joint pain, feeling nervous/tense, difficulty concentrating, depressed mood, difficulty sleeping, and night sweats ($p \leq 0.001$); for non-Maya, the PSS score was significantly associated with the intensity of the same symptoms except for night sweats. Among the Maya, the association between the PSS score and hot flashes approached significance ($p = 0.002$). $CRP_{Plasma}$ levels were not associated with symptoms among the Maya or non-Maya. EBV-Ab values were not significantly associated with any reported symptom intensity among the Maya or non-Maya.

Along with the PSS score, level of education was negatively associated with the intensity of muscle and joint pain. Cohabiting with a husband or partner was positively associated with the intensity of the loss of interest in sex. Progression through menopause was associated with the increased intensity of night sweats.

## Discussion

In this urban population of women aged 40 to 60 from Campeche, Mexico, hot flashes and night sweats were not the most commonly reported symptoms. This finding is consistent with other studies that have found aches and stiffness [32, 60, 65], lack of energy [59], and tiredness or fatigue [61, 66] to be more common than hot flashes.

Correlations between self-report measures and biological markers of stress tend to be small or moderate [38]. In the case of this Campeche sample, there were no significant relationships between self-reports of stress (PSS score) and the potentially stress-sensitive biological measures (EBV-Ab and CRP levels), although the two measures of immune function were positively and significantly correlated. None of the measures used in this study were solely measuring stress; there are many factors that can influence immune system activity, and the PSS measures perceptions of stress which can be quite variable in different individuals [38]. It may be that biological measures were elevated in relation to immunological stress, but that immunological activity did not correlate with the impact of stress on the participants within the context of their lives. It may be that these particular biomarkers were not sensitive enough, or that the biomarkers could not effectively measure stress as perceived by the person.

Self-reported PSS was found to be significantly associated with nine of the most common symptoms in bivariate analyses, and with seven symptoms after controlling for potential covariates, whereas neither CRP nor EBV-Ab were associated with symptoms. PSS scores were also associated with the intensity of ten reported symptoms, including hot flashes and night sweats. No other variable in the logistic or linear models was associated with so many midlife symptoms. Our findings are similar to the relationship reported by SWAN researchers who found that the PSS score was significantly associated with vasomotor symptoms [15].

When logistic regressions were carried out separately by ethnicity, the PSS score was significantly associated with five of the reported symptoms among Maya women, including night sweats ($n = 144$). However, among non-Maya women ($n = 121$) the PSS score was significantly associated with only three of the symptoms. These ethnic differences may reflect cultural differences in either the experience or reporting of vasomotor and other symptoms [38, 67]. For Maya women, symptoms may be a means of expressing feelings of stress [11], more so than for non-Maya women.

In results reported here, Maya and non-Maya women did not differ in mean PSS scores; however, Maya women with higher PSS scores were more likely to report a higher intensity of hot flashes ($p = 0.002$) and the presence of and a higher intensity of night sweats ($p \leq 0.001$). It is of interest to note that earlier literature found an absence of hot flash report among Maya women in the Yucatán peninsula [42, 43, 68]. In contrast, the study presented here did not find an ethnic

**Table 4** Linear regression analyses of symptom reports

| With PSS scores | | | | With CRP$_{Plasma}$ | | | | With EBV-Ab | | | |
|---|---|---|---|---|---|---|---|---|---|---|---|
| Variable | Beta | t | Signif. | Variable | Beta | t | Signif. | Variable | Beta | t | Signif. |
| **Tiredness** | | | | | | | | | | | |
| PSS Score | 0.39 | 6.8 | **<0.001** | CRP$_{Plasma}$ | 0.19 | 2.3 | <0.05 | Education | −0.20 | −2.3 | <0.05 |
| Education | −.11 | 2.0 | <0.05 | Education | −0.27 | −3.2 | <0.01 | Education | −0.26 | −2.3 | <0.01 |
| **Muscle and Joint Pain** | | | | | | | | | | | |
| PSS Score | 0.31 | 5.4 | **<0.001** | Education | −0.27 | −3.2 | <0.01 | Education | −0.26 | −2.3 | <0.01 |
| Education | −0.22 | −3.8 | **<0.001** | | | | | | | | |
| **Nervous or Tense** | | | | | | | | | | | |
| PSS Score | 0.38 | 6.8 | **<0.001** | CRP$_{Plasma}$ | 0.17 | 2.1 | <0.05 | EBV-Ab | 0.18 | 2.1 | <0.05 |
| Cohabiting | 0.10 | 1.7 | <0.1 | Cohabiting | 0.15 | 1.8 | <0.1 | Smoker | 0.19 | 2.3 | <0.05 |
| Smoker | 0.16 | 2.9 | <0.01 | Smoker | 0.20 | 2.4 | <0.05 | | | | |
| **Difficulty Concentrating** | | | | | | | | | | | |
| PSS Score | 0.33 | 5.6 | **<0.001** | BMI | 0.23 | 2.7 | <0.01 | [No variables left in model] | | | |
| Parity | 0.12 | 2.1 | <0.05 | Parity | 0.14 | 1.7 | <0.1 | | | | |
| **Depressed mood** | | | | | | | | | | | |
| PSS Score | 0.51 | 9.7 | **<0.001** | CRP$_{Plasma}$ | 0.19 | 2.3 | <0.05 | Education | −0.18 | −2.1 | <0.05 |
| Parity | 0.13 | 2.5 | <0.05 | Education | −0.18 | −2.2 | <0.05 | | | | |
| | | | | Parity | 0.18 | 2.1 | <0.05 | | | | |
| **Difficulty sleeping** | | | | | | | | | | | |
| PSS Score | 0.39 | 6.9 | **<0.001** | Menopause status | 0.27 | 3.3 | **<0.001** | Education | −0.22 | −2.6 | <0.05 |
| Menopause status | 0.13 | 2.2 | <0.05 | Education | −0.21 | −2.6 | <0.05 | | | | |
| **Head aches** | | | | | | | | | | | |
| PSS Score | 0.26 | 4.5 | **<0.001** | Ethnicity | −0.19 | −2.2 | <0.05 | [No variables left in model] | | | |
| Cohabiting | 0.12 | 2.0 | <0.05 | Smoker | −0.16 | −1.8 | <0.1 | | | | |
| Smoker | −0.12 | −2.0 | <0.1 | | | | | | | | |
| **Feeling of Ants Crawling on the Skin** | | | | | | | | | | | |
| PSS Score | 0.24 | 3.9 | **<0.001** | CRP$_{Plasma}$ | 0.21 | 2.4 | <0.05 | Education | −0.30 | −3.7 | **<0.001** |
| SES | −0.10 | −1.7 | <0.1 | BMI | −0.18 | −2.0 | <0.05 | | | | |
| Menopause status | 0.10 | 1.7 | <0.1 | | | | | | | | |

**Table 4** Linear regression analyses of symptom reports *(Continued)*

| With PSS scores | | | | With CRP$_{Plasma}$ | | | | With EBV-Ab | | | |
|---|---|---|---|---|---|---|---|---|---|---|---|
| Variable | Beta | t | Signif. | Variable | Beta | t | Signif. | Variable | Beta | t | Signif. |
| **Stress Incontinence** | | | | | | | | | | | |
| PSS Score | 0.15 | 2.4 | <0.05 | Cohabiting | 0.16 | 1.9 | <0.1 | BMI | 0.24 | 2.9 | <0.01 |
| BMI | 0.13 | 2.1 | <0.05 | | | | | Cohabiting | 0.18 | 2.1 | <0.05 |
| Cohabiting | 0.11 | 1.8 | <0.1 | | | | | Menopause status | -0.14 | -1.7 | <0.1 |
| **Loss of interest in sex** | | | | | | | | | | | |
| PSS Score | 0.18 | 2.9 | <0.01 | Cohabiting | 0.31 | 3.7 | **<0.001** | Cohabiting | 0.22 | 2.6 | <0.05 |
| Education | -0.11 | -1.8 | <0.1 | | | | | SES | -0.18 | -2.1 | <0.05 |
| Cohabiting | 0.27 | 4.6 | **<0.001** | | | | | | | | |
| Menopause status | 0.14 | 2.4 | <0.05 | | | | | | | | |
| Ethnicity | 0.10 | 1.7 | <0.1 | | | | | | | | |
| **Hot flashes** | | | | | | | | | | | |
| PSS Score | 0.23 | 3.8 | **<0.001** | [No variables left in model] | | | | SES | -0.19 | -2.3 | <0.05 |
| Menopause status | 0.13 | 2.2 | <0.05 | | | | | BMI | 0.17 | 2.0 | <0.05 |
| BMI | 0.15 | 2.6 | <0.01 | | | | | Menopause status | 0.15 | 1.8 | <0.1 |
| **Night sweats** | | | | | | | | | | | |
| PSS Score | 0.24 | 4.2 | **<0.001** | CRP$_{Plasma}$ | 0.19 | 2.4 | <0.05 | Menopause status | 0.23 | 2.8 | <0.01 |
| Menopause status | 0.22 | 3.7 | **<0.001** | Menopause status | 0.30 | 3.7 | **<0.001** | Education | -0.21 | -2.7 | <0.01 |
| Parity | 0.15 | 2.5 | <0.05 | Education | -0.22 | -2.7 | <0.01 | Cohabiting | 0.28 | 3.4 | **<0.001** |
| Cohabiting | 0.12 | 2.1 | <0.05 | Cohabiting | 0.22 | 2.7 | <0.01 | | | | |

Variables entered into the linear models: ethnicity, SES, education, cohabitation status, parity, smoking, body mass index, and menopausal status. Significance set to $p < = 0.001$

difference in hot flash report, but instead found a greater likelihood of vasomotor symptoms among the Maya in relation to higher perceived levels of stress. This bears further investigation.

This study provides only modest support for the idea that immune biomarkers applied as stress-sensitive measures are associated with the frequency of symptoms at midlife. The relationship between $CRP_{Plasma}$ levels and the occurrence of depressed mood did not reach significance, although there was a suggestion of a relationship in bivariate and linear regression analyses ($p < 0.05$). The association between CRP levels and depressed mood has been previously noted [69].

In agreement with our findings, one other previous study did not find a relationship between CRP and hot flashes [70]. In SWAN, women who had a higher frequency of hot flashes had significantly higher levels of CRP and other biological markers of inflammation, but there was no significant association between night sweat frequency and inflammatory markers [71].

EBV-Ab values were not significantly associated with hot flashes or night sweats in terms of yes/no frequency or intensity of report. To our knowledge, this is the first study to examine symptoms at midlife in relation to levels of EBV-Ab. Although $CRP_{Plasma}$ and EBV-Ab have been used as stress-sensitive biological measures in the study of stress in the past [47, 50, 51], in this study neither $CRP_{Plasma}$ nor EBV-Ab levels were associated with symptoms at midlife to the same extent as the self-reported stress measure, PSS.

Self-reports of stress have been associated with the frequency of hot flashes, both with short-term reports such as hassles scales [72] and reports of chronic stress [73]. However, there may well be differences in the association between stress and hot flashes depending upon the manner in which hot flashes are measured. For example, in a prospective study of mood and hot flashes, negative mood was associated with fewer objectively measured hot flashes but was associated with more frequent self-reported hot flashes [19]. In this study, PSS scores were significantly associated with the intensity of vasomotor symptoms when correction for multiple testing was applied, and PSS scores tended to be associated with the likelihood of vasomotor symptoms ($p = 0.007$ and $p = 0.004$ for hot flashes and night sweats), unlike the physiological measures of stress.

In general, women who reported high levels of perceived stress were also more likely to report a broad array of symptoms. Some of these symptoms are specific to menopause, such as night sweats, but many are more general concerns of men and women of a broad age range. These symptoms are associated with multiple factors. For example, not cohabiting with a husband or partner significantly decreased report of the loss of interest in sex.

Self-reported stress is clearly implicated as associated with symptoms, especially among the Maya in this sample. It is, however, unclear to what degree stress may be a causal factor in inducing these symptoms, or if instead the symptoms are a causal factor in the stress levels. There could be a reciprocal effect, with stress inducing symptoms that in turn lead to greater perceptions of stress. Few women reported either no symptoms (1.4%) or all 12 symptoms (5.4%), suggesting that there is not a simple relation between being under stress and having all symptoms; different women suffer from different symptoms, and these are likely to differ in the importance of stress levels for their occurrence. It is unclear why the stronger association between perceived stress and vasomotor symptoms is present among Maya but not non-Maya participants. The women may differ in beliefs about how stress should be reported, since ethnic differences in self-reports of stress are found in other populations [38].

This study has limitations. While the sample is likely to broadly represent the population of women at midlife in Campeche due to the multiple strategies used for contacting potential participants, it is not a random sample. The sample size is small, with 305 women providing PSS scores, and only 162 and 157 women with EBV-Ab and CRP measures, respectively. We did not find the expected relationship between the PSS and the two biomarkers. Also, this paper has relied upon self-reports of hot flashes and night sweats as well as other symptoms. As noted, a previous study has shown a difference in the relation between stress and either subjectively reported or objectively measured hot flashes [19]. Finally, this study is cross-sectional and, therefore, cannot derive causation from associations between the variables used in analyses.

## Conclusions

In support of our primary hypothesis, perceived stress was associated with the intensity of hot flashes and night sweats. In logistic and linear regressions, perceived stress was the variable most consistently associated with each of the 12 symptoms studied. This was not true for the potentially stress-sensitive biological measures of EBV-Ab or $CRP_{Plasma}$. There were ethnic differences in the associations between measures of stress and symptom frequency and intensity. Maya women demonstrated a relationship between perceived stress and five symptoms, including night sweats, while the non-Maya demonstrated no association between between perceived stress and vasomotor symptoms, suggesting that either symptoms or stress were experienced and/or reported in culture-specific ways.

## Acknowledgements

We are indebted to the women who participated and authorities of the city of Campeche. Special thanks to Drs. Alfonso Cobos Toledo, Secretario de Salud; Carlos Juárez López, Secretario Técnico del Comité de Ética en Investigación; and Liliana Montejo León, Directora Operativa del Comité de Ética de Investigación. For assistance with fieldwork, we thank Isai Delgado, Gía del Pino, Guadalupe Islas Monter, Lizbeth de las Mercedes Rodríguez, Giselle O'Connor, Elena Pasqual, and Alba Valdéz Tah. In addition, we thank Drs. Jorge Jiménez Madrigal, Diana Edith Arceo Sánchez, Miguel Briceño Dzib, Enrique Fernando Reyes Pascual; Lic. Francisco Góngora Ramírez, and especially Lic. Marlene Narváez Rosado. Authorities who facilitated the interviews by giving us the needed space include Dra. Landy del Socorro Ortíz Aldana, Ing. Jorge Marín Farías Maldonado, M. en C. Lirio Suárez Améndola, Antrop. Marco Carvajal, Dra. Lizbeth Rodríguez, Lic. Lidia Elena Berrón Osorio, Lic. Ana Verónica Lemus Castillo, Lic. José Dolores Uribe Castro, Ing. Leidy Elena Legorreta Barrancos, Ing. Rosario Suárez Améndola, Ing. José Luis Herrera Martínez, Lic. Cecilia Zúñiga Rosel, Lic. Lorenzo Alberto Can Sánchez, Lic. Yolanda Isabel Segovia Cuevas, Ing. José Raúl Ochoa Aguedo, Ing. Agustín Balvanera Aguilar, Lic. Román Acosta Estrella, Lic. Ricardo Ocampo Fernández, Lic. Margarita Alfaro Waring. Finally, we thank Prof. Martha del Carmen Preciat Castilla and Lic. Rosa Angélica Prevé Quintero for their enthusiastic support of this study.

## Funding

Supported by NSF BCS-1156368.

## Authors' contributions

LLS, LHG, and DB designed this study; data collection was carried out and supervised by LHG and DCC in collaboration with LLS and DB; DLK carried out laboratory assays; DB and LLS carried out all analyses; LLS and DB drafted the manuscript; all authors read and approved the final manuscript.

## Competing interests

The authors declare that they have no competing interests.

## Author details

[1]Department of Anthropology, Machmer Hall, 240 Hicks Way, UMass Amherst, Amherst, MA 01003-9278, USA. [2]Departamento de Sociedad y Cultura, El Colegio de la Frontera, ECOSUR, Campeche, México. [3]Department of Pharmaceutical Science, University of Hawai'i at Hilo, Hilo, HI, USA. [4]Department of Anthropology, University of Hawai'i at Hilo, Hilo, HI, USA.

## References

1. Freedman RR. Menopausal hot flashes: mechanisms, endocrinology, treatment. J Steroid Biochem Mol Biol. 2014;142:115–20.
2. World Health Organization. Research on the menopause in the 1990s, WHO technical report series, 866. Geneva: World Health Organization; 1996.
3. Kravitz HM, Ganz PA, Bromberger J, Powell LH, Sutton-Tyrrell K, Meyer PM. Sleep difficulty in women at midlife: a community survey of sleep and the menopausal transition. Menopause. 2003;10:19–28.
4. de Kruif M, Spijker AT, Molendijk ML. Depression during the perimenopause: a meta-analysis. J Affect Disord. 2016;206:174–80.
5. Ryan J, Burger H, Szoeke C, Lehert P, Ancelin M-L, Dennerstein L. A prospective study of the association between endogenous hormones and depressive symptoms in postmenopausal women. Menopause. 2009;16(3):509–17.
6. Ford K, Sowers M, Crutchfield M, Wilson A, Jannausch M. A longitudinal study of the predictors of prevalence and severity of symptoms commonly associated with menopause. Menopause. 2005;12(3):308–17.
7. Dennerstein L. Well-being, symptoms and the menopausal transition. Maturitas. 1996;23:147–57.
8. Darling CA, Coccia C, Senatore N. Women in midlife: stress, health and life satisfaction. Stress Health. 2012;28:31–40.
9. Staner L. Sleep and anxiety disorders. Dialogues Clin Neurosci. 2003;5(3):249–58.
10. Hammen C. Stress and depression. Annu Rev Clin Psychol. 2005;1:293–319.
11. Sievert LL, Obermeyer CM. Symptom clusters at midlife: a four-country comparison of checklist and qualitative responses. Menopause. 2012;19(2):133–44.
12. Sievert LL, Obermeyer CM, Saliba M. Symptom groupings at midlife: cross-cultural variation and association with job, home, and life change. Menopause. 2007;14(4):798–807.
13. Avis NE, Crawford SL, Greendale G, Bromberger JT, Everson-Rose SA, Gold EB, Hess R, Joffe H, Kravitz HM, Tepper PG, Thurston RC, Study of Women's Health Across the Nation. Duration of menopausal vasomotor symptoms over the menopause transition. JAMA Intern Med. 2015;175(4):531–9.
14. Freeman EW, Sammel MD, Lin H, Liu Z, Gracia CR. Duration of menopausal hot flushes and associated risk factors. Obstet Gynecol. 2011;117(5):1095–104.
15. Gold EB, Block G, Crawford S, Lachance L, FitzGerald G, Miracle H, Sherman S. Lifestyle and demographic factors in relation to vasomotor symptoms: baseline results from the study of Women's Health Across the Nation. Am J Epidemiol. 2004;159(12):1189–99.
16. Kuh DL, Wadsworth M, Hardy R. Women's health in midlife: the influence of the menopause, social factors and health in earlier life. Br J Obstet Gynaecol. 1997;104(8):923–33.
17. Thurston RC, Bromberger J, Chang Y, Goldbacher E, Brown C, Cyranowski JM, Matthews KA. Childhood abuse or neglect is associated with increased vasomotor symptom reporting among midlife women. Menopause. 2008;15:16–22.
18. Binfa L, Castelo-Branco C, Blümel JE, Cancelo MJ, Bonilla H, Muñoz I, Vergara V, Izaguirre H, Sarrá S, Ríos RV. Influence of psycho-social factors on climacteric symptoms. Maturitas. 2004;48(4):425–31.
19. Thurston RC, Blumenthal JA, Babyak MA, Sherwood A. Emotional antecedents of hot flashes during daily life. Psychosom Med. 2005;67(1):137–46.
20. Swartzman LC, Edelberg R, Kemmann E. Impact of stress on objectively recorded menopausal hot flushes and on flush report bias. Health Psychol. 1990;9:529–45.
21. Pollard TM, Ice GH. Measuring hormonal variation in the hypothalamic pituitary adrenal (HPA) axis: cortisol. In: Ice GH, James GD, editors. Measuring stress in humans: a practical guide for the field. Cambridge: Cambridge University Press; 2007. p. 122–57.
22. Cignarelli M, Cicinelli E, Corso M, et al. Biophysical and endocrinemetabolic changes during menopausal hot flashes: increase in plasma free fatty acid and norepinephrine levels. Gynecol Obstet Investig. 1989;27:34–7.
23. Meldrum DR, Defazio JD, Erlik Y, et al. Pituitary hormones during the menopausal hot flash. Obstet Gynecol. 1984;64:752–6.
24. Woods NF, Carr MC, Tao EY, Taylor HJ, Mitchell ES. Increased urinary cortisol levels during the menopausal transition. Menopause. 2006;13(2):212–21.
25. Cagnacci A, Cannoletta M, Caretto S, Zanin R, Xholli A, Volpe A. Increased cortisol level: a possible link between climacteric symptoms and cardiovascular risk factors. Menopause. 2011;18(3):273–8.
26. Reed SD, Newton KM, Larson JC, Booth-LaForce C, Woods NF, Landis CA, Tolentino E, Carpenter JS, Freeman EW, Joffe H, Anawalt BD, Guthrie KA. Daily salivary cortisol patterns in midlife women with hot flashes. Clin Endocrinol. 2016;84(5):672–9.
27. Rubin LH, Drogos LL, Kapella MC, Geller SE, Maki P. Cortisol awakening response differs for midlife women with objective vasomotor symptoms versus without vasomotor symptoms. Menopause. 2014;21(12):1362. [abstract]
28. Gerber LM, Sievert LL, Schwartz JE. Hot flashes and midlife symptoms in relation to levels of salivary cortisol. Maturitas. 2017;96:26–32.
29. Greenberg GP, Sievert LL. Is there a relationship between hot flashes, night sweats, and the cortisol awakening response? Am J Hum Biol. 2018;30(2): e23110. [abstract]
30. Gibson CJ, Thurston RC, Matthews KA. Cortisol dysregulation is associated with daily diary-reported hot flashes among midlife women. Clin Endocrinol. 2016;85(4):645–51.
31. Avis NE, Stellato R, Crawford S, et al. Is there a menopausal syndrome? Menopausal status and symptoms across racial/ethnic groups. Soc Sci Med. 2001;52:345–56.
32. Lerner-Geva L, Boyko V, Blumstein T, Benyamini Y. The impact of education, cultural background, and lifestyle on symptoms of the menopausal transition: the Women's Health at Midlife Study. J Women's Health (Larchmt). 2010;19:975–85.
33. Sievert LL, Morrison L, Brown DE, Reza AM. Vasomotor symptoms among Japanese-American and European-American women living in Hilo, Hawaii. Menopause. 2007;14:261–9.
34. Brown DE. Physiological stress and culture change in a group of Filipino-Americans: a preliminary investigation. Ann Hum Biol. 1982;9(6):553–63.

35. Brown DE, James GD, Nordloh L. Comparison of factors affecting daily variation of blood pressure in Filipino-American and Caucasian nurses in Hawaii. Am J Phys Anthropol. 1998;106(3):373–83.

36. Brown DE, Sievert LL, Morrison LA, Rahberg N, The RAM. Relation between hot flashes and ambulatory blood pressure: the Hilo Women's health study. Psychosom Med. 2011;73:166–72.

37. Dressler WW, Oths KS, Gravlee CC. Race and ethnicity in public health research: models to explain health disparities. Annu Rev Anthropol. 2005;34:231–52.

38. Brown DE. Stress biomarkers as an objective window on experience. In: Sievert LL, Brown DE, editors. Biological measures of human experience across the lifespan: making visible the invisible. New York: Springer; 2016. p. 117–41.

39. Beyene Y, Martin MC. Menopausal experiences and bone density of Mayan women in Yucatan, Mexico. Am J Hum Biol. 2001;13:505–11.

40. Canto-de-Cetina TE, Canto-Cetina P, Polanco-Reyes L. Encuesta de sintomas del climaterio en areas semirurales de Yucatan. Revista de Investigacion Clinica. 1998;50:133–5.

41. Gold EB, Crawford SL, Avis NE, Crandall CJ, Matthews KA, Waetjen LE, Lee JS, Thurston R, Vuga M, Harlow SD. Factors related to age at natural menopause: longitudinal analyses from SWAN. Am J Epidemiol. 2013;178:70–83.

42. Beyene Y. Cultural significance and physiological manifestations of menopause: a biocultural analysis. Cult Med Psych. 1986;10:47–71.

43. Beyene Y. From menarche to menopause: reproductive histories of peasant women in two cultures. Albany: State University of New York Press; 1989.

44. Malacara JM, Canto-de-Cetina T, Bassol S, Gonzalez N, Cacique L, Vera-Ramirez ML, Nava LE. Symptoms at pre- and postmenopause in rural and urban women from three states of Mexico. Maturitas. 2002;43:11–9.

45. Eick G, Urlacher SS, McDade TW, Kowal P, Snodgrass JJ. Validation of an optimized ELISA for quantitative assessment of Epstien-Barr virus antibodies from dried blood spots. Biodemography Soc Biol. 2016;62(2):222–33.

46. McDade TW, Stallings JF, Angold A, Costello EJ, Burleson M, Cacioppo JT, Glaser R, Worthman CM. Epstein-Barr virus antibodies in whole blood spots: a minimally invasive method for assessing an aspect of cell-mediated immunity. Psychosom Med. 2000;62(4):560–7.

47. McDade TW. Measuring immune function: markers of cell-mediated immunity an inflammation in dried blood spots. In: Ice GH, James GD, editors. Measuring stress in humans: a practical guide for the field. Cambridge: Cambridge University Press; 2007. p. 181–207.

48. Wium-Andersen MK, Orsted DD, Nielsen SF, Nordestgaard BG. Elevated C-reactive protein levels, psychological distress, and depression in 73,131 individuals. JAMA Psychiatry. 2013;70(2):176–84.

49. Black PH, Garbutt LD. Stress, inflammation and cardiovascular disease. J Psychosom Res. 2002;52:1–23.

50. Low CA, Matthews KA, Hall M. Elevated CRP in adolescents: roles of stress and coping. Psychosom Med. 2013;75(5):449–52.

51. Steptoe A, Hamer M, Chida Y. The effects of acute psychological stress on circulating inflammatory factors in humans: a review and meta-analysis. Brain Behav Immun. 2007;21:901–12.

52. McDade TW. Status incongruity in Samoan youth: a biocultural analysis of culture change, stress, and immune function. Med Anthropol Q. 2002;16(2):123–50.

53. INEGI. Anuario estadístico y geográfico de Campeche, 2014. Instituto Nacional de Estadística y Geografía. Aguascalientes: INEGI; 2014. www.inegi.org.mx

54. Huicochea Gómez L, Sievert LL, Cahuich Campos D, Brown DE. An investigation of life circumstances associated with the experience of hot flashes in Campeche, Mexico. Menopause. 2017;24(1):52–63.

55. Harlow SD, Gass M, Hall JE, Lobo R, Maki P, Rebar RW, Sherman S, Sluss PM, de Villiers TJ, STRAW+ 10 Collaborative Group. Executive summary of the Stages of Reproductive Aging Workshop+ 10: addressing the unfinished agenda of staging reproductive aging. Menopause. 2012;19(4):387–95.

56. González Ramírez MT, Landero Hernández R. Factor structure of the perceived stress scale (PSS) in a sample from Mexico. Spanish J Psychol. 2007;10:199–206.

57. Cohen S, Kamarck T, Mermelstein R. A global measure of perceived stress. J Health Soc Behav. 1983;24:386–96.

58. Cohen S, Williamson G. Perceived stress in a probability sample of the United States. In: Spacapan S, Oskamp S, editors. Social psychology of health. Newbury Park: Sage; 1988. p. 31–67.

59. Avis NE, Kaufert PA, Lock M, McKinlay SM, Vass K. The evolution of menopausal symptoms. Bailliere's Clin Endocrinol Metab. 1993;7:17–32.

60. Dennerstein L, Smith AMA, Morse C, Burger H, Green A, Hopper J, Ryan M. Menopausal symptoms in Australian women. Med J Aust. 1993;159:232–6.

61. Obermeyer CM, Reher D, Saliba M. Symptoms, menopause status, and country differences: a comparative analysis from DAMES. Menopause. 2007;14:788–97.

62. Sievert LL, Espinosa-Hernandez G. Attitudes toward menopause in relation to symptom experience in Puebla, Mexico. Women Health. 2003;38(2):93–106.

63. McDade TW, Burhop J, Dohnal J. High-sensitivity enzyme immunoassay for C-reactive protein in dried blood spots. Clin Chem. 2004;50(3):652–4.

64. Pearson TA, Mensah GA, Alexander RW, Anderson JL, Cannon RO 3rd, Criqui M, Fadl YY, Fortmann SP, Hong Y, Myers GL, Rifai N, Smith SC Jr, Taubert K, Tracy RP, Vinicor F. Markers of inflammation and cardiovascular disease: application to clinical and public health practice: a statement for healthcare professionals from the Centers for Disease Control and Prevention and the American Heart Association. Circulation. 2003;107(3):499–511.

65. Melby MK. Factor analysis of climacteric symptoms in Japan. Maturitas. 2005;52:205–22.

66. Hemminki E, Topo P, Kangas I. Experience and opinions of climacterium by Finnish women. Eur J Obstet Gynecol. 1995;62:81–7.

67. Brown DE. General stress in anthropological fieldwork. Am Anthropol. 1981;83(1):74–92.

68. Martin MC, Block JE, Sanchez SD, Arnaud CD, Beyene Y. Menopause without symptoms: the endocrinology of menopause among rural Mayan Indians. Am J Obstet Gynecol. 1993;168:1839–45.

69. Valkanova V, Ebmeier KP, Allan CL. CRP, IL-6 and depression: a systematic review and meta-analysis of longitudinal studies. J Affect Disord. 2013;150(3):736–44.

70. Bechlioulis A, Naka KK, Kalantaridou SN, Kaponis A, Papanikolaou O, Vezyraki P, Kolettis TM, Vlahos AP, Gartzonika K, Mavridis A, Michalis LK. Increased vascular inflammation in early menopausal women is associated with hot flush severity. J Clin Endocrinol Metab. 2012;97(5):E760–4.

71. Thurston RC, El Khoudary SR, Sutton-Tyrrell K, Crandall CJ, Gold E, Sternfeld B, Selzer F, Matthews KA. Are vasomotor symptoms associated with alterations in hemostatic and inflammatory markers? Findings from the study of Women's Health Across the Nation. Menopause. 2011;18(10):1044–51.

72. Gannon L, Hansel S, Goodwin J. Correlates of menopausal hot flashes. J Behav Med. 1987;10(3):277–85.

73. Gannon L, Luchetta T, Pardie L. Perimenstrual symptoms: relationships with chronic stress and selected lifestyle variables. J Behav Med. 1989;15(4):149–59.

# 15

# The challenges of midlife women: themes from the Seattle midlife Women's health study

Annette Joan Thomas[1]* ⓘ, Ellen Sullivan Mitchell[2] and Nancy Fugate Woods[3]

## Abstract

**Background:** Midlife, the period of the lifespan between younger and older adulthood, has been described as a period of transition in women's lives. Investigators studying midlife have focused on women 40 to 65 years of age, who typically experience multiple social, psychological and biological challenges, among them the menopausal transition. Investigators have reported a diverse array of stressful events, for example, health concerns, family problems, work-related issues, deaths, frustrated goal attainment, and financial worries; however, none have identified which life events midlife women experience as the most salient. The purpose of this study was to understand the meaning behind the experiences that midlife women identify as the most challenging.

**Methods:** Participants were enrolled in The Seattle Midlife Women's Health Study, a longitudinal study spanning up to 23 years. Summative content analysis, incorporating manifest and latent analysis approaches, was used to identify life experiences that women described as the most challenging looking back over 15 years of being in the study. Eighty-one women responded to the question, "Since you have been in our study (since 1990 or 1991), what has been the most challenging part of life for you?"

**Results:** Women identified the most challenging aspects of midlife as changing family relationships, re-balancing work/personal life, re-discovering self, securing enough resources, and coping with multiple co-occurring stressors. Within these themes the most frequently reported challenges were: multiple co-occurring stressors, divorce/ breaking up with a partner, health problems of self, and death of parents. Few women mentioned menopause as the most challenging aspect of their lives.

**Conclusion:** Women found themselves searching for balance in the midst of multiple co-occurring stressors while coping with losses and transitions, for some in a context of limited resources. Menopause was infrequently mentioned. Future research to identify the challenges experienced by more diverse populations of women and further understanding of the dynamics among multiple co-occurring stressors is needed to provide individualized health care appropriately to midlife women.

**Keywords:** Midlife women, Challenges, Multiple co-occurring stressors, Divorce, Health concerns, Deaths of parents, Parenting

* Correspondence: thomaann@seattleu.edu
[1]College of Nursing, Seattle University, Seattle, Washington, USA
Full list of author information is available at the end of the article

## Background

Midlife, the period of the lifespan between younger and older adulthood, has been described as a period of transition in women's lives. Investigators studying midlife have focused on women 40 to 65 years of age, who typically experience multiple social, psychological and biological transitions. Among these are the biological transition of menopause, developmental transitions related to the aging/emerging self, and situational transitions such as divorce, taking on caregiving responsibilities for parents, or launching children [1].

In an investigation of the meaning of midlife, Woods and Mitchell [2] found that participants in the Seattle Midlife Women's Health Study described experiencing a diverse array of stressful events, for example, health problems, family problems, work-related issues, deaths, frustrated goal attainment, and financial concerns [2]. Women reported health problems they were experiencing as well as those their parents experienced with similar frequency. Deaths were also a common experience for these women. Family challenges included challenges with adolescent children, domestic violence, divorce or separation from a spouse, and the ending of relationships. Work problems included difficulty finding work, workplace conflicts, and downsizing of workplaces. These midlife women also reported frustrated goal attainment, such as being unable to complete an academic program or lack of personal time while working. In addition, they experienced financial stresses such as inability to pay college tuition for a child or afford essentials. SMWHS participants also rated their perceived stress levels in a health diary throughout their participation the study [3]. Greater perceived stress levels were significantly related to employment, history of sexual abuse, depressed mood, negative appraisal of aging changes, and poorer perceived health. Although symptoms such as hot flashes, sleep disruption, difficulty concentrating, and depressed mood were associated with greater perceived stress, the menopausal transition, itself, was unrelated to perceived stress. Improvement in role burden, social support, and income adequacy were associated with significantly lower perceived stress levels. Although SMWHS participants reported stressful experiences during midlife and rated their stress levels in a variety of dimensions of their lives over an extended period of time, it was not clear which stressors were most salient to them.

One approach to understanding experiences midlife women find most salient is inquiring about challenges they face. "Challenges" refer to experiences that require great physical or mental effort and determination that test one's strength, skill, or ability. In comparison, a stressor is a stimulus or threat that places real or perceived demands on the body, emotions, mind, or spirit of an individual. The word challenge, used in this study, is a word embroidered with strength and courage, allowing for the possibility that all challenges may not be perceived as stressful or appraised as negative. Due to the design of the original survey instrument, the words "challenge" and "stressor" as well as "challenging" and "stressful" were interchangeable in this report. In recent studies, women have reported challenges due to racism such as derogatory remarks, discriminatory actions such as sexual harassment [4] as well as menopausal symptoms, such as forgetfulness or difficulty concentrating (cognitive function), mood disturbances, and sleeping problems [3].

A commonly reported challenge of midlife is managing multiple responsibilities attributable to women's multiple roles. During midlife many women have been married or partnered, have already had children (some are young, others are leaving for college or jobs), have jobs of their own, manage their household with or without any additional help, and care for their aging parents. Kenny [5] studied stressors reported by 299 women aged 18–66 years and found that midlife women had more stressors than younger or older women and that midlife women identified roles involving family, work, and eldercare as sources of stress [5], but did not identify which of these sources of stress was the most salient.

During midlife, some women experience severing a relationship with a long-term partner. In addition to being emotionally wounded, women may experience a substantially reduced household income. Women in midlife tend to experience higher rates of loneliness and distress post-divorce than do younger divorced women [6].

Women in midlife begin to experience health problems of their own, such as cardiac problems [7] and sleeping difficulties [8]. Evidence from recent studies suggests that some of these health problems are related to women's stressful experiences. Investigators for the Study of Women's Health Across the Nation (SWAN) sleep study, examined very stressful life events using an 18-item version of the Psychiatric Epidemiology Research Interview Life Events Scale (PERI), which evaluated eight areas: school, work, romantic relationships, children, family, criminal and legal matters, finances and health. Women who had high chronic stress levels had lower subjective sleep quality, more waking after sleep onset (WASO) and were more likely to report insomnia compared to women who had low to moderate chronic stress profiles [8].

Allostatic load has been proposed as the accumulation of stress over time that affects health leading to preclinical signs of disease [9]. Allostasis refers to the ability to achieve stability and to maintain homeostasis during changing conditions through physiological or behavioral means and is adaptive in the short-term [10] but can revert to chronic stress in the long-term (allostatic load). Some events in daily life can generate chronic stress resulting in "wear and tear" on a woman's body, resulting in allostatic load [11]. Physiologic responses to stress are mediated by epinephrine and/or cortisol, which in turn elevate heart rate and blood pressure. Constant elevation of these responses over time can result in atherosclerosis increasing the risk for myocardial infarction and stroke [10]. Thus, health problems and allostatic load may be a result of chronic exposure to stressors or challenges.

Some of the questions that remain unanswered about midlife women's experiences of stress include: *Which life events do midlife women experience as the most stressful? Which of these life events are the most challenging to midlife women?*

Although studies of midlife women have documented multiple sources of stress, the impact of stressful life events and perceived stress on symptoms, subclinical changes, and diagnosed disease such as cardiovascular disease, to date there are no studies that reveal the most salient challenges for midlife women. The purpose of this study was to identify the experiences that midlife women found most challenging as they reflected on their experiences over more than a decade of their lives.

## Methods
### Study design and population
Data reported here were collected as part of a longitudinal study, the Seattle Midlife Women's Health Study (SMWHS). Women entered the study between 1990 and the early part of 1992 when most were in the early stages of the menopausal transition (MT) or not yet in the transition. All households within census tracts with a wide income range and mixed ethnicity were contacted by telephone for interested and eligible women. Women who were eligible were between 35 and 55 years of age, had at least one menstrual period within the last year, had a uterus and at least one ovary, were not pregnant, and could read and understand English. Out of 11,222 telephone contacts, 820 women were eligible, and 508 women entered the study [12].

The University of Washington Institutional Review Board approved each phase of the Seattle Midlife Women's Health Study (SMWHS) and approved informed consent forms. Each participant signed informed consent forms before entering the study.

Women completed an initial in-person interview administered by a trained registered nurse interviewer. A subset of the 508 women kept a health diary and from late 1996 to 2005 provided urine samples. All women were mailed a yearly Health Questionnaire and kept a menstrual calendar.

### Sample
Eligible participants for this study ($N = 81$) provided data from the 2006 Health Questionnaire answering specifically the following question: "Since you have been in our study, what has been the most challenging part of life for you?" A total of 83 women responded to the 2006 Health Questionnaire. Two women did not answer this specific question leaving 81 women's answers for analysis. Women not eligible for this study did not answer the 2006 Health Questionnaire.

At enrollment in the parent study, women who were eligible for inclusion were midlife women with a mean age of 39.3 years (SD 3.0 years) and in the current study were approximately 53–54 years, an education of 16.6 years (SD 2.7 years), and mean family income of $38,320 (SD $14,782). Most (86%) were employed. Eligible women described themselves as African American (3.6%), Asian/Pacific Islander (8.3%), or White (88.1%). Women eligible for this study identified themselves as never married or never partnered (6%), married or partnered (76.2%), divorced or separated (16.7%) and widowed (1.2%). Most (67%) of the eligible women were parents.

As seen in Table 1, women with data included in the current analyses compared to those who were ineligible were similar with respect to family income, employment status, and marital status. They differed significantly by age, years of education, and race/ethnicity; women in the current study were younger, had more years of education, fewer were African American and more were White women, and fewer women were parents.

### Analysis
Summative Content Analysis approach as described by Hsieh and Shannon [13] was used to identify life experiences that midlife women described as challenges looking back over 15 years when they participated in the SMWHS. Summative content analysis is a method that researchers use to interpret the content of data through coding in order to identify themes about the study participants' life experiences. Consistent with the approach, content analysis of data in this study started with identifying and quantifying key words or phrases in the text with the purpose of understanding the contextual use of the words or phrases. Some of the key words and categories that were identified prior to analysis were derived from the categories of the Life Event Questionnaire [14] while others were newly identified from the text. Potter and Levine-Donnerstein [15] refer to this first level of analysis as manifest content analysis whereby the appearance of the particular word or content is analyzed rather than the meaning derived. Each response was read over initially for a first impression. Subsequent readings included circling of key words or phrases in the women's answers in order to develop a

**Table 1** Sample Characteristics at Start of Study (1990–1991) for the Eligible and Ineligible Women in the Challenges of Midlife Women from the SMWHS

| Characteristic | Eligible N = 81 | Ineligible N = 427 | p value[a] |
|---|---|---|---|
| | Mean (SD) | Mean (SD) | |
| Age (years) | 39.3 (3.0) | 42.2 (4.7) | <.0001 |
| Years of Education | 16.6 (2.7) | 15.5 (2.9) | <.0017 |
| Gross Family Income | 38, 320 (14,782) | 35, 460 (15,258) | = .1210 |
| Characteristic | % (N) | % (N) | p value[b] |
| Currently Employed | 86% | 86.3% | = .9428 |
| Race/Ethnicity % (N) | | | |
| African American | 3.6% (3) | 13% (55) | = .0152 |
| Asian/Pacific Islander | 8.3% (7) | 8.5% (36) | = .9528 |
| White | 88.1% (74) | 74.8% (317) | = .0093 |
| Other (Latina/Hispanic, Mixed/NativeAmerican) | | 3.8% | = .0749 |
| Marital status % (N) | | | |
| Never married/partnered | 6% (5) | 7.1(30) | = .7211 |
| Married/partnered | 76.2% (64) | 67.0% (284) | = .1028 |
| Divorced/separated | 16.7% (14) | 24.1% (102) | = .1469 |
| Widowed | 1.2% (1) | 1.9% (8) | = .6634 |
| Ever a parent? | | | |
| Yes | 60.7% | 72.9% | 0.0268 |
| No | 26.2% | 27.1% | 0.8673 |

[a]independent t-test
[b]Chi-square test

coding scheme. The women's responses were divided into five themes with categories listed under each main theme. The responses were listed under the appropriate category and ranged from one sub-category to five sub-categories, meaning that the women identified from one to five types of challenges. Disagreements about coding the challenges were discussed among the investigators (AJT, NFW) until a resolution was found.

In this study, counting of key words and phrases enabled the authors to identify patterns in the data and to contextualize the codes, which subsequently led the authors to discover meanings, a process which Morse and Field [16] refer to as latent content analysis, an aspect of the summative content analysis approach. Credibility or internal consistency of findings was assured by aligning the textual evidence with interpretation of data by the authors, all of whom are content experts [17].

## Results
The midlife women's challenges revealed one overarching theme, "Searching for balance in the midst of multiple co-occurring stressors while coping with losses and transitions, for some in a context of limited resources" and five themes: 1) Changing Family relationships, 2) Re-balancing Work and Personal Life, 3) Rediscovering

Self, 4) Securing Enough Resources, and 5) Coping with Multiple Co-Occurring Stressors. Each theme was further divided into categories. If a response contained more than one challenge, the challenges were each counted individually as well as placed into the Multiple Co-Occurring Stressor category. For example, if a response conveyed parenting a teenager, husband's health, and a parent's death, there would be three separate types of challenges as well as the Multiple Co-Occurring Stressor challenge.

### Searching for balance in the midst of multiple co-occurring stressors while coping with losses and transitions, for some in a context of limited resources
Data analysis revealed an overarching theme, "Searching for balance in the midst of multiple co-occurring stressors while coping with losses and transitions, for some in a context of limited resources," that encapsulated the experiences of all study participants and permeated the themes and sub-themes that emerged from the data. Women reported challenges related to changing family relationships, including those with several generations of family members, e.g. children and parents, while also striving to rebalance their work and personal life. In addition, they struggled with rediscovering

themselves, in the context of changing relationships. Securing sufficient financial resources posed challenges for many. A noteworthy set of challenges is related to coping with multiple co-occurring stressors. Each of these is discussed in greater detail below.

### Changing family relationships

The theme of *Changing Family Relationships* refers to the changing relationships that women had with different family members: husband/partner, children, aging parents, siblings, and in-laws.

#### Changing relationships with partner

A number of women described changes in their long-term relationship with their partners as a primary life stressor. These changes ranged from a declining partner's health and necessity to provide caregiving, to separation or divorce after many years together, to the untimely death of a partner. Some women, especially those who reported divorce/breaking up with partner, reported more than one challenge. For example, one woman explained that an all-encompassing life challenge was a combination of events she summed up as "my divorce, my children leaving home and my parents dying all in the same 2-year period." Like others, another woman wrote, "The death of my brother in [year] and my divorce the same year" presented the most challenge. A partner's declining health was another new life challenge for many study participants. Women disclosed having to deal with their partners' declining health, including heart attacks, depression, disability, surgery, high blood pressure, reluctance to be more active, and alcoholism as a challenge. Like others, one study participant explained, "The most challenging has been watching my husband sink more and more into alcoholism and not being able to stop him." Another woman shared, "The challenges have changed from year to year- [year] I had an ectopic pregnancy- and infertility before/after- 0 kids. [years]- Graduate school and full-time work was challenging. [year]- currently, my husband's health problems and disability are most challenging."

For other midlife women the most challenging experiences were around the transition from an old to a new partner relationship. Similar to others, for one woman the life-midlife turmoil included "Losses and transitions –death of both parents, divorce from long term partner, beginning a new life with a new partner and his child."

#### Changing relationships with children

For many women in the study, changes in relationships included challenges with parenting that ranged from foster-parenting, parenting step-children, leaving children, children moving back in, to children moving out (Empty Nest), death of a child, or dealing with infertility.

For some of the women many of these issues were intertwined. For most women in the study, problems with parenting teenage children presented a new challenge. For others, step-parenting or foster parenting was most difficult. One woman explained, "Foster-parenting teens, most often teens who have been victims of abuse." Another one reflected parenting step-children was a new life challenge for her. She explained, "Dealing with being a blended family. Trying to parent stepchildren who would rather not have me around..." was quite difficult. For others, dealing with more than simply parenting teens added to the complexity of the parenting experience. Like many other women, one study participant listed multiple challenges, "My current job, my daughter from age 15-18, my mother's death, my husband's unemployment."

Children leaving home (e.g., for college) and children moving back home were also challenging for some women. One woman explained, "Family life – Change from having little children to them all growing up and leaving – changing relationship with husband because of that and personal changes" was strenuous. A woman whose child came back home said, "getting older, stiffer, clumsier. Seeing my finances shift, caring for 2 elderly parents and having a grown child move home w/ no finances" was wearisome. One woman in the study shared, "My son dying in [year] from suicide" was her greatest midlife challenge.

For childless women in the study, a midlife challenge represented a realization that biological parenthood will never be part of their life experience. One woman reflected, "The challenges have changed from year to year – [year] I had an ectopic pregnancy – and infertility before/after resulting in 0 kids. [years]– Graduate school and full-time work was challenging. Currently my husband's health problems and disability is the greatest challenge." Another woman indicated, "accepting that I would never be a biological parent, never have my 'own' kids, and possibly never become 'important' to my two step-children (now grown and living away). Everyone else's pregnancies, baby showers, and 'kid talk' is also a challenge."

#### Changing relationships with aging parents

Caregiving for parents, death of parents, parents' health problems, and relationships with parents encompassed the women sharing about their relationships with aging parents. Like others, one woman shared, "Caregiving for parents and losses are challenging – Losing father [year], father-in-law [year], mother-in-law [year], and only having my mother still living." For some study participants, death of a parent was the most challenging part of their midlife experience. Others described, "Losing my Dad to brain cancer," and "Experiencing my parents' death" as the most challenging part of midlife. One woman remembered, "Within four months, my mother had a severe stroke, my father died and a month later (to the day) my mother passed away." For other study participants who still had their parents, "parents getting old" and "Dad's health" were cited as the most challenging.

### Changing sibling relationships

The issues surrounding women's changing relationships with siblings consisted of three key narratives: death of a sibling, relationship problems with siblings, and seeking harmonious sibling relationships. Women recounted, "the death of my brother in [year] and my divorce the same year" and "Dealing with not getting along with my older sister" as some examples of the most challenging part of midlife.

### Changing relationships with in-laws

With aging in-laws, for some women in the study challenges came from having to move in together. One woman reported, "Moving in and living with all of my In-Laws" was the most challenging thing she had to do.

### Re-balancing work and personal life

For many women in the current study, stressful job/career, unemployment, balancing multiple roles, job change/ career change, job loss/ unemployment, finding a job with health benefits, and facing retirement necessitated re-balancing work and personal life. Only three out of 81 women in the study cited their job as the most challenging part of midlife. For the majority of women, feeling overworked, and having to balance multiple roles was difficult. Like others, one woman explained: "Balancing all aspects of my life - as a mother, as a wife, as a teacher and as a woman and as the major head of the household (cooking, cleaning, etc.) currently is the greatest challenge of my life." For others, the greatest challenges came from "Getting into a more interesting career," dealing with personal health issues such as a breast cancer diagnosis, going through a divorce, or losing a partner, losing a job and seeking new employment with benefits. One woman elaborated,

"Finding and sustaining suitable employment with health care benefits. Having intermittent medical coverage caused me to postpone a surgery (hyperparathyroid) for 3 years" as the most significant issue she had to deal with in midlife.

### Re-discovering self

Re-discovering self was important to many women in the current study. Health problems, existential issues, self-esteem/ self-acceptance, returning to school, the menopausal transition, and personal changes were the five sub-themes related to the self. Many women commented about health problems they had. Health problems included heart surgery, arthritis, physical disability due to arthritic pains, chronic pain, breast cancer, motor vehicle accident resulting in the diminished use of the woman's right hand, blot clot in the leg, and as one woman summarized: "getting older, stiffer, clumsier."

Women focused on making meaning of or appraising various aspects of their lives. Some of the women focused on accepting not being able to achieve their goals in life, realizing that the number of active years is limited, others on seeking new relationships. A number of women remarked about the newly found comfort with whom they were and self-acceptance. Similar to others, one study participant concluded, "Becoming more comfortable with myself. Accepting myself & having better self-esteem..." was most challenging. In order to re-discover oneself, some women returned to graduate school or decided to finish the university degree they once started. Surprisingly, only four out of 81 women in the current study commented on their menopausal transition symptoms as being the most challenging aspect of midlife, which included hot flashes, mood swings, difficulty remembering things, and excessive uterine bleeding.

### Securing enough resources

Generating enough resources was an all-encompassing task for many study participants. The women found financial challenges, partner's unemployment, and lack of health insurance as very stressful life issues.

Some women revealed financial challenges such as supporting children in private schools with a partner's sporadic job situation, financing college, and becoming financially secure as stressful. Many of them described how they coped with such situations in life. For example, one woman enumerated, "I have to work 2 jobs and long hours to support my children, but never seem to get ahead..." Another woman explained, "having to close a business, including laying off people, not paying business debts, selling off furniture, etc., and then having to sell our home to pay off a bank loan" as most challenging. For some women the difficult financial decisions were related to their partner's unemployment. One example was "...Constant threat of strikes or job lay off for my husband and eventually job loss was difficult."

Lack of health insurance was also a great concern to women. One woman related that "Finding and sustaining suitable employment with health care benefits" and "Having intermittent medical coverage" were the greatest challenges for her.

### Coping with multiple co-occurring stressors

As stated in the preceding paragraphs many women in the current study had to deal with multiple life stressors in their midlife years, many of them occurring at or around the same time. The majority of women identified multiple co-occurring stressors as they described their most challenging experiences. One woman commented, "Dealing with stress – job stress, health stress, social stress, family stress, etc. For a time, it seemed to snowball with no end in site." Some women explained that being overworked and balancing multiple roles were the most challenging part of midlife. Two examples were, "Fulfilling obligations of work and family" and "Balancing all aspects of my life - as a mother, as a wife, as a teacher and as a woman and as the major head of the household (cooking, cleaning, etc.)."

## Discussion

Seattle Midlife Women's Health Study participants found themselves searching for balance in the midst of multiple co-occurring stressors while coping with losses and transitions, for some in a context of limited resources. Themes of challenges for this group of midlife women included 1) changing family relationships, 2) re-balancing work and personal life, 3) re-discovering self, 4) securing enough resources, and 5) coping with multiple co-occurring stressors.

Research about self-in-relation to others [18] provides a useful framework for understanding the salience of these categories of challenging experiences. Taking care of family members with whom women have affiliations or connections is central to the lives of many women. Women's affiliations are organized around being able to make and maintain relationships with others. Taking care of others (partners, children, parents) is one way of describing how women's connections are formed. For many women, the threat of terminating a connection is viewed not only as a loss of connection, but as a total loss of self. Losses were exemplified in this study as many women identified divorce and losing their parents as the most challenging aspect of midlife in *Changing family relationships*. In an ethnographic qualitative research study from Australia [19], Dare and colleagues found that while many midlife women cope with the menopausal transition and their children leaving the house, the aging and death of their parents [20] and the effect of divorce [6] present more serious long-term challenges to these women.

In addition to relational issues, the workplace continues to provide many challenges for women. Overwork is a common experience, detailed well in Hochshild's "Second Shift" [21]. The combination of responsibilities women assume beyond their employment remain daunting for U.S. women, with many not having access to help with child care and household maintenance. Indeed, Hochshild's observations were that women worked the equivalent of a 'second shift' after they returned home after employment. Thus, launching children may be emancipatory for both the late adolescent and young adult children as well as their midlife mother.

Recent study of women's multiple roles, including work-family conflicts, has largely focused on younger, reproductive age women with preschool or school-aged children. Recognition of the continuity of the challenge of balancing competing demands of work and family for midlife women, and the addition of caring responsibilities for their parents, points to increased complexity of achieving balance and leading to the use of the term "sandwich generation" [22] to describe the compression of midlife women's lives by their children's and parents' needs.

In addition to rebalancing work and personal life, women faced challenges of re-discovering themselves in the context of their changing relationships. Miller and Stiver [18], proposed that a woman's sense of self and self-worth is often grounded in her ability to make and maintain relationships, and that these connections, not separations, can lead to strong, healthy development. Individual development, seen in the category of *Re-discovering Self*, proceeds by means of connection. Women connect with other women by finding relationships that foster mutual growth or mutuality. Mutuality benefits both people to grow and develop in and as a result of the relationship. This mutuality may manifest itself in a woman with breast cancer connecting with a breast cancer support group or with others who have a different health problem. Women may develop further by questioning their existence, their purpose, or raising other existential questions that surface in midlife and relating these questions to someone with whom they share mutuality. According to Miller and Stiver [18], the inclination toward connection that women feel in themselves is a strength. Any matter in question in relation to the self may enable women to develop themselves further by sharing with another person; this forwardness of mutuality increases the strength of the relationship.

Women's descriptions of challenges related to re-discovering themselves reflected their interest in the next stage of their lives. Current literature about women's experiences of aging emphasize the "third chapter:" Sarah Lawrence-Lightfoot coined this term to designate the years when one is neither old nor young, a period that can be transformative in women's lives. In her case studies of adults, Lawrence-Lightfoot explores themes of engagement over retreat, labor over leisure, and reinvention over retirement, emphasizing the importance of active engagement, purposefulness, and new learning as themes in the stories that people write about in the third chapter of their lives [23]. Mary Catherine Bateson [24] also examines the middle years, revising Erik Erickson's model of human development to include a second stage of adulthood in which the challenges include engagement over withdrawal. Her discussion of lifelong learning as part of human developmental processes emphasizes the achievement of wisdom and humility as one confronts the challenges of aging. Both Lawrence-Lightfoot [23] and Bateson [24] invite consideration of midlife as a period during which it is possible to actively compose a life story or narratives into which we can live as we age.

Often before a woman has the opportunity for self-introspection, she may find that dealing with concerns about material resources, such as financial worries, employment and health insurance take precedence. Although the majority of women in this study were not living in poverty, women experience disproportionately lower incomes than men. For the fourth quarter of 2017, the Bureau of Labor Statistics reported weekly median earnings for women who were full-time wage or salary workers as $771.00, which was 82% of the $944.00 median weekly earnings for men [25]. During midlife, both men and women reach their peak earning capacity. Women who leave the labor force to raise their children or those women who have been laid off, struggle with access to benefits from employment, such as healthcare and often lag behind in their cumulative retirement benefits in comparison to men. A woman's exposure to securing enough resources is also impacted by her partner's employment status. For example, when a woman's partner faces unemployment, the family experiences the consequences, especially if the employment benefits, such as health insurance, are from the partner's employer. If a woman's income is the primary household income, job loss can also result in loss of healthcare if the healthcare benefits are from her employer.

The most commonly experienced challenges for midlife women across all themes were identified as *Coping with Multiple Co-occurring Stressors*. Midlife women reported multiple co-occurring stressors when asked what was the most challenging for them during the past 15 years. Midlife is marked by women who are overworked with multiple roles and responsibilities. Lanza di Scalea et al. [26] investigated role stress, role reward, and mental health in a cross-sectional sample of 2549 women, who were 45–55 years with roles such as being employed, married, a mother, and/or a caregiver, revealing 34% of the sample were involved in 2 roles and 50% of the sample were involved in 3 roles [26]. The roles reported [26] were similar to those reported in this study as challenges in a woman's job, being married/partnered, being a parent, and taking care of elderly parents.

Only four women (4/81 = 5%) in the SMWHS sample reported the menopausal transition as being part of the most challenging aspects of midlife, identifying hot flashes, mood swings, difficulty remembering, and excessive uterine bleeding. Thus, their challenges were not with experiencing the menopausal transition itself, but, experiencing symptoms. This finding is surprising given that 85% of midlife women report one or more symptoms, such as hot flashes, depressed mood, and/or sleep disturbances [27]. In

the Penn Ovarian Aging Study, 26 % of women disclosed moderate to severe hot flashes and 9 % revealed having daily hot flashes [28]. Also, The Study of Women's Health Across the Nation (SWAN) identified 60–80% of women experience hot flashes at some point during the menopausal transition [29]. Despite the prevalence of symptoms, it is possible that the stressful nature of the menopausal transition has been over-emphasized [30].

This study has several limitations. First, the sample size consisted of responses from only 81 women, most of whom were White, employed, and married or partnered. The average age was 39 years at enrollment (approximately 53–54 years at the time of the current study) with an average of 17 years of education and 61% were parents. The participants included in this component of the SMWHS differed from those in the parent study who, at enrollment, were older, made less money, were more ethnically diverse, were less likely to be married, and more likely to be parents. Additionally, the women's answers to the Health Questionnaire usually included only 2–3 sentences, and their responses to a written questionnaire vs interview made further clarification of their responses impossible. Future investigations should include more ethnic diversity. Geronimus and colleagues [31] studied weathering on Black and White adults aged 18 to 64 years using logistic regression and odds ratios and found that Black women have a larger allostatic load compared to either Black men or White women and that marked differences were between non-poor Black women and non-poor White women suggesting that race is a key component in the impact of chronic stress on health [31].

The current investigation had several strengths. This study is the first to examine midlife women's descriptions of their challenges over an extended reference period of 15 years while participating in the Seattle Midlife Women's Health Study. Results of this study included the most commonly reported challenges over the past 15 years of midlife explained by the women themselves. These findings are important as they reveal the challenges most salient to midlife women and may also help providers to identify women at high risk for allostatic overload (e.g., sustained high blood pressure, sustained high levels of cortisol as a result of chronic high levels of stress), which may lead to heart disease, stroke, or sleeping problems. Further, providers will find these results informative in order to individualize care, so that they can determine resources and interventions to help this specific age group of women who perform so many roles with all their associated responsibilities.

## Conclusion
The over-arching theme of searching for balance in the midst of multiple co-occurring stressors, while coping with losses and transitions, for some in a context of

limited resources, spanned five categories. The most frequently reported challenges identified were multiple co-occurring stressors. Further study of multiple co-occurring stressors is warranted. Perhaps a single stressor, e.g., divorce, precipitates several related stressors. For example, loss of life partner precipitates loss of income, loss of children and separation from a relational network of mutual friends of the couple. Also, experience of a single stressor, such as development of a chronic illness, may precede other stressors such as job loss, a need to relocate living arrangements and the financial stressors of paying for medications. Inquiring about a focal stressor and its consequences may help women elaborate a series of stressors that more fully illuminates midlife women's experiences.

## Acknowledgements

We acknowledge all the women who participated in the SMWHS. Only the authors of this paper contributed to this manuscript.

## Authors' contributions

AJT conducted the literature review, analyzed the data and had primary responsibility for writing the manuscript. NFW contributed to the design and literature review, analyzed the data and edited the manuscript. ESM edited the manuscript. ESM and NFW were PIs of the Seattle Midlife Women's Health Study and collected all data. All authors read and approved the final manuscript.

## Author's information

Annette Joan Thomas, College of Nursing, Seattle University,
Ellen Sullivan Mitchell, Department of Family and Child Nursing, University of Washington School of Nursing,
Nancy Fugate Woods, Department of Biobehavioral Nursing and Health Informatics, University of Washington School of Nursing,

## Competing interests

NFW is guest editor of this journal. Peer review and all decisions made regarding this manuscript were made by an associate editor at a different institution. AJT and ESM have no competing interests.

## Author details

[1]College of Nursing, Seattle University, Seattle, Washington, USA. [2]Family and Child Nursing, University of Washington, Seattle, Washington, USA. [3]Biobehavioral Nursing and Health Informatics, University of Washington, Seattle, Wahsington, USA.

## References

1. Smith-DiJulio K, Woods N, Mitchell E. Well-being during the menopausal transition and early postmenopause: a longitudinal analysis. Menopause. 2008;15(6):1095–102.
2. Woods NF, Mitchell ES. Women's images of midlife: observations from the Seattle midlife Women's health study. Health Care Women Int. 1997;18:439–53.
3. Woods NF, Mitchell ES, Percival DB, Smith-DeJulio K. Is the menopausal transition stressful? Observations of perceived stress from the Seattle midlife Women's health study. Menopause. 2009;16(1):90–7.
4. Woods-Giscombé CL, Lobel M. Race and gender matter: a multidimensional approach to conceptualizing and measuring stress in African American women. Cult Divers Ethn Minor Psychol. 2008;14(3):173–82.
5. Kenny J. Women's inner balance: a comparison of stressors, personality traits and health problems by age groups. J Adv Nurs. 2000;31:639–50.
6. Sakraida TJ. Common themes in the divorce transition experience of midlife women. J Divorce and Remarriage. 2005;43(1,2):69–88.
7. Stevens S, Thomas SP. Recovery of midlife women from myocardial infarction. Health Care for Women Int. 2012;33(12):1096–113.
8. Hall MH, Casement MD, Troxel WM, et al. Chronic stress is prospectively associated with sleep in midlife women: the SWAN sleep study. Sleep. 2014; 10(38):1645–55.
9. McEwen BS, Wingfield JC. The concept of allostasis in biology and biomedicine. Horm Behav. 2003;43(1):2–15.
10. McEwen BS. Physiology and neurobiology of stress and adaptation: central role of the brain. Physiol Rev. 2007;87:873–904.
11. McEwen BS. Protective and damaging effects of stress mediators. N Engl J Med. 1998;338:171–9.
12. Mitchell ES, Woods NF. Symptom experiences of midlife women: observations from the Seattle midlife women's health study. Maturitas. 1996; 25:1–10.
13. Hsieh H-F, Shannon S. Three approaches to qualitative content analysis. Qual Health Res. 2005;15(9):1277–88.
14. Norbeck JS. Modification of life event questionnaires with female respondents. Res Nurs Health. 1984;7(1):61–71.
15. Potter WJ, Levine-Donnerstein D. Rethinking validity and reliability in content analysis. J Appl Commun Res. 1999;27:258–84.
16. Morse JM, Field PA. Qualitative research methods for health professionals. 2nd ed. Thousand Oaks, CA: Sage; 1995.
17. Weber RP. Content analysis. Beverly Hills, CA: Sage; 1990.
18. Miller JB, Stiver IP. The healing connection: how women form connections in therapy and in life. Boston: Beacon Press; 1997.
19. Dare JS. Transitions in midlife: contemporary experiences. Health Care for Women Int. 2011;32:111–33.
20. Perrig-Chiello P, Hopflinger F. Aging parents and their middle-aged children: demographic and psychosocial challenges. European J Aging. 2005;2:183–91.
21. Hochshild AR, Machung A. The second shift: working parents and revolution at home. New York: Avon Books; 1989.
22. Raphael D, Schlesinger B. Caring for elderly parents and adult children being at home: interactions of the sandwich generation family. Soc Work Res and Abstr. 1993;29(1):1–10.
23. Lawrence-Lighfoot S. The third chapter: passion, risk, and adventure in the 25 years after 50. New York: Sarah Crichton Books; 2009.
24. Bateson MC. Composing a further life: the age of active wisdom. New York: Vintage Books; 2010.
25. Bureau of Labor Statistics, U.S. Department of Labor, The Economics Daily, Median weekly earnings 767 for women, 937 for men, in third quarter 2017 on the Internet athttps://www.bls.gov/opub/ted/2017/median-weekly-earnings-767-for-women-937-for-men-in-third-quarter-2017.htm. Accessed 29 Mar 2018.
26. Lanza di Scalea T, Matthews KA, Avis NE, et al. Role stress, role reward, and mental health in a multiethnic sample of midlife women: results from the study of women's health across the nation (SWAN). J Women's Health. 2012;21(5):481–9.
27. Woods NF, Mitchell ES. Symptoms during the perimenopause: prevalence, severity, trajectory and significance in women's lives. Proceeding of the NIH State-of-the-Science Conference on management of menopause-related symptoms. Am J Med. 2005;118(Suppl 2):14–24.
28. Freeman EW, Grisso JA, Berlin J, et al. Symptom reports from a cohort of African American and white women in the late reproductive years. Menopause. 2001;8(1):33–42.
29. Gold E, Colvin A, Avis N, et al. Longitudinal analysis of vasomotor symptoms and race/ethnicity across the menopausal transition: study of women's health across the nation (SWAN). Am J Public Health. 2006;96(7):1226–35.
30. Judd FK, Hickey M, Bryant C. Depression and midlife: are we overpathologising the menopause? J Affect Disord. 2012;136:199–211.
31. Geronimus AT, Hicken M, Keene D, Bound J. "Weathering" and age patterns of allostatic load scores among blacks and whites in the United States. Am J Pub Health. 2006;96(5):826–33.

# 16

# Neighborhood disorder, exposure to violence, and perceived discrimination in relation to symptoms in midlife women

Linda M Gerber[1,2]* and Lynnette Leidy Sievert[3]

## Abstract

**Background:** Some symptoms at midlife are associated with stress, such as hot flashes, trouble sleeping, headaches, or depressed mood. Hot flashes have been studied in relation to laboratory stressors, physiological biomarkers, and self-reported stress, but less is known about hot flashes in relation to the larger context of women's lives. This study examined the risk of symptoms in relation to neighborhood disorder, exposure to neighborhood violence, social cohesion and perceived discrimination. We hypothesized that women exposed to more negative neighborhood characteristics and discrimination would be more likely to report hot flashes and other midlife symptoms.

**Methods:** Participants were black and white women, aged 40 to 60, drawn from a cross-sectional investigation of race/ethnicity, socioeconomic status, and blood pressure in New York City (n = 139). Demographic information, medical history, menopausal status, and symptoms were measured by questionnaire. Likert scales were used to measure neighborhood characteristics, specifically, the Neighborhood Disorder Scale, the Exposure to Violence Scale, the Perceived Violence Subscale, the Neighborhood Social Cohesion and Trust Scale, and the Everyday Discrimination Scale. Ten symptoms were included in analyses: lack of energy, feeling blue/depressed, backaches, headaches, aches/stiffness in joints, shortness of breath, hot flashes, trouble sleeping, nervous tension, and pins/needles in hands/feet. Each scale with each symptom outcome was examined using logistic regression analyses adjusting for significant covariates.

**Results:** Black women reported higher scores on all negative neighborhood characteristics and discrimination, and a lower score on the positive Neighborhood Social Cohesion and Trust. Neighborhood Disorder was associated with feeling blue/depressed, aches/stiffness in joints, and hot flashes, and Perceived Violence was associated with aches/stiffness in joints, after controlling for model-specific covariates. There was a lower risk of backaches with increasing Neighborhood Social Cohesion and Trust score. The Everyday Discrimination Scale was associated with lack of energy. Lack of energy, feeling blue/depressed, aches/stiffness in joints, and hot flashes appeared to be most vulnerable to negative neighborhood context and discrimination.

**Conclusions:** This study adds to the literature linking neighborhood environments to health outcomes. The associations between negative neighborhood contexts and discrimination with diverse symptoms, and the association between social cohesion and back pain, point to the need to expand analyses of stress to multiple physiological systems.

**Keywords:** Menopause, Hot flashes, Aches, Stress, Neighborhood disorder, Violence, Discrimination

* Correspondence: lig2002@med.cornell.edu
[1]Department of Healthcare Policy & Research, Division of Biostatistics and Epidemiology, Weill Cornell Medical College, 402 E. 67th St., LA-231, New York, NY 10065, USA
[2]Department of Medicine, Division of Nephrology and Hypertension, Weill Cornell Medical College, New York City, NY, USA
Full list of author information is available at the end of the article

## Background

Multiple symptoms have been associated with the menopausal transition. Some, such as hot flashes, are clearly associated with hormonal changes [1–4]. Other symptoms, such as joint pain and headaches, may be associated with hormonal changes, but the evidence is less straight forward [5, 6]. Social, rather than hormonal, changes may be responsible for depressed mood or trouble sleeping in some women [7, 8]. Although not well established, certain studies suggest that stress may be associated with hot flashes [3, 9, 10], trouble sleeping, headaches, and depressed mood [11–13].

"Stress" can have multiple meanings, and has been measured in multiple ways. In relation to hot flashes, stress has been measured both inside the laboratory [14–16] and outside of the laboratory in relation to perceived stress scores [3, 9, 10], cortisol levels [17–21], measures of blood pressure [22–25], and C-reactive protein [10, 26]. Missing from these analyses is a consideration of the larger context of women's lives, specifically at the level of problems in the neighborhood and the social challenge of perceived discrimination.

A broad range of research links neighborhood social and economic environments to the health of residents [27–29]. Neighborhoods with high levels of poverty, violence, and disorder have been associated with detrimental effects on individuals residing in these areas [27, 30, 31]. Stress is related to the chronic difficulties encountered within neighborhoods, and this neighborhood stress has been reported to increase vulnerability to immune disorders and cardiovascular disease [32, 33]. Exposure to events known to elicit stressful emotions such as fear, anger, or depression have been assessed by two subscales (Neighborhood Disorder and Exposure to Violence) of the City Stress Inventory [34]. Studies among caregivers of children with asthma have shown an increase in asthma morbidity and depression in association with increasing levels of perceived violence [35, 36].

Neighborhoods with low levels of social cohesion have been associated with increased rates of depression in the Multi-Ethnic Study of Atherosclerosis (MESA) Study [37], coronary calcification in the CARDIA study [38], and to increased risk of acute myocardial infarction mortality in Scania, Sweden [39]. Additionally, the Jackson Heart Study found that, in disadvantaged neighborhoods, low social cohesion was associated with higher levels of cumulative biological risk among African American men [27].

Racial disparities in health have been posited to be linked to exposures of discrimination [40]. Self-reported unfair treatment or perceived discrimination has been reported to contribute to broad-based morbidity [41, 42]. Brondolo et al. [43] have reported that racial discrimination may also influence cardiovascular disease risk. It has been suggested that among African Americans, the experience of everyday unfair treatment leads to a cumulative biological "wear and tear" (or allostatic load [44]) as measured across 22 biomarkers, representing seven system levels, of biological disintegration [45]. The results of that study, conducted among midlife African Americans, adds to the literature linking the stress of discrimination to effects on multiple downstream physiological systems [45]. There is also evidence from the Study of Women's Health Across the Nation (SWAN) linking higher levels of discrimination to higher levels of allostatic load [46]. In addition, in SWAN, the Everyday Discrimination Scale was administered at baseline and at each of the 13 follow-up periods. Chronic everyday discrimination was associated with more bodily pain, in fully adjusted models, among African-American, Chinese, and non-Hispanic white women [47]. Higher allostatic load levels, in addition to contributing to increased risk for many health outcomes [48], may also contribute to greater reporting of midlife symptoms among both black and white women during this period of increased vulnerability.

The purpose of the study presented here was to examine the risk of symptoms at midlife in relation to neighborhood disorder, exposure to neighborhood violence, and perceived discrimination among black and white women living in New York City. We focused on hot flashes and night sweats because of previous studies that suggest a relationship between stress and vasomotor symptoms [3, 9, 10]. An additional reason for this focus was the suggestion that hot flashes and night sweats may be markers of cardiovascular disease risk [49, 50]. In addition, we examined other possible symptoms at midlife that could be associated with increasingly negative neighborhood characteristics and levels of discrimination. We hypothesized that women who report higher levels of neighborhood disorder, violence, and increasing experience of personal discrimination would be more likely to report hot flashes and other symptoms at midlife, even after controlling for age, ethnicity, BMI, and menopausal status. To our knowledge, this is the first study of symptoms at midlife among black and white women in relation to neighborhood context, beyond discrimination.

## Methods

The Neighborhood Study of Blood Pressure and Sleep, conducted from September 1999 through July 2003, was a cross-sectional investigation of race/ethnicity, socioeconomic status, and diurnal blood pressure (BP) patterns [18, 51]. Data for this study were drawn from this parent study. Because this study examined both neighborhood characteristics and symptom experience at midlife, these data offer a unique opportunity to test our hypothesis that hot flashes are more frequently reported among those residing in a stressful environment.

Participants were recruited through fliers and word of mouth from Weill Cornell Medical College, Mount Sinai School of Medicine, Harlem Hospital, and North General Hospital using a common protocol and consent form approved by the institutional review committee at each of the four institutions. At recruitment, women were 18 to 65 years old, white or black, had no previous cardiovascular disease, and no major medical problems other than hypertension ($n = 211$). Those who were eligible and chose to participate completed informed consent before initiating study procedures. The analyses here focus on women aged 40 to 60 ($n = 139$) at the time of interview in order to better assess symptoms at midlife; thus, this is a subset of a larger study.

## Data collected

Participants completed a self-administered demographic and medical history questionnaire that included questions about education, smoking habits, and menstruation. Age and race/ethnicity were self-reported. Questions about menopausal status queried the last menstrual cycle, whether menstruation had occurred in the previous 12 months, menstrual regularity, and whether cycles had changed in length. Post-menopausal status was defined as having had at least 12 months of amenorrhea. Peri-menopausal status was defined by missed menstrual periods and significant changes in menstrual cycle regularity and length. Pre-menopausal status was defined as having regular menstruation. These categories were used in lieu of the STRAW+ 10 stages [52] because of the cross-sectional nature of the study and the small number of women in the peri-menopausal group. Because of the small number of women in the peri-menopause category, women were grouped into two groups: pre- vs. peri/postmenopause for analyses. Height and weight were measured twice by a technician. The average of the two measurements was used, and body mass index (BMI) was calculated as weight divided by the square of height (kg/m$^2$).

The following Likert scales were used to measure neighborhood characteristics: (1) The Neighborhood Disorder (ND) Scale [34] assessed perceptions of neighborhood disorder with 11 items that served as a subset of City Stress Inventory, scaled as 0–33 (e.g., I heard neighbors complaining about crime in our neighborhood; People in the neighborhood complained about being harassed by police). (2) The Exposure to Violence (EV) Scale, [34], is a 7 items subset of the City Stress Inventory, scaled as 0–21 (e.g., A family member was attacked or beaten; A friend was robbed or mugged). (3) The Perceived Violence (PV) Subscale is from the Project on Human Development

in Chicago Neighborhoods: Community Survey, 1994–1995 [53], scaled 5–20, (e.g., During the past 6 months, how often was there a fight in this neighborhood in which a weapon was used; How often were their sexual assaults/rape). (4) The Neighborhood Social Cohesion and Trust (NSCT) Scale is a subscale of the Collective Efficacy instrument used to assess social cohesion among neighbors with 5 items, scaled 0–15 (e.g., This is a close-knit neighborhood; People around here are willing to help their neighbors) [54]. (5) The Everyday Discrimination Scale (EDS), scaled 0–45 [55] is a scale of 9 items that assesses chronic and routine experiences of unfair treatment (e.g., You are treated with less courtesy than other people; people act as if they are afraid of you; you are called names or insulted.)

Symptoms associated with menopause were queried with a frequently used questionnaire that embeds menopausal symptoms into a list of everyday complaints [56, 57]. Each participant was asked whether or not she had been bothered by each of 23 symptoms during the past 2 weeks, e.g., hot flashes, trouble sleeping, or feeling blue or depressed. Answers were assessed as yes/no.

We selected symptoms for study by first excluding 8 symptoms that were placed in the list to make the instrument less obviously about menopausal symptoms (diarrhea, persistent cough, upset stomach, sore throat, loss of appetite, menstrual problems, fluid retention, urinary tract/bladder infections). We also excluded one symptom, vaginal dryness, which was not expected to vary with contextual stress.

## Statistical analysis

Exploratory factor analyses were carried out with the 14 remaining symptoms to examine how symptoms grouped in the entire sample. Our assumption was that symptoms clustering with hot flashes were our best candidates for the study of midlife symptoms. Scree plots were examined to identify the point at which eigenvalues began to level off. It was decided that three was the most informative number of factors. Three factors were extracted using the method of unweighted least squares with varimax rotation. Unweighted least squares was applied to achieve more conservative results (i.e., fewer symptoms with factor scores > 0.300).

We repeated the factor analyses and each time excluded one symptom that did not cluster with hot flashes. In this way, difficulty concentrating, rapid heartbeat, dizzy spells, and cold sweats were excluded. With each change, the total variance explained increased. The final 10 symptoms were: lack of energy, feeling blue/depressed, backaches, headaches, aches/stiffness in joints, shortness of breath, hot flashes, trouble sleeping, nervous tension, and pins/needles in hands/feet. With fewer than 10 symptoms, the total variance explained started to decline.

Bivariate Spearman correlations were examined among the scores for neighborhood disorder, violence, and discrimination. Spearman correlations were applied because scores were not normally distributed. We examined race/ethnicity in relation to neighborhood characteristics, and each symptom in relation to neighborhood characteristics using Mann-Whitney U tests. Symptoms significantly associated with neighborhood characteristics at the level of $p < 0.20$ were chosen for logistic regression analyses.

In those occasional situations where a participant was missing a subset of the items used to compute a scale score, we used a regression-based approach to estimate the expected value of the scale based on the non-missing items, and replaced/imputed the missing value with its expected value if the $R^2$ for the regression $\geq 70\%$. By definition, the resulting equation is the optimal linear function of the available items for estimating the scale score based on data from those who answered all items.

We examined race/ethnicity, smoking, menopausal status, and education ($\leq 12$, 13–16, > 16 years) in relation to each symptom by chi-square analysis, and age and BMI in relation to each symptom by t-test and included race/ethnicity, smoking, education, and/or BMI as covariates in logistic regression models if the relationship between the variable and the symptom was $p < 0.20$ in unadjusted analyses. We did not include all possible covariates in our models in order to increase the power of each model.

Logistic regression analyses were carried out with the symptom (yes/no) as the dependent variable, with each neighborhood or discrimination scale as the primary independent variable controlling for any significant covariate(s). In addition, linear regression was used to examine derived factor scores as outcome variables with each neighborhood or discrimination scale as a predictor variable while controlling for covariates. All analyses were conducted with IBM SPSS Statistics for Windows, Version 24.0. Armonk, NY: IBM Corp.

## Results

Table 1 shows the sample characteristics for the total sample ($n = 139$), and for the white (45%) and black (55%) women. Mean age was 49.1 years and did not vary by race/ethnicity. White women had higher levels of education, but did not significantly differ with regard to smoking, BMI, or menopausal status. All of the neighborhood and discrimination scales differed by race/ethnicity so that black women reported higher scores on negative neighborhood characteristics and discrimination, and a lower score on the positive neighborhood social cohesion and trust scale.

**Table 1** Sample characteristics

|  | Total sample N = 139 | White women N = 62 | Black women N = 77 | p-value |
|---|---|---|---|---|
| Mean age (s.d.) | 49.1 (5.7) | 49.7 (6.0) | 48.7 (5.5) | 0.31 |
| % Level of education |  |  |  |  |
| ≤ 12 | 16.3% | 6.7% | 24.6% | < 0.001 |
| 13–16 | 58.9% | 50.0% | 66.7% |  |
| 17+ | 24.8% | 43.3% | 8.7% |  |
| % Smoking | 22.1% | 15.0% | 28.2% | 0.07 |
| Mean BMI (s.d.) | 29.6 (6.4) | 28.5 (6.1) | 30.6 (6.5) | 0.06 |
| % Menopause status |  |  |  |  |
| Pre- | 48.0% | 39.6% | 55.6% | 0.09 |
| Peri- | 6.9% | 4.2% | 9.3% |  |
| Post- | 45.1% | 56.3% | 35.2% |  |
| Neighborhood Disorder |  |  |  |  |
| Scale range 0–28 |  |  |  |  |
| Means (s.d.) | 8.3 (7.4) | 5.1 (5.6) | 11.1 (7.6) | < 0.001 |
| Medians | 6.00 | 3.23 | 10.00 | < 0.001 |
| Exposure to Violence |  |  |  |  |
| Scale range 0–15 |  |  |  |  |
| Means (s.d.) | 1.9 (3.0) | 0.8 (1.5) | 2.9 (3.5) | < 0.001 |
| Medians | 1.00 | 0.00 | 2.00 | < 0.001 |
| Perceived Violence |  |  |  |  |
| Subscale range 5–18 |  |  |  |  |
| Means (s.d.) | 9.4 (3.6) | 8.4 (3.1) | 10.4 (3.8) | 0.002 |
| Medians | 9.00 | 7.10 | 10.25 | 0.004 |
| Neighborhood Social Cohesion and Trust |  |  |  |  |
| Scale range 1–14 |  |  |  |  |
| Means (s.d.) | 8.4 (2.5) | 9.3 (1.9) | 7.6 (2.7) | < 0.001 |
| Medians | 8.63 | 10.00 | 8.00 | < 0.001 |
| Everyday Discrimination |  |  |  |  |
| Scale range 0–39 |  |  |  |  |
| Means (s.d.) | 8.7 (8.2) | 6.2 (5.9) | 11.1 (9.4) | 0.001 |
| Medians | 6.00 | 5.00 | 7.50 | 0.002 |

There were no significant differences between white and black women with regard to symptom report. Only nervous tension approached significance ($p = 0.05$) (Table 2).

### Factor analysis

After selecting the 10 symptoms of interest, among all women, the first factor comprised psychosomatic symptoms. Hot flashes loaded onto the second factor along with three somatic symptoms (backaches, aches/stiffness in joints, and pins/needles in hands/feet). A third factor captured some remaining somatic symptoms, including headaches and shortness of breath. Although sample

**Table 2** Frequency of symptoms by race/ethnicity

|  | Total sample | White women | Black women | p-value |
|---|---|---|---|---|
|  | (n), % | (n), % | (n), % |  |
| Lack of energy | (66), 55.0% | (31), 57.4% | (35), 53.0% | 0.632 |
| Feeling blue/ depressed | (42), 34.7% | (18), 32.7% | (24), 36.4% | 0.676 |
| Backaches | (58), 47.9% | (23), 42.6% | (35), 52.2% | 0.291 |
| Headaches | (66), 53.7% | (27), 49.1% | (39), 57.4% | 0.361 |
| Aches/stiffness in joints | (71), 58.7% | **(27), 50.9%** | **(44), 64.7%** | 0.127 |
| Shortness of breath | (22), 18.2% | (8), 14.8% | (14), 20.9% | 0.389 |
| Hot flashes | (49), 39.8% | **(18), 33.3%** | **(31), 44.9%** | 0.192 |
| Trouble sleeping | (58), 47.5% | **(30), 55.6%** | **(28), 41.2%** | 0.114 |
| Nervous tension | (42), 34.4% | **(24), 43.6%** | **(18), 26.9%** | 0.052 |
| Pins and needles in hands/feet | (30), 24.4% | **(10), 18.2%** | **(20), 29.4%** | 0.149 |

Differences with a p value < 0.20 bolded for inclusion as a covariate in logistic regressions

sizes were small, there were differences in factor loadings between white and black women. White women reflected the total sample findings. Among black women, hot flashes clustered with lack of energy, feeling blue/depressed, backaches, and nervous tension in addition to aches/stiffness in joints and pins/needles in hands/feet. Of the 10 symptoms in Table 3, headaches, shortness of breath, and trouble sleeping did not group into a factor with hot flashes (Table 3).

### Spearman correlations

The neighborhood scales were correlated with each other in the expected directions. Neighborhood Disorder correlated positively with Exposure to Violence ($r = .649$, $p < 0.001$), Perceived Violence ($r = .679$, $p < 0.001$), and Everyday Discrimination Scale ($r = .495$, $p < 0.001$), and correlated negatively with Neighborhood Social Cohesion and Trust ($r = -.300$, $p = 0.001$). Exposure to

Violence correlated positively with Perceived Violence ($r = .489$, $p < 0.001$) and Everyday Discrimination Scale ($r = .422$, $p < 0.001$), and negatively with Neighborhood Social Cohesion and Trust ($r = -.232$, $p = 0.009$). Neighborhood Social Cohesion and Trust correlated negatively with Perceived Violence ($r = -.283$, $p = 0.002$) and Everyday Discrimination Scale ($r = -.318$, $p < 0.001$).

### Bivariate results

The following associations were found between symptoms and women's characteristics (data not shown). With regard to age at interview, women reporting aches/stiffness in joints ($p < 0.001$), hot flashes ($p < 0.001$) and nervous tension ($p = 0.04$) were older than women not reporting those symptoms. Women reporting headaches were younger ($p = 0.006$) than women not reporting headaches. With regard to menopausal status, peri- and post-

**Table 3** Factor analyses of symptoms included in study

|  | Total sample | | | White women | | | Black women | | |
|---|---|---|---|---|---|---|---|---|---|
|  | 1 | 2 | 3 | 1 | 2 | 3 | 1 | 2 | 3 |
| Lack of energy | .712 | .252 | .270 | .739 | .160 | .326 | .712 | .367 | −.012 |
| Feeling blue/ depressed | .842 | .084 | −.144 | .776 | −.073 | −.071 | .533 | .490 | .366 |
| Backaches | .344 | .510 | .352 | .326 | .741 | −.212 | .533 | .544 | −.182 |
| Headaches | −.058 | .040 | .803 | .104 | .098 | .609 | .162 | −.020 | −.844 |
| Aches/stiffness in joints | .119 | .808 | .221 | .093 | .828 | .186 | .761 | .030 | .016 |
| Shortness of breath | .280 | .190 | .467 | −.005 | .111 | .775 | .072 | .801 | −.051 |
| Hot flashes | .055 | .720 | −.283 | −.152 | .631 | .221 | .485 | −.097 | .557 |
| Trouble sleeping | .653 | .060 | .211 | .752 | .194 | −.046 | .205 | .720 | .073 |
| Nervous tension | .717 | .250 | .002 | .597 | .045 | .456 | .713 | .283 | .329 |
| Pins and needles in hands/feet | .359 | .493 | .157 | .315 | .377 | .248 | .652 | .209 | −.108 |
| Variance explained (rounded) | 25% | 18% | 13% | 23% | 19% | 15% | 29% | 20% | 13% |
| Cumulative variance explained | 56.31% | | | 56.70% | | | 61.78% | | |

menopausal women (combined) were more likely to report a lack of energy ($p = 0.007$), aches/stiffness in joints ($p = 0.004$), and hot flashes ($p < 0.001$). Finally, with regard to BMI, women with aches/stiffness in joints ($p = 0.06$), and backaches ($p = 0.07$) tended to have a higher BMI than women not reporting those symptoms. No symptom frequencies differed by smoking status or level of education ($\leq 12$, $13–16$, $> 16$ years) at $p < 0.20$.

Looking across bivariate results for symptoms (yes/no) in relation to measures of neighborhood disorder, violence, cohesion, and discrimination, Table 4 shows that the measures of Neighborhood Disorder were associated with 7 symptoms at the $p < 0.2$ level. In all instances, women with the symptoms had higher median levels of neighborhood disorder. The two measures of neighborhood violence (Exposure to Violence and Perceived Violence) were associated with 4 and 3 symptoms, respectively, at the $p < 0.20$ level. The Neighborhood Social Cohesion and Trust was associated with 2 symptoms so that women with more social cohesion and trust in the neighborhood were less likely to report backaches ($p < 0.05$) and aches/stiffness in joints ($p < 0.20$). The Everyday Discrimination Scale was associated with 4 symptoms at the $p < 0.20$ level.

### Logistic regression results

Neighborhood Disorder remained significantly associated with feeling blue/depressed, aches/stiffness in joints, and hot flashes (OR 1.084, 95% CI 1.007–1.165) after controlling for model-specific independent variables (Table 5). Exposure to Violence did not remain associated with any symptom (Table 6), but aches/stiffness in joints remained associated with Perceived Violence after controlling for age, race/ethnicity, BMI and menopausal status (Table 7). There was a lower risk of backaches as the neighborhood cohesion score increased (Table 8). Finally, discrimination (Everyday Discrimination Scale) remained associated with lack of energy after controlling for model-specific independent variables (Table 9).

Looking across Tables 5, 6, 7, 8 and 9, in addition to neighborhood context and discrimination, increasing age reduced the risk of headaches, but elevated the risks of aches/stiffness in joints. Peri/post-menopausal status was associated with an increased likelihood of lack of energy in two models (OR 7.324 and OR 8.071) and an increased likelihood of hot flashes in three models (OR 4.734, OR 3.611, and OR 4.265). BMI was not associated with any symptom in logistic regression models after controlling for age, race/ethnicity, menopausal status, and neighborhood characteristics.

### Linear regression results

Both Neighborhood Disorder and Everyday Discrimination scores were significantly associated with derived Factor 1 scores (data not shown). Symptoms loading onto Factor 1 included "Feeling blue or depressed" and "Lack of energy." These results are consistent with our logistic regression results where the associations were significant between "Feeling blue or depressed" and Neighborhood Disorder ($p = 0.011$) and between "Lack of energy" and Everyday Discrimination ($p = 0.006$).

### Discussion

The results of this study suggest that neighborhood context and discrimination may be associated with midlife symptoms in a cohort of black and white women residing in a large urban environment. To our knowledge, this is one of very few studies to extend the investigation of perceived social features of neighborhoods to symptoms among women at midlife. A major strength of this study is the many measures of neighborhood context collected in relation to the broad range of symptoms examined. A novel approach used factor analysis to focus our examination on ten symptoms, clustered on three factors. Of those ten symptoms, five were found to be significantly associated with neighborhood context or discrimination.

As is often the case with midlife symptoms [58–61], the ten symptoms of interest did not separate cleanly

**Table 4** Median level of each scale by symptom occurrence (yes/no)

|  | Lack of energy | | Feeling blue/depressed | | Backaches | | Headaches | | Aches/stiffness in joints | | Short of breath | | Hot flashes | | Trouble sleeping | | Nervous tension | | Pins and needles in hands/feet | |
|---|---|---|---|---|---|---|---|---|---|---|---|---|---|---|---|---|---|---|---|---|
|  | No | Yes | No | Yes | No | Yes | No | Yes | No | Yes | No | Yes | No | Yes | No | Yes | No | Yes | No | Yes |
| ND | 5.09 | 6.00& | 5.00 | 9.00* | 6.00 | 6.00 | 4.50 | 8.00# | 4.00 | 8.00# | 5.04 | 9.00# | 5.04 | 9.00* | 5.54 | 6.00 | 6.00 | 6.00 | 5.09 | 10.00* |
| EV | 0.00 | 1.00& | 0.00 | 1.00& | 1.00 | 1.00 | 1.00 | 1.00 | 0.00 | 1.00 | 1.00 | 1.00 | 0.50 | 2.00& | 1.00 | 1.00 | 1.00 | 1.00 | 0.00 | 2.00* |
| PV | 9.00 | 9.89 | 9.00 | 10.13 | 9.12 | 9.59 | 9.00 | 10.00 | 7.58 | 10.40* | 9.16 | 9.33 | 8.43 | 10.00# | 10.18 | 9.08& | 9.00 | 10.13 | 9.00 | 10.00 |
| NSCT | 8.00 | 8.51 | 8.00 | 9.00 | 9.00 | 8.00# | 8.00 | 8.57 | 9.00 | 8.00& | 8.57 | 8.00 | 8.30 | 8.00 | 8.79 | 8.00 | 8.00 | 8.51 | 8.00 | 8.03 |
| EDS | 5.00 | 7.00* | 6.00 | 7.00 | 6.00 | 7.00 | 5.00 | 7.00& | 6.00 | 7.00* | 6.50 | 6.50 | 7.00 | 6.50 | 6.00 | 7.50 | 6.00 | 8.00 | 6.00 | 9.00# |

*$p < 0.05$; #$p \leq 0.1$; &$p < 0.20$ using Mann-Whitney U test
*ND* Neighborhood Disorder Scale, *EV* Exposure to Violence Scale, *PV* Perceived Violence Scale, *NSCT* Neighborhood Social Cohesion and Trust, *EDS* Everyday Discrimination Scale

**Table 5** Logistic regression results for Neighborhood Disorder (ND)[a]

| | Lack of energy | Feeling blue/depressed | Headaches | Aches/ stiffness in joints | Short of breath | Hot flashes | Pins and needles in hands/feet |
|---|---|---|---|---|---|---|---|
| | AOR[f] (95% CI) | AOR (95% CI) | AOR (95% CI) | AOR (95% CI) | AOR (95% CI) | AOR (95% CI) | AOR (95% CI) |
| Age | .92 (.82–1.03) | | .86 (.77–.96)[c] | 1.13 (.99–1.28) | | 1.05 (.94–1.18) | 1.04 (.97–1.13) |
| Black | | | | 2.62 (.89–7.73) | | 1.70 (.62–4.69) | 1.41 (.54–3.68) |
| BMI | 1.04 (.97–1.12) | | | 1.04 (.955–1.126) | 1.04 (.06–1.12) | | |
| Peri/Post[b] | 7.32 (1.80–29.76)[d] | | 1.88 (.55–6.38) | 2.66 (.62–11.36) | | 4.73 (1.25–17.93)[e] | |
| ND | 1.07 (.997–1.145) | 1.07 (1.02–1.13)[f] | 1.06 (.99–1.12) | 1.11 (1.01–1.21)[g] | 1.06 (.997–1.13) | 1.08 (1.01–1.17)[h] | 1.06 (.99–1.13) |

[a]Symptoms selected for logistic regression were those associated with the neighborhood characteristic in Table 4
[b]Pre is the reference
[c]$p = .007$; [d]$p = .005$; [e]$p = .022$; [f]$p = 0.011$; [g]$p = 0.030$; [h]$p = 0.031$
[f]AOR adjusted odds ratio

into distinct groups through factor analyses. Also consistent with other studies [58, 61], there is population variation in how symptoms cluster. In the study presented here, depressed mood and hot flashes grouped together among the Black sample, but not the White sample or in the sample as a whole.

Lack of energy, feeling blue/depressed, aches/stiffness in joints, and hot flashes were the symptoms most vulnerable to the effect of negative neighborhood context. Each of these four symptoms remained significantly associated with different neighborhood characteristics after adjusting for model-specific covariates. All but lack of energy were associated with Neighborhood Disorder.

Why these symptoms would be most affected by neighborhood context is not immediately clear. Looking at the factor analyses, aches/stiffness in joints consistently clustered together with hot flashes, but feeling blue/depressed only clustered with hot flashes among Black women. Backaches and pins/needles also clustered with hot flashes, but backaches were only significantly associated with the Neighborhood Social Cohesion and Trust, and pins/needles were not associated with any measure of neighborhood context or discrimination. The factor analyses did not help us predict how symptoms would be associated with neighborhood stress.

Neighborhood Disorder remained significantly associated with feeling blue/depressed, aches/stiffness in joints, and hot flashes after controlling for model-specific independent variables. This suggests that stress related to neighborhood disorder may be expressed as emotional, somatic, and vasomotor experience. Somatization of emotional symptoms may at times serve as psychosomatic "idioms of distress," calling attention to difficulties that are hard to verbally express [62–64].

Aches/stiffness in joints remained associated with Perceived Violence, but not Exposure to Violence, after controlling for age, race/ethnicity, BMI and menopausal status. Because of differences in the scales, as well as the relatively modest correlation between them ($r = .489$), it is not surprising that they are not similarly associated with midlife symptoms.

Only backaches were associated with the neighborhood cohesion score, decreasing the risk of backaches as the score increased (Table 8). Women were 15% less likely to report having had backaches for each unit increase (1 point on a 0–15 point scale) on the Neighborhood Social Cohesion and Trust scale. Backaches may also be indicative of depression and somatization [65, 66]. The Multi-Ethnic Study of Atherosclerosis (MESA) found that neighborhoods with low levels of social

**Table 6** Logistic regression results for Exposure to Violence (EV)[a]

| | Lack of Energy | Feeling blue/depressed | Hot flashes | Pins and needles in hands/feet |
|---|---|---|---|---|
| | AOR[c] (95% CI) | AOR (95% CI) | AOR (95% CI) | AOR (95% CI) |
| Age | .93 (.83–1.04) | | 1.07 (.96–1.20) | 1.05 (.97–1.13) |
| Black | | | 2.02 (.74–5.47) | 1.47 (.57–3.77) |
| BMI | 1.05 (.97–1.13) | | | |
| Peri/Post[a] | 5.82 (1.52–22.38)[d] | | 3.61 (1.01–12.92)[e] | |
| EV | 1.13 (.96–1.33) | 1.06 (.94–1.20) | 1.11 (.95–1.304) | 1.13 (.99–1.30) |

[a]Symptoms selected for logistic regression were those associated with the neighborhood characteristic in Table 4
[b]Pre is the reference
[c]AOR adjusted odds ratio
[d]$p = 0.010$; [e]$p = 0.048$

**Table 7** Logistic regression results for Perceived Violence (PV)[a]

| | Aches/ stiffness in joints AOR[e] (95% CI) | Hot flashes AOR (95% CI) | Trouble sleeping AOR (95% CI) |
|---|---|---|---|
| Age | 1.13 (.99–1.29) | 1.05 (.93–1.18) | |
| Black | 2.55 (.85–7.63) | 2.54 (.90–7.20) | .69 (.31–1.54) |
| BMI | .998 (.91–1.09) | | |
| Peri/Post[b] | 1.57 (.35–7.05) | 4.27 (1.09–16.68)[c] | |
| PV | 1.17 (1.01–1.36)[d] | 1.10 (.96–1.25) | .95 (.85–1.06) |

[a]Symptoms selected for logistic regression were those associated with the neighborhood characteristic in Table 4
[b]Pre is the reference
[c]$p = 0.037$; [d]$p = 0.035$
[e]AOR adjusted odds ratio

cohesion had increased rates of depression [37], but that was not the case here. It should be noted that the Neighborhood Social Cohesion and Trust scale in the MESA study was evaluated as tertiles, and a different measure of depressed mood (the Centers of Epidemiologic Studies Depression scale) was used.

Finally, the Everyday Discrimination Scale remained associated with lack of energy after controlling for model-specific independent variables (Table 9). A number of studies have documented associations between discrimination and physical symptoms The SWAN study found everyday discrimination was significantly associated with bodily pain in all ethnic groups [47]. In contrast, data from the Midlife Development in the United States study (MIDUS) did not show a significant association in whites, but demonstrated a significant positive relationship between perceived discrimination and frequency of back pain among African Americans, with a stronger association observed among African-American women [67].

In examining the relation between neighborhood social environments and discrimination with midlife symptoms, there were also contributions of age, race/ethnicity, and menopausal status. Older women had a reduced risk of headaches compared to younger women, in contrast to

**Table 8** Logistic regression results for the Neighborhood Social Cohesion and Trust (NSCT) Scale[a]

| | Backaches AOR[*] (95% CI) | Aches/ stiffness in joints AOR (95% CI) |
|---|---|---|
| Age | . | 1.14 (1.01–1.29)[c] |
| Black | | 3.40 (1.16–9.97)[d] |
| BMI | 1.05 (.98–1.12) | 1.03 (.95–1.12) |
| Peri/Post[b] | | 2.03 (.49–8.46) |
| NSCT | .85 (.72–.99)[e] | .94 (.78–1.13) |

[*]AOR adjusted odds ratio
[a]Symptoms selected for logistic regression were those associated with the neighborhood characteristic in Table 4
[b]Pre is the reference
[c]$p = 0.042$; [d]$p = 0.026$; [e]$p = 0.035$

studies of tension-related headaches [68]. Older women had an elevated risk of aches/stiffness in joints, as would be expected [69]. Although higher rates of reported pain among African-Americans was noted in Dugan et al. [47], the differences of 65% among black women vs 50% among white women in the frequency of aches/stiffness of joints observed in this study did not reach statistical significance, perhaps due to small numbers. Nervous tension was reported less frequently among black than white women (27% vs 44%, respectively), approaching statistical significance ($p = 0.052$). It is interesting to note, however, in models where neighborhood context or discrimination were significantly associated with a midlife symptom, race/ethnicity did not significantly add risk.

Peri/post-menopausal status was associated with an increased likelihood of lack of energy and, in three models, an increased likelihood of hot flashes. Lack of energy is frequently one of the most commonly reported symptoms among women at menopause [56, 70, 71], and it is well established that the loss of estrogen during the late menopausal transition is associated with hot flashes [1].

This study has several limitations. There is limited assessment of symptoms (i.e., presence in past 2 weeks, without assessment of frequency or bothersomeness.) Given the cross-sectional design of this study, we are unable to determine the temporal sequence of the reported relationships. This study posited that the effects of neighborhood context would be related to symptoms at midlife; however, a depressed person might perceive her neighborhood more negatively than a person without depressive symptoms [72]. Longitudinal studies are needed to address the direction of any causal association.

There is a potential for spurious associations given the multiplicity of outcomes. We were careful, however, to limit just those covariates into multivariable models that were significant or marginally significant in bivariate analyses. An additional limitation is the potential lack of power to detect significant findings due to the small sample size. Among the strengths of this study is the fact that participants were drawn

**Table 9** Logistic regression results for Everyday Discrimination Scale (EDS)[a]

| | Lack of energy | Headaches | Aches/ stiffness in joints | Pins and needles in hands/feet |
|---|---|---|---|---|
| | AOR[*] (95% CI) | AOR (95% CI) | AOR (95% CI) | AOR (95% CI) |
| Age | .92 (.82–1.04) | .87 (.78–.97)[c] | 1.14 (.998–1.29) | 1.05 (.97–1.13) |
| Black | | | 2.75 (.94–8.07) | 1.80 (.71–4.55) |
| BMI | | | 1.03 (.95–1.12) | |
| Peri/Post[b] | 8.07 (1.93–33.81)[d] | 1.63 (.48–5.54) | 2.26 (.51–9.98) | |
| EDS | 1.10 (1.03–1.18)[e] | 1.05 (.99–1.11) | 1.08 (.996–1.17) | 1.05 (.997–1.11) |

[*]AOR adjusted odds ratio
[a]Symptoms selected for logistic regression were those associated with the neighborhood characteristic in Table 4
[b]Pre is the reference
[c]$p = 0.010$; [d]$p = 0.004$; [e]$p = 0.006$

from four distinct sites from a large and diverse city. Additionally, standardized data collection protocols were used across sites to assess multiple measures of neighborhood characteristics.

## Conclusions

This study adds to the literature linking neighborhood environments to health outcomes. We have extended this literature to a number of women's midlife symptoms that have not been previously examined. In our sample comprised of both black and white women, we found that negative neighborhood context increased the risk of self-reported depression, aches/stiffness in joints, and hot flashes while greater social cohesion lowered the risk of backaches. The association between discrimination and lack of energy is intriguing, and points to the need to further examine links between exposure to everyday discrimination, and other measures of neighborhood context, and multiple physiological systems.

### Acknowledgments
The authors thank the other investigators, and particularly Joseph E. Schwartz, PhD, for his valuable contributions. We also thank the participants of the Neighborhood Study of Blood Pressure and Sleep for their cooperation.

### Funding
The study was supported by grants NIH P01HL47540, R24HL76857, and M01RR00047.

### Authors' contributions
LMG designed this study and supervised data collection; LMG and LLS carried out all analyses, drafted the manuscript, and approved the final manuscript.

### Competing interests
The authors declare that they have no competing interests.

### Author details
[1]Department of Healthcare Policy & Research, Division of Biostatistics and Epidemiology, Weill Cornell Medical College, 402 E. 67th St., LA-231, New York, NY 10065, USA. [2]Department of Medicine, Division of Nephrology and Hypertension, Weill Cornell Medical College, New York City, NY, USA. [3]Department of Anthropology, UMass Amherst, Amherst, MA, USA.

### References
1. Freedman RR. Pathophysiology and treatment of menopausal hot flashes. Semin Reprod Med. 2005;23:117–25.
2. Freeman EW, Sammel MD, Lin H. Temporal associations of hot flashes and depression in the transition to menopause. Menopause. 2009;16:728–34.
3. Gold EB, Block G, Crawford S, Lachance L, FitzGerald G, Miracle H, Sherman S. Lifestyle and demographic factors in relation to vasomotor symptoms: baseline results from the Study of Women's Health Across the Nation. Am J Epidemiol. 2004;159(12):1189–99.
4. Randolph JF, Sowers M, Bondarenko I, Gold EB, Greendale GA, Bromberger JT, Brockwell SE, Matthews KA. The relationship of longitudinal change in reproductive hormones and vasomotor symptoms during the menopausal transition. J Clin Endocrinol Metab. 2005;90:6106–12.
5. Sacco S, Ricci S, Degan D. Carolei. Migraine in women: the role of hormones and their impact on vascular diseases. J Headache Pain. 2012; 13(3):177–89.
6. Szoeke CE, Cicuttini F, Guthrie J, Dennerstein L. Self-reported arthritis and the menopause. Climacteric. 2005;8(1):49–55.
7. Bromberger JT, Kravitz HM. Mood and menopause: findings from the Study of Women's Health Across the Nation (SWAN) over ten years. Obstet Gynecol Clin N Am. 2011;38(3):609–25.
8. Tom SE, Kuh D, Guralnik JM, Mishra G. Self-reported sleep difficulty during the menopausal transition: results from a prospective cohort study. Menopause. 2010;17(6):1128–35.
9. Freeman EW, Sammel MD, Lin H, Liu Z, Gracia CR. Duration of menopausal hot flushes and associated risk factors. Obstet Gynecol. 2011;117(5):1095–104.
10. Sievert LL. Huicochea-Gómez L, Cahuich-Campos D, Koomoa D-L, Brown DE. Stress and the menopausal transition in Campeche. Mexico Women's Midlife Health. 2018. http://doi.org/10.1186/s40695-018-0038-x.
11. Han KS, Kim L, Shim I. Stress and sleep disorder. Exp Neurobiol. 2012;21(4): 141–50.
12. Martin PR, Lae L, Reece J. Stress as a trigger for headaches: relationship between exposure and sensitivity. Anxiety Stress & Coping. 2007;20(4): 393–407.
13. Tafet GE, Nemeroff CB. The links between stress and depression: psychoneuroendocrinological, genetic, and environmental interactions. J Neuropsychiatry Clin Neurosci. 2016;28(2):77–88.
14. Cignarelli M, Cicinelli E, Corso M, et al. Biophysical and endocrinemetabolic changes during menopausal hot flashes: increase in plasma free fatty acid and norepinephrine levels. Gynecol Obstet Investig. 1989;27:34–7.
15. Meldrum DR, Defazio JD, Erlik Y, et al. Pituitary hormones during the menopausal hot flash. Obstet Gynecol. 1984;64:752–6.
16. Swartzman LC. Impact of stress on objectively recorded menopausal hot flushes and on flush report bias. Health Psychol. 1990;9(5):529–45.
17. Cagnacci A, Cannoletta M, Caretto S, Zanin R, Xholli A, Volpe A. Increased cortisol level: a possible link between climacteric symptoms and cardiovascular risk factors. Menopause. 2011;18(3):273–8.
18. Gerber LM, Sievert LL, Schwartz JE. Hot flashes and midlife symptoms in relation to levels of salivary cortisol. Maturitas. 2017;96:26–32.
19. Gibson CJ, Thurston RC, Matthews KA. Cortisol dysregulation is associated with daily diary-reported hot flashes among midlife women. Clin Endocrinol. 2016;85:645–51.

20. Reed SD, Newton KM, Larson JC, Booth-LaForce C, Woods NF, Landis CA, Tolentino E, Carpenter JS, Freeman EW, Joffe H, Anawalt BD, Guthrie KA. Daily salivary cortisol patterns in midlife women with hot flashes. Clin Endocrinol. 2016;84(5):672–9.

21. Woods NF, Carr MC, Tao EY, Taylor HJ, Mitchell ES. Increased urinary cortisol levels during the menopause transition. Menopause. 2006;13(2):212–21.

22. Brown DE, Sievert LL, Morrison LA, Rahberg N, Reza A. Relationship between hot flashes and ambulatory blood pressure: the Hilo Women's health study. Psychosom Med. 2011;73(2):166–72.

23. Gerber LM, Sievert LL, Warren K, Pickering TG, Schwartz JE. Hot flashes are associated with increased ambulatory systolic blood pressure. Menopause. 2007;14(2):308–15.

24. Jackson EA, El Khoudary SR, Crawford SL, Matthews K, Joffe H, Chae C, Thurston RC. Hot flash frequency and blood pressure: data from the Study of Women's Health Across the Nation. J Women's Health. 2016;25(12):1204–9.

25. James GD, Sievert LL, Flanagan E. Ambulatory blood pressure and heart rate in relation to hot flash experience among women of menopausal age. Ann Hum Biol. 2004;31(1):49–58.

26. Thurston RC, El Koudary SR, Sutton-Tyrrell K, Crandall CJ, Gold E, Sternfeld B, Selzer F, Matthews KA. Are vasomotor symptoms associated with alterations in hemostatic and inflammatory markers? Findings from the Study of Women's Health Across the Nation. Menopause. 2011;18(10):1044–51.

27. Barber S, Hickson DA, Kawachi I, Subramanian SV, Earls F. Double-jeopardy: the joint impact of neighborhood disadvantage and low social cohesion on cumulative risk of disease among African American men and women in the Jackson Heart Study. Soc Sci Med. 2016;153:107–15.

28. Diez Roux AV, Mair C. Neighborhoods and health. Ann N Y Acad Sci. 2010; 1186(1):125–45.

29. Diez-Roux AV, Merkin SS, Arnett D, Chambless L, Massing M, Nieto FJ, Watson RL. Neighborhood of residence and incidence of coronary heart disease. N Engl J Med. 2001;345(2):99–106. https://doi.org/10.1056/NEJM200107123450205.

30. Sternthal MJ, Jun H-J, Earls F, Wright RJ. Community violence and urban childhood asthma: a multilevel analysis. Eur Respir J. 2010;36(6):1400–9.

31. Ewart CK, Elder GJ, Smyth JM. How neighborhood disorder increases blood pressure in youth: agonistic striving and subordination. J Behav Med. 2014; 37(1):113–26.

32. Suchday S, Kapur S, Ewart CK, Friedberg JP. Urban stress and health in developing countries: development and validation of a neighborhood stress index for India. Behav Med. 2006;32(3):77–86.

33. Gallo LC, Fortmann AL, de los Monteros KE, Mills PJ, Barrett-Connor E, Roesch SC, Matthews KA. Individual and neighborhood socioeconomic status and inflammation in Mexican-American women: what is the role of obesity? Psychosom Med. 2012;74(5):535–42.

34. Ewart CK, Suchday S. Discovering how urban poverty and violence affect health: development and validation of a Neighborhood Stress Index. Health Psychol. 2002;21(3):254–62.

35. Wright RJ, Mitchell H, Visness CM, Cohen S, Stout J, Evans R, Gold DR. Community violence and asthma morbidity: the Inner-City Asthma Study. Am J Public Health. 2004;94(4):625–32.

36. Tonorezos ES, Breysse PN, Matsui EC, McCormack MC, Curtin-Brosnan J, Williams D, et al. Does neighborhood violence lead to depression among caregivers of children with asthma? Soc Sci Med. 2008;67(1):31–7.

37. Echeverría S, Diez-Roux AV, Shea S, Borrell LN, Jackson S. Associations of neighborhood problems and neighborhood social cohesion with mental health and health behaviors: the multi-ethnic study of atherosclerosis. Health & Place. 2008;14(4):853–65.

38. Kim D, Diez Roux AV, Kiefe CI, Kawachi I, Liu K. Do neighborhood socioeconomic deprivation and low social cohesion predict coronary calcification?: the CARDIA study. Am J Epidemiol. 2010;172(3):288–98.

39. Chaix B, Lindström M, Rosvall M, et al. Neighbourhood social interactions and risk of acute myocardial infarction. J Epidemiol Comm Health. 2008;62: 62–8.

40. Colen CG, Ramey DM, Cooksey EC, Williams DR. Racial disparities in health among nonpoor African Americans and Hispanics: the role of acute and chronic discrimination. Soc Sci Med. 2018;199:167–80.

41. Krieger N. Embodying inequality: a review of concepts, measures, and methods for studying health consequences of discrimination. International J Health Services. 1999;29:295–352.

42. Williams DR, Mohammed SA. Discrimination and racial disparities in health: evidence and needed research. J Behavioral Med. 2009;32(1):20–47.

43. Brondolo E, Libby DJ, Denton E, Thompson S, Beatty DL, Schwartz J, et al. Racism and ambulatory blood pressure in a community sample. Psychosom Med. 2008;70(1):49–56.

44. McEwen BS, Seeman T. Protective and damaging effects of mediators of stress: elaborating and testing the concepts of allostasis and allostatic load. Ann N Y Acad Sci. 1999;896:30–47.

45. Ong AD, Williams DR, Nwizu U, Gruenewald TL. Everyday unfair treatment and multisystem biological dysregulation in African American adults. Cult Divers Ethn Minor Psychol. 2017;23(1):27–53.

46. Upchurch DM, Stein J, Greendale GA, Chyu L, Tseng CH, Huang MH, Seeman T. A longitudinal investigation of race, socioeconomic status, and psychological mediators of allostatic load in midlife women: findings from the study of women's health across the nation. Psychosom Med. 2015;77:402–12.

47. Dugan SA, Lewis TT, Everson-Rose SA, Jacobs EA, Harlow SD, Janssen I. Chronic discrimination and bodily pain in a multiethnic cohort of midlife women in the Study of Women's Health Across the Nation. Pain. 2017; 158(9):1656–65.

48. Seeman TE, Crimmins E, Huang MH, Singer B, Bucur A, Gruenewald T, Reuben DB. Cumulative biological risk and socio-economic differences in mortality: MacArthur studies of successful aging. Soc Sci Med. 2004; 58:1985–97.

49. Gast GC, Grobbee DE, Pop VJ, Keyzer JJ, Wijnands-van Gent CJ, Samsioe GN, Nilsson PM, van der Schouw YT. Menopausal complaints are associated with cardiovascular risk factors. Hypertention. 2008;51:1492–8.

50. Thurston RC, Chang Y, Barinas-Mitchell E, Jennings JR, Landsittel DP, Santoro N, von Känel R, Matthews KA. Menopausal hot flashes and carotid intima media thickness among midlife women. Stroke. 2016;47(12):2910–5.

51. Spruill TM, Gerber LM, Schwartz JE, Pickering TG, Ogedegbe G. Race differences in the physical and psychological impact of hypertension labeling. Am J Hypertens. 2012;25(4):458–63.

52. Harlow SD, Gass M, Hall JE, Lobo R, Maki P, Rebar RW, Sherman S, Sluss PM, de Villiers TJ. STRAW+10 collaborative group. Executive summary of the stages of reproductive aging workshop + 10: addressing the unfinished agenda of staging reproductive aging. Menopause. 2012;19(4):387–95.

53. Earls FJ, Brooks-Gunn J, Raudenbush SW, Sampson RJ. Project on human development in Chicago neighborhoods (PHDCN): master file, wave 1, 1994–1997 [Computer file]. ICPSR13580-v3. Boston, MA: Harvard Medical School [producer], 2002d. Ann Arbor, MI: Inter-university Consortium for Political and Social Research [distributor], 2005:12–06.

54. Sampson RJ, Raudenbush SW, Earls F. Neighborhoods and violent crime: a multilevel study of collective efficacy. Science. 1997;277:918–24.

55. Williams DR, Yu Y, Jackson JS, Anderson NB. Racial differences in physical and mental health socio-economic status, stress and discrimination. J Health Psychol. 1997;2(3):335–51.

56. Avis NE, Kaufert PA, Lock M, McKinlay SM, Vass K. The evolution of menopausal symptoms. Baillieres Clin Endocrinol Metab. 1993;7:17–32.

57. Obermeyer CM, Reher D, Saliba M. Symptoms, menopausal status, and country differences: a comparative analysis from the DAMeS project. Menopause. 2007;14(4):788–97.

58. Lerner-Geva L, Boyko V, Blumstein T, Benyamini Y. The impact of education, cultural background, and lifestyle on symptoms of the menopausal transition: the Women's health at midlife study. J Women's Health. 2010;19: 975–85.

59. Melby MK. Factor analysis of climacteric symptoms in Japan. Maturitas. 2005; 52:205–22.

60. Sievert LL, Obermeyer CM. Symptom clusters at midlife: a four-country comparison of checklist and qualitative responses. Menopause. 2012;19(2): 133–44.

61. Sievert LL, Obermeyer CM, Saliba M. Symptom groupings at midlife: cross-cultural variation and association with job, home, and life change. Menopause. 2007;14(4):798–807.

62. Gureje O, Simon GE, Ustun TB, Goldberg DP. Somatization in crosscultural perspective: a World Health Organization study in primary care. Am J Psychiatry. 1997;154:989–95.

63. Keyes CL, Ryff CD. Somatization and mental health: a comparative study of the idiom of distress hypothesis. Soc Sci Med. 2003;57:1833–45.

64. Kleinman A, Kleinman J. Somatization: the interconnections in Chinese society among culture, depressive experiences, and the meanings of pain. In: Kleinman A, Good B, editors. Culture and depression. Berkeley, CA: University of California Press; 1985. p. 429–90.

Neighborhood disorder, exposure to violence, and perceived discrimination in relation to symptoms...

163

65. Licciardone JC, Gatchel RJ, Kearns CM, Minotti DE. Depression, somatization, and somatic dysfunction in patients with nonspecific chronic low back pain: results from the OSTEOPATHIC trial. J Am Osteopath Assoc. 2012;112(12): 783–91.

66. Pincus T, Burton AK, Vogel S, Field AP. A systematic review of psychological factors as predicators of chronicity/disability in prospective cohorts of low back pain. Spine. 2002;27(5):E109–20.

67. Edwards RR. The association of perceived discrimination with low back pain. J Behav Med. 2008;31:379–89.

68. Neri I, Granella F, Nappi R, Manzoni G, Facchinetti F, Genazzani A. Characteristics of headache at menopause: a clinico-epidemiologic study. Maturitas. 1993;17(1):31–7.

69. Gao HL, Lin SQ, Chen Y, Wu ZL. The effect of age and menopausal status on musculoskeletal symptoms in Chinese women aged 35-64 years. Climacteric. 2013;16(6):639–45.

70. Dennerstein L, Smith AMA, Morse C, Burger H, Green A, Hopper J, Ryan M. Menopausal symptoms in Australian women. Med J Aust. 1993;159:232–6.

71. Sievert LL, Anderson D, Melby MK, Obermeyer CM. Methods used in cross-cultural comparisons of somatic symptoms and their determinants. Maturitas. 2011;70:127–34.

72. Mair C, Diez Roux AV, Shen M, Shea S, Seeman T, Echeverria S, O'Meara ES. Cross-sectional and longitudinal associations of neighborhood cohesion and stressors with depressive symptoms in the multiethnic study of atherosclerosis (MESA). Ann Epidemiol. 2009;19(1):49–57.

# 17

# Recent evidence exploring the associations between physical activity and menopausal symptoms in midlife women: perceived risks and possible health benefits

Kelley Pettee Gabriel[1,2,3*], Jessica M. Mason[1,2,3] and Barbara Sternfeld[4]

## Abstract

Although the health benefits of physical activity are well established, the prevalence of midlife women accumulating sufficient physical activity to meet current physical activity guidelines is strikingly low, as shown in United States (U.S.) based surveillance systems that utilize either (or both) participant-reported and device-based (i.e., accelerometers) measures of activity. For midlife women, these low prevalence estimates may be due, in part, to a general lack of time given more pressing work commitments and family obligations. Further, the benefits or "*reward*" of allocating limited time to physical activity may be perceived, by some, as too distant for immediate action or attention. However, shifting the health promotion message from the long term benefits of physical activity to the more short-term, acute benefits may encourage midlife women to engage in more regular physical activity. In this article, we review the latest evidence (i.e., past 5 years) regarding the impact of physical activity on menopausal symptoms. Recent studies provide strong support for the absence of an effect of physical activity on vasomotor symptoms; evidence is still inconclusive regarding the role of physical activity on urogenital symptoms (vaginal dryness, urinary incontinence) and sleep, but consistently suggestive of a positive impact on mood and weight control. To further advance this field, we also propose additional considerations and future research directions.

**Keywords:** Physical activity, Menopause, Midlife, Women

## Introduction

The aging of the baby boomer cohort, born in the United States (U.S.) between mid-1946 and mid-1964 [1], has resulted in increased interest in strategies to optimize the health and well-being of midlife adults (ages 45 to 64 years). Indeed, research efforts specifically targeting midlife women, in particular, has increased exponentially in recent years. This interest may be due, in part, to the relatively recent recognition that sex differences exist, not only with regards to the incidence and/or prevalence of various health outcomes, but also with the prevalence of health behaviors (e.g., not meeting

* Correspondence: Kelley.P.Gabriel@uth.tmc.edu
[1]Division of Epidemiology, Human Genetics and Environmental Sciences, University of Texas Health Science Center at Houston: School of Public Health – Austin Regional Campus, Austin, TX, USA
[2]School of Public Health, Austin Regional Campus, 1616 Guadalupe Street, Suite 6.300, Austin, TX 78701, USA
Full list of author information is available at the end of the article

physical activity guidelines) that increase one's disease and/or mortality risk.

Physical activity is a viable strategy to reduce the burden of chronic disease and disability. Strategies to increase physical activity at the individual- and population- level are particularly appealing given the strong evidence demonstrating the multiplicity of health benefits, including reduced risk of premature death, coronary heart disease (CHD), stroke, hypertension, hyperlipidemia, type 2 diabetes, metabolic syndrome, breast and colon cancer, and depression [2]. Further, since physical activity is a behavior and, thus, is modifiable, it is an excellent target for health promotion interventions focused on prevention.

Yet, despite the well-established health benefits of regular, habitual physical activity, few midlife women are accumulating sufficient levels to meet physical activity guidelines. Current U.S. based aerobic guidelines encourage: (1) ≥150 min per week of moderate intensity physical activity, (2) ≥75 min per week of vigorous intensity physical activity or (3) an equivalent combination of moderate and vigorous intensity physical activity (MVPA) [3]. The guidelines also recommend that adults participate in muscle-strengthening activities, across all major muscle groups, on ≥2 days per week. Based on 2013 Behavioral Risk Factor Surveillance System (BRFSS) data [4], 28.2 % (Standard Error (SE) ± 0.41) of women aged 45 to 54 years met the aerobic physical activity guidelines only, 6.0 % (SE ± 0.20) met muscle-strengthening guidelines only, and 14.8 % (SE ± 0.30) met both the aerobic and muscle-strengthening guidelines. Among women aged 55 to 64 years, the prevalence estimates for meeting guidelines were similar: 28.5 % (SE ± 0.37), 5.6 % (SE ± 0.19), and 13.7 % (SE ± 0.26) met aerobic guidelines only, muscle-strengthening guidelines only, or met both guidelines, respectively [4]. In the 2003–04 and 2005–06 cycles of the National Health and Nutrition Examination Survey (NHANES) [5], physical activity levels of a U.S. representative sample were also directly measured via accelerometers. The prevalence estimates for meeting physical activity guidelines were strikingly lower than those obtained in BRFSS using self-reported methods (as reported above). Using NHANES 2003–06 accelerometer data, only 26.7 % (SE ± 2.4) and 18.0 % (SE ± 2.6) of midlife women, aged 45–54 and 55 to 56 years, respectively, met aerobic guidelines. To be consistent with the wording of the *2008 Physical Activity Guidelines for Americans* [3], meeting physical activity guidelines was defined as *any* accumulated time (minutes per day) spent above the moderate-intensity threshold (1952 counts per minute [6]), and did not necessarily occur in prolonged activity bouts. It is important to note that these low prevalence estimates may be due, in part, to functional limitations that emerge during midlife. Previous studies have found that 20–40 % of midlife women reported moderate to severe physical limitations [7, 8], which could serve as a significant barrier to engaging in sufficient, higher intensity physical activity to meet current physical activity guidelines.

Previous studies have suggested that another barrier to engaging in sufficient physical activity is a *"lack of time"* [9–11]. This is certainly a tangible barrier for midlife women given that during this stage of adulthood, women often find themselves *"sandwiched"* between caring for both dependent children and aging parents [12]. In addition, many midlife women are working outside the home; according to 2013 BRFSS data [4], 56.6 % (SE ± 0.46) and 43.1 % (SE ± 0.41) women aged 45 to 54 and 55 to 64 years, respectively, reported being employed for wages. Additionally, self-employment was reported in 8.6 % (SE ± 0.28) and 7.1 % (SE ± 0.21) of women aged 45 to 54 years and 55 to 64 years, respectively. Work demands and family obligations, therefore, frequently compete with the desire for leisure time activities such as physical activity, given the limited amount of time (i.e., leisure time) available during a day.

Principles of behavioral economics posit that decisions about being physically active involve trade-offs relative to fixed resources [13]. Thus, allocating time to recreational physical activity, given other competing demands, may be perceived as a *"risk"* for midlife women. However, individuals may undertake this risk, if the perceived *"rewards"* are sufficiently adequate and/or valued. The risk of developing the top three leading causes of death in women (i.e., coronary heart disease, cancer, and stroke) [14] increases with age, with risk escalating after age 65 [15, 16]. While midlife women are at immediate risk for developing these conditions, they may not perceive that a reduction in disease risk, that may be manifested in the future, is an adequate reward given the immediate risk of needing to allocate ≥ 30 min per day for physical activity in their already full schedules.

One potential strategy to alter the risk/benefit ratio and increase the prevalence of midlife women meeting physical activity guidelines may be to target health promotion messages centered on the benefit of physical activity for more acute health outcomes or concerns, such as a reduction in- or relief from- menopausal symptoms. A 2005 review paper by Woods and Mitchell [17] summarized the prevalence of menopausal symptoms from published community-based longitudinal studies of the menopausal transition by Staging Reproductive Aging Workshop (STRAW) criteria, whenever possible. The prevalence of reported vasomotor symptoms ranged from 6 to 13 % in the late reproductive phase to as high as 79 % among postmenopausal women. The prevalence of reported vaginal dryness ranged from 3 % of women in the reproductive stage to 47 % among women who were 3 years postmenopausal. According to data from the Study of Women's Health Across the Nation (SWAN), Sampselle et al. [18] found that 57 % of study participants reported urinary incontinence with 15 % reporting it as moderate and 10 % as severe. The prevalence of reported sleep disturbances ranged from 31 % of women in the reproductive phase to 45 % among women who are 3 years postmenopausal. With regards to reported depressed mood symptoms, the prevalence estimates ranged from 19 to 29 %. Several other longitudinal investigations have reported significant increases in mean body weight and other markers of adiposity (e.g., waist circumference and fat mass) during the menopausal transition [19–22]. In addition to the moderate to high prevalence of reported menopausal symptoms in mid-life women, other studies [23, 24] suggest that these symptoms may persist for a substantial portion of the menopausal transition. For example, a recent (2015) longitudinal SWAN analysis found that vasomotor symptoms persisted for a median duration of 7.4 years [25], and even longer among some demographic groups such as Black women.

Therefore, if women were convinced that physical activity would improve their most salient and disturbing symptoms, they might accept the *"risk"* of allocating valuable time to be physically active in exchange for the *"reward"* of symptom relief. They would also, as a secondary, longer-term reward, gain additional benefit in relation to chronic disease and disability prevention. The purpose of this paper is to evaluate whether this health promotion message is tenable by reviewing the recent literature (i.e., past 5 years) reporting on the effect of physical activity on menopausal symptoms. The selection of menopausal symptoms included in this review were based on the prevalence estimates reported by Woods et al. [17] We also provide commentary on the strengths and limitations of the existing research, and propose future research directions.

## Review

The recent literature, published with the past 5 years (i.e., January 01, 2010 to February 28, 2015), exploring the association of physical activity with menopausal symptoms that are frequently reported by midlife women was reviewed and summarized [26]. Menopausal symptoms targeted in this literature review include those related specifically to hormonal changes that characterize the menopausal transition (i.e., vasomotor symptoms, including hot flashes and night sweats, and vaginal dryness) and more general symptoms that are characteristic of midlife and/or the normal aging process (i.e., urinary incontinence, sleep quality and/or sleep disturbances, psychological distress, and weight gain). While all selected studies for this review are included in the summary tables, investigations utilizing prospective cohort-, quasi-experimental-, or experimental- study designs are highlighted in the text. Studies were not included in this review if more general symptom categories (e.g., urogenital symptoms versus urinary incontinence) were ascertained and/or reported by study investigators. This literature review summarizes the major findings from 14 cross-sectional studies [27–40], 2 longitudinal studies [41, 42], 7 prospective cohort studies [43–49], 1 non-randomized intervention studies [50], and 9 randomized controlled trials (RCT) [51–59] (see Tables 1, 2, 3, 4, 5 and 6).

## Potential biological mechanisms: physical activity and menopausal symptoms

Physical activity has both acute and chronic physiological and psychological effects, many of which could help to alleviate menopausal symptoms and other complaints of midlife women. Even though the specific etiology of vasomotor symptoms remains unclear, hot flashes and night sweats are the result of neuroendocrine processes at the level of the hypothalamus [60]. One hypothesis for how physical activity might alleviate vasomotor symptoms is through the impact of physical activity on neurotransmitters (e.g., β-endorphins) which regulate thermoregulation [61]. Similarly, physical activity, which increases sympathetic nervous system activity, could alleviate the vaginal dryness which results from the declines in circulating estrogen characteristic of menopause [62] by increasing sexual arousal and lubrication [63]. However, it is unclear if this is an acute effect of physical activity or if the increased lubrication persists at rest. The benefit of physical activity for reduced risk of urinary incontinence is likely mediated through obesity. Previous studies have indicated that obesity is a risk factor for urinary incontinence and studies have shown that weight loss can result in urinary incontinence remission [64]. The mechanisms by which physical activity may improve sleep quality include associated reductions in anxiety and depression. More directly, physical activity has been shown to promote increases in slow wave sleep, which is indicative of good sleep quality. Physical activity may also impact sleep through favorable influences on circadian functioning [65]. As reported by Dugan et al., the proposed biological mechanisms supporting the beneficial role of physical activity for preventing or reducing depression include: reduced inflammation, increased neurotransmitter (i.e., dopamine and serotonin) levels, and increased endorphin secretion [46]. Finally, physical activity contributes to prevention of weight gain and promotion of weight loss and reduces risk of adiposity-related outcomes because physical activity is a key component of total energy expenditure (i.e., ~20 % of total energy expenditure) [66].

## Physical activity and vasomotor symptoms

Table 1 summarizes the recent evidence examining the association between physical activity and vasomotor symptoms, including hot flashes and night sweats. In a 15-day longitudinal study, Elavsky et al. [41] found an acute bout of exercise (30 min of moderate intensity exercise) decreased subjective and objectively determined hot flashes, but had no impact on night sweats. Also, daily physical activity estimates (detected via accelerometry during the 15-day observation period) were not associated with reported hot flash frequency, although less fit participants reported more hot flashes on days when they engaged in more activity than usual. In another longitudinal study by Elavsky and colleagues [42], participants concurrently wore an accelerometer and reported daily hot flashes via an electronic personal digital assistant for 30 consecutive days. Statistically significant

**Table 1** Selected studies of physical activity and vasomotor symptoms (includes hot flashes and night sweats)

| Reference | Sample | Physical activity measure | Menopausal symptom measure | Other measures | Detailed findings | Summarized findings: observed association | | | |
|---|---|---|---|---|---|---|---|---|---|
| | | | | | | Null | Positive | Negative | Mixed |
| **Cross-sectional studies** | | | | | | | | | |
| Canário et al. 2012 [27] | Population-based sample of 370 women from Natal, Brazil aged 40-65 | International Physical Activity Questionnaire with three categories of classification: sedentary, moderately active and very active (vigorous) | Blatt–Kupperman Menopausal Index with three categories of classification: mild (≤19), moderate (20–35), or severe (>35) | Socio-demographic and behavioral characteristics | Bivariate analysis revealed a statistically significant inverse association between physical activity and hot flashes | | | x | |
| Haimov-Kochman et al. 2013 [28] | 151 healthy women aged 45-55 who attended the menopause clinic at the Hadassah Hebrew University Medical Center (Jerusalem, Israel) | Physical activity was quantified by self-reported frequency of exercise (1–7 times a week), and categorized into 3 groups: 1–2; 3–4; 5–7 times per week | The Greene climactic scale, estimates include total score. Subscores for psychological, somatic/physical, sexual, and vasomotor symptoms also reported | Demographic, anthropometric, and lifestyle (behavioral) variables | There was no association between physical activity frequency and the vasomotor subscale | x | | | |
| Kandish et al. 2010 [29] | Female employees at a Mid-Western University were invited to participate in an on-line survey. The analytic sample included 196 women aged ≥40 years that did not smoke or use hormone therapy | Usual physical activity per week reported via 30 min intervals of aerobic and strength activity. Intensity of activity was reported as mild, moderate, or heavy | Usual daily frequency and severity (10-point scale, ranging from 'very mild' to 'very severe') of hot flashes were ascertained | Socio-demographic characteristics, alcohol and caffeine consumption | Adjusted analyses, suggested higher frequency of aerobic physical activity significantly increased the frequency of hot flashes. Yet, higher intensity of aerobic physical activity was associated with decreased frequency and severity of hot flashes | | | | x |
| Mansikkamäki et al. 2015 [30][a] | Random sample of 5000 women born in 1963 was obtained from the Finnish Population Register Centre. Analytic sample included 2606 women aged 49 years old that responded to a postal survey in 2012 | A single item pertaining to usual exercise (frequency and duration) per week during past 12-months. Women were classified as 'active' if they reported ≥ 150 min per week of moderate intensity or ≥75 min of vigorous intensity, with strength training and balance training | Women's Health Questionnaire addressing nine domains of physical and emotional experiences, including vasomotor symptoms | Socio-demographic factors, anthropometrics, self-rated health | In the unadjusted models, inactive women had a higher odds of vasomotor symptoms (POR 1.9; 95 % CI: 1.03–1.36). However, after adjustment for BMI and education level, results were no longer statistically significant | x | | | |
| Moilanen et al. 2010 [31] | Participants drawn from Finnish Health 2000 Study ($n = 7,977$), data collection included a home interview, 3 self-administered questionnaires, and a clinical exam. Analytic sample included 1427 women, ages 45–64; | Physical activity was assessed via a single item on the questionnaire, "How much do you exercise or strain yourself physically in your leisure time" with four response options ranging from 'sedentary' (reading, watching television) to | Severity of general symptoms, including vasomotor symptoms, were assessed via two items on the questionnaire | Socio-demographics, health behaviors, anthropometrics, menopausal status and hormone therapy use | Low active women reported significantly more vasomotor symptoms ($\beta = 0.18$; 95 % CI: 0.10, 0.27) than the high active group after adjustment for baseline age, menopausal status, education, chronic disease, and hormone therapy use | | | x | |

**Table 1** Selected studies of physical activity and vasomotor symptoms (includes hot flashes and night sweats) (Continued)

| Study | Sample | PA assessment | VMS measure | Covariates | Results | |
|---|---|---|---|---|---|---|
| | known menopausal status) who completed the home interview, first questionnaire | 'competitive sports'. Participants were classified based on low, moderate, and high physical activity | | | | x |
| Pimenta et al. 2011 [32] | Community-based sample of 243 women (Lisbon, Portugal) that reported vasomotor symptoms in the past month; aged 42–60 years old | Physical exercise was assessed using reported frequency and duration of exercise sessions per week. Summary scores were computed using the mean frequency and duration values | Menopause Symptoms' Severity Inventory was used to assess the frequency and intensity of night sweats through classification on a 5-point Likert scale which ranged from 'never' to 'daily' and from 'not intense' to 'extreme intensity'. Severity for each symptom was computed as the mean frequency and intensity values | Socio-demographic characteristics, health and menopausal related variables and lifestyle factors | Physical exercise was not associated with perceived severity of hot flashes or night sweats | x |
| Tan et al. 2014 [33] | 305 Turkish (District of Izmir) menopausal women who went to their primary care physician between August and October 2009 | International Physical Activity Questionnaire (IPAQ)-short version. Women were classified as: low, moderate, or high active | Turkish version of the Menopause Rating Scale (MRS), which includes 11 items assessing assess somato-vegetative, psycho logical and urogenital symptoms; scores range from 'not present' to 'very severe' | Socio-demographic factors, health behaviors, anthropometrics | There was no difference in the reported frequency of hot flashes/night sweating by physical activity groups | x |

Short-term (≤30 days) Longitudinal Studies

| Study | Sample | PA assessment | VMS measure | Covariates | Results | |
|---|---|---|---|---|---|---|
| Elavsky et al. 2012 [41] | Community-dwelling midlife women (N = 121; age range, 40–60 years) not using hormone therapy for at least 6 months. Prospective monitoring across a 15-day period. The analytic sample included 92 participants that reported a menopausal-related vaso motor symptom (i.e., night sweats or hot flashes) within the last 2 weeks | To examine the acute effects of PA, participants attended a second visit during week 1, where they completed a 30-min moderate intensity exercise bout. Daily PA was also assessed objectively using an ActiGraph (GT1M) accelerometer placed over the participants' nondominant hip for 15 consecutive days | Hot flash and night sweat data were collected using Purdue Momentary Assessment platform in which participants self-reported hot flashes and night-sweats in real-time using a personal digital assistant (PDA). Objective data were obtained via skin conductance monitoring (Biolog Hot Flash Monitor), a battery-powered, portable device. Participants wore the monitor for 24 h, twice during data collection. In addition to continuous monitoring, participants were asked to flag perceived events | Basic demographic and health history information. Psychological symptoms through questionnaires | An acute bout of moderate-intensity of aerobic exercise decreases both reported and objective and subjective hot flashes<br><br>There was no significant change in night sweats as a result of the acute exercise bout<br><br>Daily physical activity was not associated with reported hot flash frequency. Yet, less fit women reported more hot flashes on days when they engaged in more moderate-intensity physical activity than usual | x |

**Table 1** Selected studies of physical activity and vasomotor symptoms (includes hot flashes and night sweats) *(Continued)*

| Study | Sample | PA assessment | VMS assessment | Covariates | Findings | |
|---|---|---|---|---|---|---|
| Elavsky et al. 2012 [42] | 24 symptomatic peri- and post-menopausal women not on HT were picked from volunteers who responded to advertisements | Participants used accelerometers across a menstrual cycle or for 30 days if postmenopausal. Accelerometer count data were classified as % time sedentary, and in light, moderate and vigorous 2intensity physical activity (Matthews cutpoints) | Daily HFs were reported using an electronic PDA across one menstrual cycle or 30 days | Socio-demographic and health history. Psychosocial questionnaires, including depression, chronic stress, and anxiety. Reproductive hormones via blood draw | The association between physical activity and hot flashes was statistically significant in half the participants (n = 10 of 20). Same day, as well as cross-lagged (effects of previous day's physical activity on hot flashes the next day), were examined. Yet, the direction and magnitude of the association varied across participants. The associations between daily PA and night sweats were not reported | x |
| **Prospective cohort studies** | | | | | | |
| Gibson et al. 2014 [43] | Analytic sample included Study of Women's Health across the Nation (SWAN) participants (n = 51); Pittsburgh site, only. At enrollment (1996–97), participants were aged 42–52 years old. Hot flashes were assessed in 2008–09 | PA was measured using accelerometer-derived activity counts from the Biolog monitor. The mean activity count in the 10 min before a hot flash were classified as "pre-flash" physical activity. The other data were classified as "control" physical activity. Habitual physical activity assessed via the Kaiser Physical Activity Survey (KPAS) | Self-reported hot flashes were assessed using a portable electronic diary. Physiologically detected hot flashes were measured using Biolog sternal skin conductance monitors | Socio-demographic and health behavior information, anthropometrics, depression & anxiety | There was no relationship of daily physical activity with physiologic hot flashes, self-reported hot flashes, or physiologically monitored hot flashes (not confirmed by self-report). Yet, higher habitual PA, higher BMI, more depressive symptoms and anxiety were associated with higher levels of self-reported hot flashes not corroborated by a physiologic hot flash | x |
| Gjelsvik et al. 2011 [44] | Analytic sample included 2229 women aged 40–44 years, randomly selected from national survey in Hordaland County, Norway. Baseline data were collected in 1997–98 and follow-up occurred every second year and continued to 2010 | A short follow-up question naire included items pertaining to physical exercise. Participants were classified as inactive based on <1 h hard activity and/or <2 | A short follow-up question naire included items pertaining to the reported frequency ('daily to 'never/almost never') and burden ('very much' to 'not bothered') | Sociodemographic factors, health behaviors, menopausal status and symptoms | When compared to inactive women, women with >3 h of hard exercise per day were 1.5 times (1.1–1.9) more likely to report daily hot flashes | x |
| de Azevedo Guimaraes et al. 2011 [45] | 120 Brazilian women aged 45–59 years old volunteered for the 12-week study (re cruited through work or other institutions) | Habitual PA was assessed through the short form of the International PA Questionnaire (IPAQ); Participants were classified as: maintained <30 min/day, | Hot flashes were assessed using the Kupperman Menopausal Index | Socio-demographic factors, anthropometrics, menopausal status and symptoms, and QOL | Women classified in the highest active group (maintained or increased to 60 min per day) had reported significantly fewer hot flashes after 12-weeks | x |

**Table 1** Selected studies of physical activity and vasomotor symptoms (includes hot flashes and night sweats) *(Continued)*

| | Sample | Intervention | Measures | Results | |
|---|---|---|---|---|---|
| | 104 women completed the 12-week study. | maintained or increased to 30–60 min/day, or maintained or increased to >60 min/day | | than the other two active groups after adjustment for baseline values | X |
| **Non-randomized intervention studies** | | | | | |
| Karacan, 2010 [50]^a | 112 women aged 46–55. The analytic sample included 65 participants that regularly participated in the 3- and 6-month exercise program | The 6-month exercise program included aerobic activity (75–80 % heart rate capacity) with calisthenics for 3 days a week for 55 min each session | The menopause rating scale (MRS) was composed of 11 items assessing menopausal symptoms divided into three groups: psychological, somatic-vegetative and urogenital | Physical characteristics (height, weight, and age at menopause), resting heart rate and blood pressure, lower back flexibility, hand grip strength, and body composition (skin folds) | There was a significant decrease in hot flushes and night sweats from baseline to 6-months |
| **Randomized controlled trials** | | | | | |
| Agil et al. 2010 [51] | 42 Turkish postmenopausal women (aged 45–60 years old) who agreed to participate in the 8-week study after presenting to the Department of Obstetrics and Gynecology (Bayindir Hospital) between March and December 2009. Participants were randomly assigned to the aerobic or resistance training group | Aerobic and Resistance Groups: Supervised sessions 3 × per week. The resistance group used elastic belt; no other details provided for either group | Vasomotor symptoms were assessed using the Menopause-specific Quality of Life Questionnaire (MENQOL) | Socio-demographics and health behaviors | Both the aerobic and resistance groups had a significant reduction in vasomotor symptoms following the exercise program. | X |
| Luoto et al. 2012 [52]^a | 176 Finnish white women were recruited for the study by newspaper advertisements. The analytic sample included 154 inactive participants were randomly assigned to the exercise (n = 74) or control group (n = 77) that completed the 6-month study protocol | Exercise Group: Unsupervised aerobic training intervention; 4 × per week at 64–80 % maximal heart rate for 50 min each time | Hot flashes were assessed via the Women's Health Questionnaire (primary). Hot flashes were also collected 2 × per day using a mobile phone-administered questionnaire | Socio-demographic factors, anthropometrics, and menopausal symptoms | WHQ assessed hot flashes did not differ by group. There was no group × time differences in daily reported daytime hot flashes. X |
| Moilanen et al. 2012 [53]^a | 176 Finnish white women were recruited for the study by newspaper advertisements. The analytic sample included 154 inactive participants were randomly assigned to the exercise (n = 74) or control group (n = 77) that completed the 6-month study protocol | Exercise Group: Unsupervised aerobic training intervention; 4 × per week at 64–80 % maximal heart rate for 50 min each time | The frequency of night sweats were collected 2 × per day using a mobile phone-administered questionnaire | Socio-demographic factors, anthropometrics, and menopausal symptoms | The prevalence of night sweats decreased pre- to post-intervention | X |

**Table 1** Selected studies of physical activity and vasomotor symptoms (includes hot flashes and night sweats) *(Continued)*

| Study | Participants/design | Intervention | Vasomotor measure | Other measures | Results | |
|---|---|---|---|---|---|---|
| Newton et al. 2014 [54][a] | Women aged 40–62 recruited from 3 sites in US (IN, CA, WA) and randomly assigned to a 12-week yoga (n = 107), exercise (n = 106), or usual activity (n = 142) group. Participants were and also randomly assigned to the omega-3 (n = 177) or placebo (n = 178) group. Participants were followed for 12-weeks | Yoga Group: Supervised: 1 × per week for 90 min; Unsupervised: 6 × per week for 20 min. Usual Activity: Instructed to follow usual physical activity plan; asked not to initiate yoga or a new exercise regimen. | Frequency and intensity of vasomotor were recorded in daily diaries by the participants. VMS bother was rated each day on a scale ranging from 1 'none' to 4 'a lot'. Baseline frequency was calculated from the mean number of vasomotor symptoms reported in a 24-h period during the 14 days prior to the 1st visit. Vasomotor frequency during weeks 6 and 12 were computed similarly using the corresponding diaries | Socio-demographics, anthropometrics, daily diaries assessing vasomotor symptoms, sleep quality, health history, and anxiety | After 12-weeks, based on intent-to-treat analysis, yoga had no effect on vasomotor frequency or bother when compared to usual activity | x |
| Reed et al. 2014 [55][a] | Women aged 40–62 recruited from 3 sites in US (IN, CA, WA) and randomly assigned to a 12-week yoga (n = 107), exercise (n = 106), or usual activity (n = 142) group. Participants were and also randomly assigned to the omega-3 (n = 177) or placebo (n = 178) group. Participants were followed for 12-weeks | Yoga Group: Supervised: 1 × per week for 90 min; Unsupervised: 6 × per week for 20 min. Exercise Group: Supervised: 3 × per week, 50–60 % HRR during month 1, 60–70 % HRR during months 2 & 3. Usual Activity: Instructed to follow usual physical activity plan; asked not to initiate yoga or a new exercise regimen | Menopausal Quality of Life Questionnaire (MENQOL; range, 1–8) is a 29-item assessment of menopause-related QOL. Total score and 4 domain-specific scores (vasomotor, physical, psychosocial, & sexual functioning). Frequency of vasomotor symptoms were also assessed via daily diaries | Socio-demographics, anthropometrics, daily diaries assessing vasomotor symptoms, sleep quality, health history, and anxiety | After 12-weeks, compared to the usual activity group, yoga group participants had significant improvements in vasomotor symptoms (as reported via MENQOL). There was no difference in pre- to post- vasomotor symptoms between the exercise and usual activity groups | |
| Sternfeld et al. 2014 [56][a] | Women aged 40–62 recruited from 3 sites in US (IN, CA, WA) and randomly assigned to a 12-week yoga (n = 107), exercise (n = 106), or usual activity (n = 142) group. Participants were and also randomly assigned to the omega-3 (n = 177) or placebo (n = 178) group. Participants were followed for 12-weeks | Exercise Group: Supervised: 3 × per week, 50–60 % HRR during month 1, 60–70 % HRR during months 2 & 3. Possible modes included, treadmill, elliptical trainer, or stationary bicycle. Trained staff recorded heart rate, workload, and perceived 7 exertion every 5–10 minutes | Frequency and intensity of vasomotor were recorded in daily diaries by the participants. VMS bother was rated each day on a scale ranging from 1 'none' to 4 'a lot'. Baseline frequency was calculated from the mean number of vasomotor symptoms reported in a 24-h period during the 14 days prior to the 1st visit. Vasomotor frequency during weeks 6 and 12 were computed similarly using the corresponding diaries | Socio-demographics, anthropometrics, daily diaries assessing vasomotor symptoms, sleep quality, health history, and anxiety | After 12-weeks, compared to the usual activity group, exercise group participants had no change in frequency or burden of vasomotor symptom, compared to the usual activity group | x |

[a]Physical activity dose reflective of 2008 Physical Activity Guidelines for Americans [3]

**Table 2** Selected studies of physical activity and vaginal dryness

| Reference | Sample | Physical activity measure | Menopausal symptom measure | Other measures | Detailed findings | Summarized findings: observed association | | | |
|---|---|---|---|---|---|---|---|---|---|
| | | | | | | Null | Positive | Negative | Mixed |
| **Cross-sectional studies** | | | | | | | | | |
| Aydin et al. 2014 [34] | 1071 Islamic postmenopausal women (of 1328 women that expressed interest) who attended an outpatient clinic from 2005–12 | Questionnaire included an item on regular exercise, defined as 30-min for ≥2 times per week (yes/no) | Validated questionnaire assessing genitourinary symptoms, including presence or absence of vaginal dryness | Socio-demographics, health behaviors, anthropometrics, length of menopausal status (months) | The prevalence of vaginal dryness was higher in participants reporting regular exercise | | | x | |
| Tan et al. 2014 [33] | 305 Turkish (District of Izmir) menopausal women who went to their primary care physician between August and October 2009 | International Physical Activity Questionnaire (IPAQ)-short version. Women were classified as: low, moderate, or high active | Turkish version of the Menopause Rating Scale (MRS), which includes 11 items assessing assess somato-vegetative, psychological and urogenital symptoms; scores range from 'not present' to 'very severe' | Socio-demographic factors, health behaviors, anthropometrics | High active women had a lower prevalence of vaginal dryness symptoms than low and moderate active women | | x | | |
| **Prospective cohort studies** | | | | | | | | | |
| de Azevedo Guimaraes et al. 2011 [45] | 120 Brazilian women aged 45–59 years old volunteered for the 12-week study (recruited through work or other institutions)<br><br>104 women completed the 12-week study | Habitual PA was assessed through the short form of the International PA Questionnaire (IPAQ); Participants were classified as: maintained <30 min/day, maintained or increased to 30–60 min/day, or maintained or increased to >60 min/day | Vaginal dryness was assessed using the Kupperman Menopausal Index | Socio-demographic factors, anthropometrics, menopausal status and symptoms, and QOL | There was no difference in reported vaginal dryness by activity group | x | | | |
| **Non-randomized intervention studies** | | | | | | | | | |
| Karacan, 2010 [50][a] | 112 women aged 46–55. The analytic sample included 65 participants that regularly participated in the 3- and 6-month exercise program | The 6-month exercise program included aerobic activity (75–80 % heart rate capacity) with calisthenics for 3 days a week for 55 min each session | The menopause rating scale (MRS) was composed of 11 items assessing menopausal symptoms divided into three groups: psychological, somatic-vegetative and urogenital | Physical characteristics (height, weight, and age at menopause), resting heart rate and blood pressure, lower back flexibility, hand grip strength, and body composition (skin folds) | There was no pre- to post- exercise program difference in vaginal dryness | x | | | |

**Table 2** Selected studies of physical activity and vaginal dryness (*Continued*)

Randomized controlled trials

| | | | | | |
|---|---|---|---|---|---|
| Moilanen et al. 2012 [53][a] | 176 Finnish white women were recruited for the study by newspaper advertisements. The analytic sample included 154 inactive participants were randomly assigned to the exercise (n = 74) or control group (n = 77) that completed the 6-month study protocol | Exercise Group: Unsupervised aerobic training intervention; 4 × per week at 64–80 % maximal heart rate for 50 min each time | The presence of vaginal dryness were collected 2 × per day using a mobile phone-administered questionnaire | Socio-demographic factors, anthropometrics, and menopausal symptoms | The prevalence of vaginal dryness decreased pre- to post- intervention |
| | | | | | x |

[a]Physical activity dose reflective of 2008 Physical Activity Guidelines for Americans [3]

**Table 3** Selected studies of physical activity and urinary incontinence

| Reference | Sample | Physical activity measure | Menopausal symptom measure | Other measures | Main findings | Summarized findings: observed association | | | |
|---|---|---|---|---|---|---|---|---|---|
| | | | | | | Null | Positive | Negative | Mixed |
| *Cross-sectional studies* | | | | | | | | | |
| Aydin et al. 2014 [34] | 1071 Islamic postmenopausal women (of 1328 women that expressed interest) who attended an outpatient clinic from 2005–12 | Questionnaire included an item on regular exercise, defined as 30-min for ≥2 times per week (yes/no) | Validated questionnaire assessing genitourinary symptoms, including presence or absence of urinary symptoms (dysuria, frequency, urgency, nocturia, and incontinence) | Sociodemographic factors, health behaviors, anthropometrics, length of menopausal status (months) | There was no significant difference in urinary symptoms in regular exercisers versus non-exercisers | x | | | |
| *Prospective cohort studies* | | | | | | | | | |
| de Azevedo Guimaraes et al. 2011 [45] | 120 Brazilian women aged 45–59 years old volunteered for the 12-week study (recruited through work or other institutions)<br><br>104 women completed the 12-week study | Habitual PA was assessed through the short form of the International PA Questionnaire (IPAQ); Participants were classified as: maintained <30 min/day, maintained or increased to 30-60 min/day, or maintained or increased to >60 min/day | Urinary complaints (exertion-induced urinary incontinence or difficult micturition) assessed using the Kupperman Menopausal Index | Sociodemographic factors, anthropometrics, menopausal status and symptoms, and QOL | Women classified in the highest active group (maintained or increased to 60 min per day) had reported significantly less instances of leaking urine | | x | | |
| *Non-randomized intervention studies* | | | | | | | | | |
| Karacan, 2010 [50][a] | 112 women aged 46–55. The analytic sample included 65 participants that regularly participated in the 3- and 6-month exercise program | The 6-month exercise program included aerobic activity (75–80 % heart rate capacity) with calisthenics for 3 days a week for 55 min each session | The menopause rating scale (MRS) was composed of 11 items assessing menopausal symptoms divided into three groups: psychological, somatic-vegetative and urogenital | Physical characteristics (height, weight, and age at menopause), resting heart rate and blood pressure, lower back flexibility, hand grip strength, and body composition (skin folds) | There was a significant reduction in urinary symptoms from baseline to 6-months | | x | | |

**Table 3** Selected studies of physical activity and urinary incontinence (Continued)

Randomized controlled studies

| | | | | |
|---|---|---|---|---|
| Moilanen et al. 2012 [53][a] | 176 Finnish white women were recruited for the study by newspaper advertisements. The analytic sample included 154 inactive participants were randomly assigned to the exercise (n = 74) or control group (n = 77) that completed the 6-month study protocol | Exercise Group: Unsupervised aerobic training intervention; 4 × per week at 64-80 % maximal heart rate for 50 min each time | The frequency of urinary symptoms were collected 2 × per day using a mobile phone-administered questionnaire | Socio-demographic factors, anthropometrics, and menopausal symptoms | There was no change in urinary symptoms as a result of the exercise intervention          × |

[a]Physical activity dose reflective of 2008 Physical Activity Guidelines for Americans [3]

**Table 4** Selected studies of physical activity and sleep quality and/or sleep disturbances

| Reference | Sample | Physical activity measure | Menopausal symptom measure | Other measures | Detailed findings | Summarized findings: observed association | | | |
|---|---|---|---|---|---|---|---|---|---|
| | | | | | | Null | Positive | Negative | Mixed |
| Cross-sectional studies | | | | | | | | | |
| Canário et al. 2012 [27] | Population-based sample of 370 women from Natal, Brazil aged 40–65 | International Physical Activity Questionnaire with three categories of classification: sedentary, moderately active and very active (vigorous) | Blatt-Kupperman Menopausal Index with three categories of classification: mild (≤19), moderate (20–35), or severe (>35) | Socio-demographic and behavioral characteristics | Bivariate analysis revealed a statistically significant inverse association between physical activity and insomnia | | | x (insomnia) | |
| Casas et al. 2012 [38][a] | 48 month follow-up data from the Women on the Move through Activity and Nutrition (WOMAN) Study. The analytic sample included 393 postmenopausal women, aged 62 ± 3 years | Modifiable Activity Questionnaire (past year version). Participants were also classified as high or low active based on sample-determined median (11.8 MET-hr-wk$^{-1}$) | Pittsburgh Sleep Quality Index (PSQI) | Socio-demographic factors, anthropometrics, hormone therapy status, cardiovascular risk factors | Bivariate analysis suggest that sleep quality and duration did not vary in participants classified as high vs. low active | x (sleep quality & duration) | | | |
| Lambiase et al. 2013 [39] | Sub-sample of 52 Study of Women's Health Across the Nation (SWAN) participants (Pittsburgh site only) attending the 10th annual visit (2008–09) | Kaiser Physical Activity Survey, including four indices of physical activity: (a) household/caregiving, (b) occupational, (c) active living, and (d) sport/exercise activity. Each index was calculated as the average score (ranged from 1 to 5) | Minimitter Actiwatch-64 (dominant wrist) and sleep diary. In the diary, participants reported times in and out of bed and number of awakenings. Participants were also asked to report their global sleep quality in the past month on a 4-point scale (very bad to very good) | Demographic factors, medical history, medication use, and health behaviors | Participants with higher physical activity levels reported better sleep quality and recorded fewer nighttime awakenings. Reported physical activity was not significantly associated with objectively-determined sleep estimates | | | | x |
| Kline et al. 2013 [40] | 339 participants from the Study of Women's Health Across the Nation (SWAN) Sleep Study, an ancillary study located at 4 of 7 SWAN clinical sites (Chicago, IL; Detroit Area, MI; Oakland, CA; Pittsburgh, PA). Data were collected from 2003–05 | Kaiser Physical Activity Survey, including four indices of physical activity: (a) household/caregiving, (b) occupational, (c) active living, and (d) sport/exercise activity. Each index was calculated as the average score (ranged | In-home polysomnography (PSG), daily sleep diaries, and the Pittsburgh Sleep Quality Index (PSQI) | Sociodemographic factors, medication use, menopausal status, vasomotor symptoms and other health behaviors | Higher sports/exercise index scores were significantly related with greater sleep quality and continuity (via diary) and greater sleep depth (PSG). Those with a higher sports/exercise index had a significantly lower odds of meeting diagnostic | | x (sleep quality) | | |

**Table 4** Selected studies of physical activity and sleep quality and/or sleep disturbances (Continued)

| Study | Sample | Physical activity measure / Intervention | Outcome measures | Covariates | Results | Sleep quality | Sleep disturbances |
|---|---|---|---|---|---|---|---|
| | | from 1 to 5). Recent (KPAS scores from preceding SWAN visit) and historical (2–4 KPAS assessments in the 5–6 years prior to the SWAN Sleep Study) physical activity estimates were created. Participants were further classified as, "consistently active", "inconsistent/ moderate" or "consistently inactive" based on the historical estimates | | | criteria for insomnia. The associations with the household or active living index were not statistically significant | | |
| Mansikkamäki et al. 2015 [30] | Random sample of 5000 women born in 1963 was obtained from the Finnish Population Register Centre. Analytic sample included 2606 women aged 49 years old that responded to a postal survey in 2012 | A single item pertaining to usual exercise (frequency and duration) per week during past 12-months. Women were classified as 'active' if they reported ≥ 150 min per week of moderate intensity or ≥75 min of vigorous intensity, with strength training and balance training | Women's Health Questionnaire addressing nine domains of physical and emotional experiences, including sleep problems | Socio-demographic factors, anthropometrics, self-rated health | There was no difference in reported sleep problems in active vs. inactive | x (sleep problems) | |
| **Non-randomized intervention studies** | | | | | | | |
| Karacan, 2010 [50][a] | 112 women aged 46–55. The analytic sample included 65 participants that regularly participated in the 3- and 6-month exercise program | The 6-month exercise program included aerobic activity (75–80 % heart rate capacity) with calisthenics for 3 days a week for 55 min each session | The menopause rating scale (MRS) was composed of 11 items assessing menopausal symptoms divided into three groups: psychological, somatic-vegetative and urogenital | Physical characteristics (height, weight, and age at menopause), resting heart rate and blood pressure, lower back flexibility, hand grip strength, and body composition (skin folds) | There was a significant decrease in reported sleeping problems from baseline to 3- and 6-months | x (sleep problems) | |
| **Randomized controlled studies** | | | | | | | |
| Kline et al. 2012 [58][a] | 437 sedentary, overweight/obese participants from the | Exercise Training Groups: The supervised exercise | Medical Outcomes Study (MOS) Sleep Scale was used to | Socio-demographic factors, anthropometric | After adjustment: (1) a significant effect of the intervention was | x (sleep quality) | x (sleep disturbances) |

**Table 4** Selected studies of physical activity and sleep quality and/or sleep disturbances (Continued)

| Study | Sample and intervention | Sleep assessment | Other measures | Results | Sleep quality | Insomnia symptoms |
|---|---|---|---|---|---|---|
| | Dose-response to Exercise in postmenopausal Women (DREW) Study, randomized to no exercise (n = 102), 50 % (n = 155), 100 % (n = 104), or 150 % (n = 103) of the NIH Consensus Panel physical activity recommendations program (3–4 times per week) included aerobic activity at varying doses (i.e., 4-, 8-, or 12- kcal per kilogram of body weight per week (KKW). For the 1st week all exercise training groups expended 4 KKW. Then, the 8- and 12- KKW groups increased energy expenditure by 1 KKW until they reached the appointed dose | assess sleep quality during the previous 4-weeks. A modified Sleep Problems Index (SPI) was also used to assess overall sleep quality. SPI scores >25 were used to indicate significant sleep disturbance | measures, medication use, health behaviors, diet, cardiorespiratory fitness, heart rate variability | found with reported sleep quality, (2) a linear dose-response effect was found with reported sleep quality across treatment groups, (3) compared to the control group, the exercise groups all had a lower odds of having significant sleep disturbance, and (4) the odds of having significant sleep disturbance decreased across increasing exercise doses | | |
| Mansikkamäki et al. 2012 [59][a] | 176 inactive women, aged 40–63 years with no current or recent (<3 months) hormone therapy use, and 6 to 36 months since last menstruation Exercise Program: aerobic training, 4 times per week for 50 min each time for 6-months. Participants were asked to include at least 2 sessions of walking or Nordic walking per week | Reported sleep was obtained via 1-item included on a mobile phone administered questionnaire. Participants responded to the question, "how well did you sleep last night" via 5 response options ranging from poor to good | Socio-demographic factors, health behaviors, anthropometrics | Sleep quality improved significantly more in the exercise vs. control group. The odds for sleep improvement were 2 % in the exercise group compared to −0.5 % in the control group. Women randomized to the intervention also reported significantly fewer hot flushes disturbing their sleep than the control group | x (sleep quality) | |
| Sternfeld et al. 2014 [56][a] | Women aged 40-62 recruited from 3 sites in US (IN, CA, WA) and randomly assigned to a 12-week yoga (n = 107), exercise (n = 106), or usual activity (n = 142) group. Participants were also randomly assigned to the omega-3 (n = 177) or placebo (n = 178) group. Participants were followed for 12-weeks Exercise Group: Supervised: 3 × per week, 50-60 % HRR during month 1, 60-70 % HRR during months 2 & 3. Possible modes included; treadmill, elliptical trainer, or stationary bicycle. Trained staff recorded heart rate, workload, and perceived exertion every 5–10 min | Sleep quality and sleep disturbances were ascertained via the Pittsburgh Sleep Quality Index (PSQI) and insomnia symptoms were collected using the Insomnia Severity Index (ISI) | Socio-demographics, anthropometrics, daily diaries assessing vasomotor symptoms, health history, and anxiety | After 12-weeks, compared to the usual activity group, exercise group participants reported greater improvement in sleep quality and insomnia symptoms | x (sleep quality) | x (insomnia symptoms) |

[a]Physical activity dose reflective of 2008 Physical Activity Guidelines for Americans [3]

**Table 5** Selected studies of physical activity and psychological symptoms

| Reference | Sample | Physical activity measure | Menopausal symptom measure | Other measures | Detailed findings | Summarized findings: observed association | | | |
|---|---|---|---|---|---|---|---|---|---|
| | | | | | | Null | Positive | Negative | Mixed |
| Cross-sectional studies | | | | | | | | | |
| Canário et al. 2012 [27] | Population-based sample of 370 women from Natal, Brazil aged 40-65 | International Physical Activity Questionnaire with three categories of classification: sedentary, moderately active and very active (vigorous) | Blatt–Kupperman Menopausal Index with three categories of classification: mild (≤19), moderate (20–35), or severe (>35) | Socio-demographic and behavioral characteristics | Bivariate analysis revealed a statistically significant inverse association between physical activity and depression | | | x (depression) | |
| Mansikkamäki et al. 2015 [30] | Random sample of 5000 women born in 1963 was obtained from the Finnish Population Register Centre, 2606 women aged 49 years old responded that responded to a postal survey in 2012 | A single item pertaining to usual exercise (frequency and duration) per week during past 12-months. Women were classified as 'active' if they reported ≥ 150 min per week of moderate intensity or ≥75 min of vigorous intensity, with strength training and balance training | Women's Health Questionnaire addressing nine domains of physical and emotional experiences, including anxiety/depressed mood | Sociodemographic factors, anthropometrics, self-rated health | In the unadjusted and adjusted models, inactive women had a statistically significant increased probability of anxiety/ depression [Unadjusted POR: 1.44 (95 % CI: 1.26, 1.65); Adjusted POR: 1.31 (95 % CI: 1.14, 1.51)] | | | x (anxiety, depression) | |
| Moilanen et al. 2010 [31] | Participants drawn from Finnish Health 2000 Study (n = 7,977), data collection included a home interview, 3 self-administered questionnaires, and a clinical exam. Analytic sample included 1427 women, ages 45–64; known menopausal status) who completed the home interview, first questionnaire | Physical activity was assessed via a single item on the questionnaire, "How much do you exercise or strain yourself physically in your leisure time" with four response options ranging from 'sedentary' (reading, watching television) to 'competitive sports'. Participants were classified based on low, moderate, and high physical activity | Severity of general symptoms, including psychological symptoms (e.g., depression), were assessed via two items on the questionnaire | Socio-demographics, health behaviors, anthropometrics, menopausal status and hormone therapy use | Compared to the high active group, low active women were significantly more likely to report psychological symptoms | | | x (psychological symptoms) | |
| Timur et al. 2010 [35] | Community-based randomly selected sample of 685 Turkish (Malatya) women aged 45–59 years. Data were collected from February to May, 2008 | A single item to assess regular exercise, operationalized as:≥3 times per week or not (yes or no) | The Beck Depression Inventory, a 21 question survey that uses a Likert scale from 0 to 3 to assess severity of depressive symptoms | Socio-demographics, anthropometrics, health behaviors, parity, menopausal status and hormone therapy use | No significant difference in depression by regular exercise status | x | | | |

**Table 5** Selected studies of physical activity and psychological symptoms (*Continued*)

| Study | Sample | Physical activity measure | Psychological symptom measure | Covariates | Findings | | |
|---|---|---|---|---|---|---|---|
| Vallance et al. 2010 [36]a | 297 post-menopausal women from the Palliser Region of Alberta, Canada | Godin Leisure-Time Exercise Questionnaire which assesses the frequency and duration of mild-, moderate-, and strenuous- leisure-time physical activity. Participants also wore a pedometer (DigiWalker SC-01) for 3 days, average steps per day were computed. Estimates reflecting meeting physical activity recommendations were also computed for both reported and pedometer-based (>7500 steps per day) estimates. | Depression was assess via the 20-item Center for Epidemiologic Studies-Depression scale. For each item, responses ranged from 0 '<1 day in the past week' to 3 '5–7 days in the past week'. Anxiety was assessed via the 10-item Spielberger's state Anxiety Inventory (SAI). For each item, responses ranged from 1 'not all' to 4 'very much so' | Socio-demographic factors, anthropometrics, health history, menopausal symptoms | Unadjusted and adjusted analyses found that participants meeting physical activity recommendations reported significantly fewer depression symptoms than those who did not | x (depression symptoms) | |
| Chang et al. 2013 [37] | Secondary data analysis of 481 multi-racial/ethnic women who completed questions on menopausal symptoms that were part of a larger Internet survey study | Kaiser Physical Activity Survey, including four indices of physical activity: (a) household/ caregiving, (b) occupational, (c) active living, and (d) sport/exercise activity. Each index was calculated as the average score (ranged from 1 to 5) | Midlife women's Symptoms Index, which measured psychological symptoms based on their prevalence 'yes' or 'no' and severity '1 = not at all and 5 = extremely' | Sociodemographic factors, self-rated health, menopausal status, hormone therapy use | After adjustment, there was a statistically significant association between the household/ caregiving index and psychological symptoms in Non-Hispanic Asians and Blacks, only. Associations were not statistically significant for any other race/ethnic group or indices of physical activity | | x |
| *Prospective cohort studies* | | | | | | | |
| Dugan et al. 2015 [46] | Included 2891 participants from the Study of Women's Health Across the Nation. Women were recruited in 1995–97. Included data from follow-up, 3, 6 & 9 | Kaiser Physical Activity Survey, including four indices of physical activity: (a) household/ caregiving, (b) occupational, (c) active living, and (d) sport/exercise activity. | Depression was assess via the 20-item Center for Epidemiologic Studies-Depression scale. For each item, responses ranged from 0 '<1 day in the past week' to 3 '5–7 days in the | Socio-demographic factors, health behaviors, anthropometrics, menopausal status, hormone therapy use, antidepressant medication use | After adjustment for covariates, participants classified as 'meeting physical activity guidelines' or 'below guidelines' had a significantly lower odds for depressive symptoms than those | x (depressive symptoms) | |

**Table 5** Selected studies of physical activity and psychological symptoms (Continued)

| Reference | Sample | PA / intervention | Psychological symptom measure | Other measures / covariates | Results | Association |
|---|---|---|---|---|---|---|
| | | Each index was calculated as the average score (ranged from 1 to 5). Participants were then classified as: meeting physical activity guidelines, below physical activity guidelines or Inactive | past week. High depressive symptoms were classified as ≥16 | | classified as inactive. This association persisted over 10 years of observation | |
| de Azevedo Guimaraes et al. 2011 [45] | 120 Brazilian women aged 45–59 years old volunteered for the 12-week study (recruited through work or other institutions) 104 women completed the 12-week study | Habitual PA was assessed through the short form of the International PA Questionnaire (IPAQ); Participants were classified as: maintained <30 min/day, maintained or increased to 30–60 min/day, or maintained or increased to >60 min/day | Psychological symptoms were assessed using the World Health Organization Quality of Life Brief Version Questionnaire; higher scores reflect less severe psychological symptoms | Socio-demographic factors, anthropometrics, menopausal status and symptoms, and QOL | Women classified in the highest active group (maintained or increased to 60 min per day) had increased psychological domain QOL scores after 12-weeks than the other two active groups after adjustment for baseline values | x (better psycho-social symptoms) |
| Non-randomized Intervention Studies | | | | | | |
| Karacan, 2010 [50][a] | 112 women aged 46–55. The analytic sample included 65 participants that regularly participated in the 3- and 6-month exercise program | The 6-month exercise program included aerobic activity (75–80 % heart rate capacity) with calisthenics for 3 days a week for 55 min each session | The menopause rating scale (MRS) was composed of 11 items assessing menopausal symptoms divided into three groups: psychological, somatic-vegetative and urogenital | Physical characteristics (height, weight, and age at menopause), resting heart rate and blood pressure, lower back flexibility, hand grip strength, and body composition (skin folds) | There was a significant reduction in psychological symptoms, including depressive mood, irritability, and anxiety after 3- and 6-months of the exercise program. Reported exhaustion also significantly decreased from baseline to 3- and baseline to 6- months | x (psychosocial symptoms) |
| Randomized Controlled Studies | | | | | | |
| Agil et al. 2010 [51] | 42 Turkish, postmenopausal women aged 45–60 years old, presented to the Department of Obstetrics and Gynecology of Bayindir Hospital | Participants were randomly assigned to either an aerobic (n = 18) or resistance (n = 18) physical activity intervention. Both groups were | Menopause Rating Scale (MRS) assessed psychological symptoms, the Beck Depressive Inventory (BDI) was used to assess depressive symptoms | Socio-demographic factors, health behaviors | Psychological symptoms decreased significantly in both groups post exercise programs according to the MRS subscale. The BDI showed a decrease in | x (psychosocial symptoms) |

**Table 5** Selected studies of physical activity and psychological symptoms (*Continued*)

| Study | Sample | Intervention | Measures | Psychological assessment | Results | Symptoms |
|---|---|---|---|---|---|---|
| | between March and December 2009 and volunteered to participate in an 8-week physical activity intervention. The analytic sample included 36 participants; intent to treat analysis was not done | supervised, 3 days per week. No other details were provided | | | depressive symptoms for both groups, but was higher in the resistance exercise group than the aerobic exercise group | x |
| Moilanen et al. 2012 [53][a] | 176 Finnish white women were recruited for the study by newspaper advertisements. The analytic sample included 154 inactive participants were randomly assigned to the exercise (n = 74) or control group (n = 77) that completed the 6-month study protocol | Exercise Group: Unsupervised aerobic training intervention; 4 × per week at 64–80 % maximal heart rate for 50 min each time | Socio-demographic factors, anthropometrics, and menopausal symptoms | The frequency of psychological symptoms (i.e., mood swings, depressive moods, irritability) were collected 2 × per day using a mobile phone- administered questionnaire | The prevalence of mood-swings decreased pre- to post- intervention. No other reductions were noted | |
| Sternfeld et al. 2014 [56][a] | 248 women aged 40–62 recruited from 3 sites in US (IN, CA, WA) and randomly assigned to a 12-week yoga (n = 107), exercise (n = 106), or usual activity (n = 142) group. Participants were and also randomly assigned to the omega-3 (n = 177) or placebo (n = 178) group. Participants were followed for 12-weeks | Exercise Group: Supervised: 3 × per week, 50–60 % HRR during month 1, 60–70 % HRR during months 2 & 3. Possible modes included, treadmill, elliptical trainer, or stationary bicycle. Trained staff recorded heart rate, workload, and perceived exertion every 5–10 min | Socio-demographics, anthropometrics, daily diaries assessing vasomotor symptoms, sleep quality, and health history | Depressive symptoms were assessed using the Patient Health Questionnaire-8 (PHQ-8) and anxiety symptoms using the Generalized Anxiety Disorder-7 (GAD-7) | Compared to the usual activity group, the exercise group had a greater decrease in depressive symptoms (p = 0.028), but did not meet the set alpha level of p < 0.0125 for multiple comparisons. Change in anxiety symptoms did not differ between the exercise and usual activity groups | x |
| Villaverde Gutiérrez et al. 2012 [57][a] | 330 postmenopausal women, aged 60–70, were recruited from a healthcare clinic in Granada, Spain. Of those, 60 (19.1 %) meet eligibility criteria | Exercise group: During the first 8 weeks of the supervised program, 2 × per week, 50 min each time, 50–70 % | Anthropometrics | Depressive symptoms were assessed via the 30-item Geriatric Depression Scale (GDS). Participants were classified as: moderate depression | Unadjusted results suggest that among the exercise group, women initially classified with moderate or severe depression had | x (severe depression, depressive symptoms & anxiety) |

**Table 5** Selected studies of physical activity and psychological symptoms *(Continued)*

| | | |
|---|---|---|
| and were willing to participate. Women were randomly selected to the exercise (n = 30) or control (n = 30) group and followed for 6-months. Three women from the exercise group were excluded for not completing at least 80 % of the exercise intervention | heart rate reserve. During weeks 8–12, 3 × per week, 60 min each time, 50–70 % heart rate reserve and muscle training exercises were added. Weeks 12–24, intensity was increased to 60–85 % heart rate reserve; all other components were similar to weeks 8–12<br><br>Control group: Received no exercise treatment | (11–14) or severe depression (15–30). Anxiety was assessed via the 14-itemHamilton Anxiety Scale (HRSA). Responses ranged from 0 'absence of symptoms' to 4 'total incapacitated'. Participants were classified as: minor anxiety (6–15) or major anxiety (>15) | significantly reduced depressive symptoms after 6-months. Similarly, participants in the exercise group, classified with minor or major anxiety had significantly reduced anxiety symptoms after 6-months. In the Control group, women initially classified with moderate depression had a slight increase in depressive symptoms after 6 months. This slight increase was also shown in the control group among participants initially classified with minor anxiety |

aPhysical activity dose reflective of 2008 Physical Activity Guidelines for Americans [3]

**Table 6** Selected studies of physical activity and weight gain

| Reference | Sample | Physical activity measure | Menopausal symptom measure | Other measures | Detailed findings | Summarized findings: observed association | | | |
|---|---|---|---|---|---|---|---|---|---|
| | | | | | | Null | Positive | Negative | Mixed |
| Prospective cohort studies | | | | | | | | | |
| Choi et al. 2012 [47] | 346 women, aged 40–50 years with regular menstrual cycles were enrolled in the Biobehavioral Health in Diverse Midlife Women Study in 1996–1997. The analytic sample included 232 pre (n = 175) and peri (n = 57) menopausal women that completed physical activity data at baseline and after 2 years | Paffenbarger Physical Activity Questionnaire was assessed every 6-months for 2 years. Leisure time physical activity estimates are MET · hr · wk$^{-1}$ and are computed as the product of the duration and frequency, weighted by the corresponding MET value for each reported activity. After 2-years, change physical activity status was classified as: increase (≥300 MET · hr · wk$^{-1}$), maintain (−300 to 300 MET · hr · wk$^{-1}$), or decrease (<300 MET · hr · wk$^{-1}$) | Trained study staff measured body weight (via electronic scale) and waist circumference (specialized tape to the nearest 0.1 cm), every 6 months | Sociodemographic factors and Menopausal status (via urinary levels of FSH) | Unadjusted results suggest that after 2-years, participants who maintained their physical activity had an average weight gain of 3.3 ± 12.2 lbs. Participants who decreased physical activity gained the most weight over time 5.3 ± 8.9 lbs. Participants who increased physical activity gained the least amount of weight 0.8 ± 12.2 lbs. Similar group differences were also shown for waist circumference. Compared to those who decreased physical activity over time, those that increased physical activity had statistically significant less weight gain ($p < 0.05$) and waist circumference increase ($p < 0.01$), after adjustment for covariates | | | x | |
| Lusk et al. 2010 [48] | 18,414 Nurses' Health Study (NHS) II participants, recruited in 1989. Follow-up through 2005 and completed the 1989 and 2005 questionnaires | The NHS II Physical Activity Questionnaire includes reported frequency and duration (10 response options from 'zero' to ≥11 h per week' of 9 specific activity types over the past year. Usual walking pace was also reported (responses range from 'unable to walk' to 'very brisk (≥4 miles per hour). Average number of flights of stairs climbed daily were also reported. Inactivity via reported sitting time was also assessed | Height and weight were participant reported On the baseline and follow-up questionnaires. BMI was computed from these self-reported values | Socio-demographic factors, dietary patterns (i.e, sugar-sweetened beverages, trans-fats, and dietary fiber), health behaviors, parity, oral contraceptive use, antidepressant use | A 30 min per day increase in overall physical activity levels between 1989 and 2005 was associated with less weight gain [−1.31 kg (95 % CI: −1.44, −1.18)]. A 30 min increase in brisk walking and bicycling, specifically, was associated with less weight gain [−1.81 kg (95 % CI: −2.05, −1.56) and −1.59 kg (95 % CI: −2.09, −1.08), respectively]. Further, women that reported no bicycling in 1989 and increased to ≥5 min per day in 2005, gained significantly less weight [−0.74 (95 % CI: −1.41, −0.07)] than those who reported no bicycling in 2005 | | | x | |

Recent evidence exploring the associations between physical activity and menopausal symptoms in midlife...

185

**Table 6** Selected studies of physical activity and weight gain (*Continued*)

| Study | Participants | Physical activity measure | Outcome measure | Covariates | Results | |
|---|---|---|---|---|---|---|
| Sims et al. 2012 [49] | Participants were drawn from the Women's Health Initiative (WHI) Study (40 clinical sites) and included 58,610 postmenopausal women aged 50–79 years old that took part in either the diet modification or hormone therapy arms. Participants enrolled in 1993–98 and were followed annually for 8 years | The WHI Physical Activity Questionnaire includes reported frequency and duration within moderate- and strenuous- physical activity categories. Walking was also assessed. Participants were further classified into four groups: sedentary (≤100 MET·hr·wk⁻¹), low activity (>100 to 500 MET·hr·wk⁻¹), moderate activity (>500 to 1200 MET·hr·wk⁻¹), and high activity (≥1200 MET·hr·wk⁻¹) | Trained clinical staff measured body weight and height with a calibrated balance beam or digital scale and a wall-mounted stadiometer. BMI was calculated from these measures. Waist (midpoint between last floating rib and upper part of the iliac crest at the end of expiration)-to-hip (maximum extension of the buttocks) ratio (WHR) was also measured using a conventional measuring tape | Sociodemographic factors, dietary intake, smoking, alcohol, hormone use, and sleep | In the fully adjusted models, in the 50–59 year age group, women in the moderate activity group experienced a significant weight loss [−0.30 (95 % CI: −0.53, −0.07) compared to the sedentary group. In women aged 70–79 years, higher physical activity was significantly associated with less weight loss [0.34 (95 % CI: 0.04, 0.63) | x |
| **Non-randomized intervention studies** | | | | | | |
| Karacan, 2010 [50][a] | 112 women aged 46–55. The analytic sample included 65 participants that regularly participated in the 3- and 6-month exercise program | The 6-month exercise program included aerobic activity (75–80 % heart rate capacity) with calisthenics for 3 days a week for 55 min each session | Height and weight were assessed with a metal meter and scale; BMI was also computed. Body fat percentage was also measured via skinfold calipers using the Sloan and Weir formula (triceps and suprailiac) | Menopausal symptoms, physical characteristics (age at menopause), resting heart rate and blood pressure, lower back flexibility, hand grip strength, and body composition (skin folds) | There was a significant decrease in body weight, BMI, and body fat percentage from baseline to 6-months | x |

[a]Physical activity dose reflective of 2008 Physical Activity Guidelines for Americans [3]

same-day and cross-lagged (previous day's physical activity compared to hot flashes the next day) associations were highly variable in both magnitude and direction. Three recent prospective cohort studies have also been conducted, including one showing a null association [43], another showing an increased risk of hot flashes among women classified as active [44], and the third reporting significantly fewer hot flashes in women classified in the highest active group (i.e., maintained or increased to >60 min per day over 12-weeks) [45]. A non-randomized intervention study also reported a significant decrease in reported hot flashes and night sweats following a 6-month aerobic program [50], and the same general finding was seen in a small randomized control trial of Turkish women ($n = 42$) [51].

In contrast, the evidence from the majority of randomized controlled trials, including results from the 2 × 3 Factorial Menopause Strategies: Finding Lasting Answers for Symptoms & Health (MsFLASH) Study, shows no association between physical activity and vasomotor symptoms [54, 56]. For MsFLASH, women were recruited from three sites: Indianapolis, IN, Oakland, CA, and Seattle, WA and were randomized (3:3:4) to 12 weeks of exercise, yoga, or usual activity and further randomized to (1:1) to omega-3 fish oil or a placebo. Women in the yoga group performed one, 90 min session of supervised yoga per week and 20 min of unsupervised yoga on all other days. The exercise group participated in an individualized, supervised aerobic program (3 times per week, 40–60 min per session) with a progressively increasing energy expenditure goal. During month 1, the prescribed workload was 50–60 % of heart rate reserve. In months 2 and 3, heart rate reserve was increased to 60–70 % heart rate reserve [55]. Activity modes included: treadmill, elliptical trainer, or stationary bike. Heart rate and perceived exertion was recorded every 5–10 min by trained supervisors [56]. The usual activity group were instructed to follow their usual activity patterns and were asked to not begin a yoga or new exercise program [55, 56]. Reed et al. [55] reported that after the 12-week program, the yoga group had significant improvements in reported vasomotor symptoms, obtained via the 29-item Menopausal Quality of Life Questionnaire (MENQOL), when compared to the usual activity group. However, when the frequency and intensity of vasomotor systems were obtained using more sophisticated daily diaries, yoga had no effect on the vasomotor symptoms when compared to the usual activity group [54]. This null association was also found when comparing the reported frequency and burden of vasomotor symptoms via daily diaries between the exercise and usual activity groups [56]. This evidence from the more rigorous RCT studies largely supports the 2014 Cochrane Report by Daley et al. [67], which concluded

there was insufficient evidence to demonstrate that physical activity is an effective treatment for management of vasomotor symptoms.

**Physical activity and vaginal dryness**
As shown in Table 2, the recent evidence from cross-sectional studies examining the association between physical activity and vaginal dryness is mixed [33, 34], while a prospective cohort study [45] of Brazilian women by de Azevedo Guimaraes and colleagues found no association between habitual physical activity and vaginal dryness. Similarly, a non-randomized intervention study found no pre- to post- exercise program difference in vaginal dryness after 6-months [50]. Yet, in a randomized controlled trial of Finnish women [53] the prevalence of vaginal dryness decreased pre- to post intervention following a 6-month, unsupervised aerobic training program (4 times per week, 50 min per session at 64–80 % of maximal heart rate) in the treatment group versus control.

**Urinary incontinence**
Table 3 presents the evidence regarding the association between physical activity and urinary symptoms, including incontinence. In the prospective cohort study of Brazilian women by de Azevedo Guimaraes et al., women classified in the highest active group (maintained or increased to >60 min per day), reported less instances of leaking urine than those classified as low or moderately active at the 12-week follow-up [45], and in the non-randomized intervention study by Karacan [50], there was a reduction in urinary symptoms following a 6-month aerobic exercise program. However, in the Finnish randomized controlled study, there was no change in urinary symptoms as a result of a 6-month aerobic exercise program [53]. When interpreting these findings it is important to note that associations were not adjusted for change in body weight, which is unfortunate given the proposed underlying biological mechanism between physical activity and urinary incontinence.

**Sleep quality and disturbances**
Cross-sectional studies have generally shown better sleep quality and/or fewer sleep disturbances among physically active women (Table 4); this association was also shown in the non-randomized intervention study by Karacan [50] and has been largely confirmed in recent evidence from randomized controlled trials. Utilizing data from the Dose–response to Exercise in postmenopausal Women (DREW) Study [58], participants randomized to any of the three exercise groups reported improvements in sleep quality when compared to the control group. Further, a dose–response effect was shown with reported sleep quality across the exercise groups, with the magnitude of the effect increasing with each increase in

exercise dose. The exercise intervention arms were designed specifically to reflect 50 %, 100 % or 150 % of the National Institutes of Health (NIH) Consensus Panel physical activity recommendations [68]. Further, the odds of reporting a significant sleep disturbance were also lower with a dose response relation in all exercise groups compared to the controls. The beneficial effect of physical activity on sleep quality was also shown in two additional randomized control studies, including the Finnish study [59] and the MsFLASH trial [56]. The Advisory Committee for the development of the *2008 Physical Activity Guidelines for Americans* [2], concluded that the evidence supporting the benefit of physical activity for improved sleep quality was moderate. These findings will likely provide additional support for the next iteration of the *Guidelines*.

### Psychological distress: depression and anxiety

As shown in Table 5, the majority of the recent evidence in midlife women supports an inverse association between physical activity and depressive symptoms, including anxiety. Indeed of six recent cross-sectional studies [27, 30, 31, 35–37], only one study [35] found no difference in depressive symptoms by regular exercise status (≥3 times per week). In the prospective cohort study of Brazilian women, de Azevedo Guimaraes et al. [45], found improved psychological symptoms after 12-weeks in the high active group. This was also shown in an analysis of SWAN participants. Here, those classified as meeting physical activity guidelines had a lower odds of depression than inactive participants and this finding persisted over 10 years [46]. Karacan [50] also reported a reduction in psychological symptoms, including depressive mood, irritability, and anxiety after 3 and 6 months of participation in an aerobic exercise program. There was also a statistically significant reduction in exhaustion from baseline to 3 and 6 months. Of the four studies detailing findings from randomized controlled studies, all demonstrated a beneficial effect of physical activity for psychological symptoms including depressive symptoms [51, 56, 57], mood swings [53], and anxiety symptoms [57] when compared to a control [51, 53, 57] or usual activity group [56]. However, the impact of the physical activity intervention on depressive symptoms did not reach statistical significance in the MsFLASH Study [56] due to a more conservative alpha level to account for multiple comparisons ($\alpha = p < 0.028$). These findings generally support the conclusions of the *2008 Physical Activity Guidelines for Americans* [2] Advisory Committee that rated the evidence pertaining to the benefit of physical activity for reduced risk of depression as strong.

### Weight gain

Table 6 outlines the recent evidence including three prospective cohort studies [47–49] and one non-randomized intervention study [50], supporting an inverse association between physical activity and weight gain Cross-sectional studies were not included in this review because the outcome was weight change or weight loss over time,. In a study by Choi and colleagues [47], 346 participants from the Biobehavioral Health in Diverse Midlife Women Study, the 2-year change in physical activity was categorized as increase, decrease, or maintained. Participants who increased physical activity levels had significantly less weight gain and less of an increase in waist circumference when compared to those who decreased physical activity levels, after controlling for age, initial physical activity and relevant outcome value (both $p < 0.05$). Similarly, in an analysis of Nurses' Health Study II participants [48], a 30-min increase in leisure-time physical activity levels between 1989 and 2005 was significantly associated with less weight gain [−1.31 kg (95 % CI: −1.44, −1.18)], and these same findings were found for the associations with weight change and walking and bicycling, specifically [−1.81 kg (95 % CI: −2.05, −1.56) and −1.59 kg (95 % CI: −2.09, −1.08), respectively]. In an analysis of 58,610 Women's Health Initiative participants [49], the associations between physical activity groups (sedentary, low-, moderate-, and high- active) and weight change were examined by age group (50–59 years, 60–69 years, and 70–79 years). Interestingly, Sims et al., reported that among the youngest age group, women in the moderate activity group experienced a significant weight loss [−0.30 (95 % CI: −0.53, −0.07) compared to the sedentary group. Yet, in women aged 70–79 years, higher physical activity was associated with the attenuation of the expected age-related weight loss due to loss of lean mass observed in this age group [0.34 (95 % CI: 0.04, 0.63). Authors posit that this attenuation in weight loss was due to the retention of lean muscle mass rather than a loss in adipose tissue [49]. Finally, Karacan [50] reported a significant decrease in body weight, body mass index (BMI), and body fat percentage (via skinfolds) after a 6-month supervised, aerobic-based physical activity program. However, these associations were not adjusted for potential confounders or other covariates. These findings generally support the conclusions of the *2008 Physical Activity Guidelines for Americans* [2] Advisory Committee that rated the evidence supporting the benefit of physical activity for the prevention of weight gain and promotion of weight loss as strong, particularly when combined with reduced dietary intake. There is also currently moderate to strong evidence to support the inverse association between physical activity and abdominal adiposity.

## Conclusions

The recent evidence, accumulated over the past 5 years, regarding the association between physical activity and hormone-related (i.e., primary) menopausal symptoms in midlife women generally mirrors previous research in this area in that the evidence remains either null or inconclusive. However, with more general health outcomes that result from biological aging, including poor sleep quality, increased depressive symptoms, and weight gain, the evidence supporting the beneficial effect of physical activity is quite conclusive. For primary menopausal symptoms, the inconsistencies across studies may be due to differences in targeted study populations. (i.e., study eligibility based on general age range, reflecting midlife versus menopausal status) as well as measurement strategies used to assess physical activity and menopausal symptom outcomes. Further, many studies did not examine and/or report the observed physical activity-menopausal symptom associations by menopausal status. This is particularly important given that the prevalence and severity of reported symptomology varies by menopausal status, as reported by Woods et al. [17]. Finally, for studies including a physical activity intervention component, there have also been distinct differences in the specific targets in terms of prescribed activity mode (i.e., aerobic versus resistance), frequency, intensity, and duration.

While it is intuitive that physical activity measurement strategies may vary across studies due to differences in the target population (e.g., race and cultural differences, menopausal status), a preponderance of studies included in this review utilized physical activity questionnaires with unreported and/or unknown measurement properties. This is despite recently published evaluation studies demonstrating the test-retest reliability and validity of physical activity questionnaires designed specifically for midlife women [69]. It is well-established that physical activity behaviors in women are quite different than in men and can vary by activity domain and/or preferred activity type [70]. For example, midlife women may accumulate the majority of their daily physical activity in domestic pursuits (e.g., caretaking) and walking or yoga during leisure-time. Therefore, it is critically important that, whenever possible, physical activity questionnaires used in this population are structured to elicit the most accurate information (i.e., reliable and valid) on the types of physical activities that are most pertinent to midlife women. This practice was implemented in a few studies included in this review that utilized more established questionnaires including, the International Physical Activity Questionnaire (IPAQ), Kaiser Physical Activity Survey (KPAS), or Modifiable Activity Questionnaire (MAQ) was used. A few additional studies included in this review used accelerometers, with known measurement properties, to quantify the physical activity exposure [41, 42].

Another weakness is that several observational studies included in this review, classified participants into physical activity groups in analyses, and did not provide details on the threshold limits used to distinguish groups. While these categories, distinguishing non-exerciser from exerciser or low and moderate active from high active, may have acceptable internal study validity, the categorization is a substantial limitation to interpreting overall study findings within the context of the entire body of literature relevant to physical activity and menopausal symptoms during midlife. Further, the practice of utilizing cut-point thresholds that are not meaningful from a clinical or public health standpoint may increase the likelihood for potential misclassification bias of the physical activity exposure and also lead to spurious findings.

Since there is currently a lack of evidence regarding the specific dose of physical activity that confers menopausal symptom risk reduction, threshold values used for analysis should be based on meaningful categories that reflect current physical activity recommendations for general health benefit [3]. This same practice should also be applied when designing physical activity interventions. The specific physical activity targets or components of interventions should allow participants to accumulate at least 150 min of moderate intensity physical activity per week to reflect current physical activity guidelines [3]. However, it is important to note that midlife women may also have pre-existing disease or disability that may preclude their ability to fully meet recommended physical activity levels. For these women, even low to moderate increases in daily physical activity may be beneficial to health, which is also noted in the *2008 Physical Activity Guidelines for Americans* [3]. Further, the intervention should include activity modes or types that are common and acceptable among midlife women, including brisk walking or bicycling. These intervention specific details should be included in the methods section of all peer-reviewed publications to facilitate the interpretation of the study findings. The MsFLASH [54–56] and DREW studies [58] provide excellent examples of how best to implement these recommendations when designing and/or reporting findings from physical activity intervention studies.

In summary, the recent evidence has not provided much clarity regarding the role of physical activity with menopausal symptoms in mid-life women beyond what was already known [67]. Yet, the evidence supporting the beneficial role of physical activity for more general health outcomes, including sleep quality, psychological distress, and weight gain, is quite conclusive. Given the considerable prevalence of sleep disturbances [71], depressive symptoms [72, 73], and overweight/obesity [74] in midlife women, health care and physical fitness professionals should encourage their patients or clients to engage in regular physical activity levels to reduce risk of these important health outcomes. For some midlife women, this may be sufficient *"reward"* to overcome the *"risk"* of allocating sufficient time, in an already busy schedule, to be physically active. In addition, midlife is a particularly vulnerable period when individuals are at immediate risk for disability, and there is moderate to strong evidence to support the beneficial role of physical activity for optimizing functional health and reducing risk of falls among older adults [3]. However, midlife women initiating a new exercise program should strive to make small, incremental increases in physical activity levels over time to reduce risk of acute musculoskeletal injuries, including sprains and strains [3]. Finally, while the evidence is still accumulating regarding the role of physical activity for specific menopausal symptoms, health care professionals should periodically remind midlife women that they will experience a reduced lifetime risk of chronic disease and disability development if they remain physically active as they age.

### Competing interests
The authors declare that they have no competing interests.

### Authors' contributions
KPG and BS participated in the design of the literature review, KPG and JMM conducted the literature review and summarized the literature, KPG drafted the manuscript, and JMM and BS provided a critical review of the manuscript. All authors read and approved the final manuscript.

### Acknowledgments
This work was supported by the Michael & Susan Dell Foundation through resources provided at the Michael & Susan Dell Center for Healthy Living, part of The University of Texas School of Public Health Austin Regional Campus (KPG). The authors would also like to thank Ms. Eun Me Cha for computing the BRFSS and NHANES prevalence estimates presented in the introduction.

### Author details
[1]Division of Epidemiology, Human Genetics and Environmental Sciences, University of Texas Health Science Center at Houston: School of Public Health – Austin Regional Campus, Austin, TX, USA. [2]School of Public Health, Austin Regional Campus, 1616 Guadalupe Street, Suite 6.300, Austin, TX 78701, USA. [3]Michael & Susan Dell Center for Healthy Living; University of Texas Health Science Center in Houston, Houston, TX, USA. [4]Division of Research, Kaiser Permanente Northern California, Oakland, CA 94612, USA.

### References
1. Hogan H, Perez D, Bell WR. Who (Really) are the first baby boomers? In: Statistical meetings proceedings, social statistics section; Alexandria, VA. 2008.
2. U.S. Department of Health and Human Services. Physical activity guidelines advisory committee report. 2008. Available from: http://www.health.gov/paguidelines/report/pcf/CommitteeReport.pdf. Accessed: June 18, 2015.
3. U.S. Department of Health and Human Services. 2008 Physical activity guidelines for Americans. 2008. Available from: http://www.health.gov/paguidelines/pdf/paguide.pdf. Accessed: June 18, 2015.
4. U.S. Department of Health and Human Services. Behavioral Risk Factor Surveillance System [database on the Internet]. Centers for Disease Control and Prevention. 2013. Available from: http://www.cdc.gov/brfss/annual_data/annual_2013.html. Accessed: January 24, 2015.
5. U.S. Department of Health and Human Services. National Health and Nutrition Examination Survey, Accelerometer Data 2003–04 & 2005–06 [database on the Internet]. Available from: http://www.cdc.gov/nchs/nhanes/nhanes_questionnaires.htm. Accessed: January 25, 2015.
6. Freedson PS, Melanson E, Sirard J. Calibration of the Computer Science and Applications, Inc. accelerometer. Med Sci Sports Exerc. 1998;30(5):777–81.
7. Sowers M, Pope S, Welch G, Sternfeld B, Albrecht G. The association of menopause and physical functioning in women at midlife. J Am Geriatr Soc. 2001;49(11):1485–92.
8. Tseng LA, El Khoudary SR, Young EA, Farhat GN, Sowers M, Sutton-Tyrrell K, et al. The association of menopause status with physical function: the Study of Women's Health Across the Nation. Menopause. 2012;19(11):1186–92.
9. Wilcox S, Castro C, King AC, Housemann R, Brownson RC. Determinants of leisure time physical activity in rural compared with urban older and ethnically diverse women in the United States. J Epidemiol Community Health. 2000;54(9):667–72.
10. King AC, Castro C, Wilcox S, Eyler AA, Sallis JF, Brownson RC. Personal and environmental factors associated with physical inactivity among different racial-ethnic groups of U.S. middle-aged and older-aged women. Health Psychol. 2000;19(4):354–64.
11. Heesch KC, Masse LC. Lack of time for physical activity: perception or reality for African American and Hispanic women? Women Health. 2004;39(3):45–62.
12. Pierret CR. The 'sandwich generation': women caring for parents and children. Mon Labor Rev. 2006;129(9):3.
13. Leonard T, Shuval K, de Oliveira A, Skinner CS, Eckel C, Murdoch JC. Health behavior and behavioral economics: economic preferences and physical activity stages of change in a low-income African-American community. Am J Health Promot. 2013;27(4):211–21.
14. U.S. Department of Health and Human Services. Centers for Disease Control and Prevention: Leading Causes of Death in Females by Age Group. 2011. http://www.cdc.gov/women/lcod/. Accessed June 9 2015.
15. Mozaffarian D, Benjamin EJ, Go AS, Arnett DK, Blaha MJ, Cushman M, et al. Heart disease and stroke statistics–2015 update: a report from the American Heart Association. Circulation. 2015;131(4):e29–322.
16. American Cancer Society. Cancer facts & figures 2015. 2015. http://www.cancer.org/acs/groups/content/@editorial/documents/document/acspc-044552.pdf. Accessed June 9 2015.
17. Woods NF, Mitchell ES. Symptoms during the perimenopause: prevalence, severity, trajectory, and significance in women's lives. Am J Med. 2005;118(Suppl 12B):14–24.
18. Sampselle CM, Harlow SD, Skurnick J, Brubaker L, Bondarenko I. Urinary incontinence predictors and life impact in ethnically diverse perimenopausal women. Obstet Gynecol. 2002;100(6):1230–8.
19. Sternfeld B, Wang H, Quesenberry Jr CP, Abrams B, Everson-Rose SA, Greendale GA, et al. Physical activity and changes in weight and waist circumference in midlife women: findings from the Study of Women's Health Across the Nation. Am J Epidemiol. 2004;160(9):912–22.
20. Sowers M, Zheng H, Tomey K, Karvonen-Gutierrez C, Jannausch M, Li X, et al. Changes in body composition in women over six years at midlife: ovarian and chronological aging. J Clin Endocrinol Metab. 2007;92(3):895–901.
21. Guthrie JR, Dennerstein L, Dudley EC. Weight gain and the menopause: a 5-year prospective study. Climacteric. 1999;2(3):205–11.
22. Lovejoy JC, Champagne CM, de Jonge L, Xie H, Smith SR. Increased visceral fat and decreased energy expenditure during the menopausal transition. Int J Obes (Lond). 2008;32(6):949–58.
23. Freeman EW, Sammel MD, Lin H, Gracia CR, Pien GW, Nelson DB, et al. Symptoms associated with menopausal transition and reproductive hormones in midlife women. Obstet Gynecol. 2007;110(2 Pt 1):230–40.
24. Dennerstein L, Dudley EC, Hopper JL, Guthrie JR, Burger HG. A prospective population-based study of menopausal symptoms. Obstet Gynecol. 2000;96(3):351–8.
25. Avis NE, Crawford SL, Greendale G, Bromberger JT, Everson-Rose SA, Gold EB, et al. Duration of menopausal vasomotor symptoms over the menopause transition. JAMA Intern Med. 2015;175(4):531–9.

26. Sowers M, Harlow S, Karvonen C, Bromberger J, Cauley JA, Gold EB et al. Menopause: Its Epidemiology. Women and Health. Academic Press; 2013.

27. Canario AC, Cabral PU, Spyrides MH, Giraldo PC, Eleuterio Jr J, Goncalves AK. The impact of physical activity on menopausal symptoms in middle-aged women. Int J Gynaecol Obstet. 2012;118(1):34–6.

28. Haimov-Kochman R, Constantini N, Brzezinski A, Hochner-Celnikier D. Regular exercise is the most significant lifestyle parameter associated with the severity of climacteric symptoms: a cross sectional study. Eur J Obstet Gynecol Reprod Biol. 2013;170(1):229–34.

29. Kandish J, Amend V. An exploratory study on perceived relationship of alcohol, caffeine, and physical activity on hot flashes in menopausal women. Health. 2010;2(9):989–96.

30. Mansikkamaki K, Raitanen J, Malila N, Sarkeala T, Mannisto S, Fredman J, et al. Physical activity and menopause-related quality of life - a population-based cross-sectional study. Maturitas. 2015;80(1):69–74.

31. Moilanen J, Aalto AM, Hemminki E, Aro AR, Raitanen J, Luoto R. Prevalence of menopause symptoms and their association with lifestyle among Finnish middle-aged women. Maturitas. 2010;67(4):368–74.

32. Pimenta F, Leal I, Maroco J, Ramos C. Perceived control, lifestyle, health, socio-demographic factors and menopause: impact on hot flashes and night sweats. Maturitas. 2011;69(4):338–42.

33. Tan MN, Kartal M, Guldal D. The effect of physical activity and body mass index on menopausal symptoms in Turkish women: a cross-sectional study in primary care. BMC Womens Health. 2014;14(1):38.

34. Aydin Y, Hassa H, Oge T, Yalcin OT, Mutlu FS. Frequency and determinants of urogenital symptoms in postmenopausal Islamic women. Menopause. 2014;21(2):182–7.

35. Timur S, Sahin NH. The prevalence of depression symptoms and influencing factors among perimenopausal and postmenopausal women. Menopause. 2010;17(3):545–51.

36. Vallance JK, Murray TC, Johnson ST, Elavsky S. Quality of life and psychosocial health in postmenopausal women achieving public health guidelines for physical activity. Menopause. 2010;17(1):64–71.

37. Chang SJ, Chee W, Im EO. Menopausal symptoms and physical activity in multiethnic groups of midlife women: a secondary analysis. J Adv Nurs. 2013;69(9):1953–65.

38. Casas RS, Pettee Gabriel KK, Kriska AM, Kuller LH, Conroy MB. Association of leisure physical activity and sleep with cardiovascular risk factors in postmenopausal women. Menopause. 2012;19(4):413–9.

39. Lambiase MJ, Thurston RC. Physical activity and sleep among midlife women with vasomotor symptoms. Menopause. 2013;20(9):946–52.

40. Kline CE, Irish LA, Krafty RT, Sternfeld B, Kravitz HM, Buysse DJ, et al. Consistently high sports/exercise activity is associated with better sleep quality, continuity and depth in midlife women: the SWAN sleep study. Sleep. 2013;36(9):1279–88.

41. Elavsky S, Gonzales JU, Proctor DN, Williams N, Henderson VW. Effects of physical activity on vasomotor symptoms: examination using objective and subjective measures. Menopause. 2012;19(10):1095–103.

42. Elavsky S, Molenaar PC, Gold CH, Williams NI, Aronson KR. Daily physical activity and menopausal hot flashes: applying a novel within-person approach to demonstrate individual differences. Maturitas. 2012;71(3):287–93.

43. Gibson C, Matthews K, Thurston R. Daily physical activity and hot flashes in the Study of Women's Health Across the Nation (SWAN) Flashes Study. Fertil Steril. 2014;101(4):1110–6.

44. Gjelsvik B, Rosvold EO, Straand J, Dalen I, Hunskaar S. Symptom prevalence during menopause and factors associated with symptoms and menopausal age. Results from the Norwegian Hordaland Women's Cohort study. Maturitas. 2011;70(4):383–90.

45. de Azevedo Guimaraes AC, Baptista F. Influence of habitual physical activity on the symptoms of climacterium/menopause and the quality of life of middle-aged women. Int J Womens Health. 2011;3:319–28.

46. Dugan SA, Bromberger JT, Segawa E, Avery E, Sternfeld B. Association between physical activity and depressive symptoms: midlife women in SWAN. Med Sci Sports Exerc. 2015;47(2):335–42.

47. Choi J, Guiterrez Y, Gilliss C, Lee KA. Physical activity, weight, and waist circumference in midlife women. Health Care Women Int. 2012;33(12):1086–95.

48. Lusk AC, Mekary RA, Feskanich D, Willett WC. Bicycle riding, walking, and weight gain in premenopausal women. Arch Intern Med. 2010;170(12):1050–6.

49. Sims ST, Larson JC, Lamonte MJ, Michael YL, Martin LW, Johnson KC, et al. Physical activity and body mass: changes in younger versus older postmenopausal women. Med Sci Sports Exerc. 2012;44(1):89–97.

50. Karacan S. Effects of a long-term aerobic exercise on physical fitness and postmenopausal symptoms with menopausal rating scale. Sci Sports. 2010;25(1):39–46.

51. Agil A, Abike F, Daskapan A, Alaca R, Tuzun H. Short-term exercise approaches on menopausal symptoms, psychological health, and quality of life in postmenopausal women. Obstet Gynecol Int. 2010;2010.

52. Luoto R, Moilanen J, Heinonen R, Mikkola T, Raitanen J, Tomas E, et al. Effect of aerobic training on hot flushes and quality of life–a randomized controlled trial. Ann Med. 2012;44(6):616–26.

53. Moilanen JM, Mikkola TS, Raitanen JA, Heinonen RH, Tomas EI, Nygard CH, et al. Effect of aerobic training on menopausal symptoms–a randomized controlled trial. Menopause. 2012;19(6):691–6.

54. Newton KM, Reed SD, Guthrie KA, Sherman KJ, Booth-LaForce C, Caan B, et al. Efficacy of yoga for vasomotor symptoms: a randomized controlled trial. Menopause. 2014;21(4):339–46.

55. Reed SD, Guthrie KA, Newton KM, Anderson GL, Booth-LaForce C, Caan B, et al. Menopausal quality of life: RCT of yoga, exercise, and omega-3 supplements. Am J Obstet Gynecol. 2014;210(3):244 e1-11.

56. Sternfeld B, Guthrie KA, Ensrud KE, LaCroix AZ, Larson JC, Dunn AL, et al. Efficacy of exercise for menopausal symptoms: a randomized controlled trial. Menopause. 2014;21(4):330–8.

57. Villaverde Gutierrez C, Torres Luque G, Abalos Medina GM, Argente del Castillo MJ, Guisado IM, Guisado Barrilao R, et al. Influence of exercise on mood in postmenopausal women. J Clin Nurs. 2012;21(7–8):923–8.

58. Kline CE, Sui X, Hall MH, Youngstedt SD, Blair SN, Earnest CP, et al. Dose–response effects of exercise training on the subjective sleep quality of postmenopausal women: exploratory analyses of a randomised controlled trial. BMJ Open. 2012;2(4):e001044.

59. Mansikkamaki K, Raitanen J, Nygard CH, Heinonen R, Mikkola T, Tomas E, et al. Sleep quality and aerobic training among menopausal women–a randomized controlled trial. Maturitas. 2012;72(4):339–45.

60. Sternfeld B, Dugan S. Physical activity and health during the menopausal transition. Obstet Gynecol Clin North Am. 2011;38(3):537–66.

61. Ivarsson T, Spetz AC, Hammar M. Physical exercise and vasomotor symptoms in postmenopausal women. Maturitas. 1998;29(2):139–46.

62. Portman DJ, Gass ML. Genitourinary syndrome of menopause: new terminology for vulvovaginal atrophy from the International Society for the Study of Women's Sexual Health and the North American Menopause Society. Maturitas. 2014;79(3):349–54.

63. Lorenz TA, Meston CM. Acute exercise improves physical sexual arousal in women taking antidepressants. Ann Behav Med. 2012;43(3):352–61.

64. Legendre G, Ringa V, Panjo H, Zins M, Fritel X. Incidence and remission of urinary incontinence at midlife, a cohort study. BJOG. 2015;122(6):816–24.

65. Youngstedt SD. Effects of exercise on sleep. Clin Sports Med. 2005;24(2):355–65. 2.

66. Ravussin E, Bogardus C. A brief overview of human energy metabolism and its relationship to essential obesity. Am J Clin Nutr. 1992;55(1 Suppl):242S–5.

67. Daley A, Stokes-Lampard H, Thomas A, MacArthur C. Exercise for vasomotor menopausal symptoms. Cochrane Database Syst Rev. 2014;11:CD006108.

68. Physical activity and cardiovascular health. NIH consensus development panel on physical activity and cardiovascular health. JAMA. 1996;276(3):241–6.

69. Pettee Gabriel K, McClain JJ, Lee CD, Swan PD, Alvar BA, Mitros MR, et al. Evaluation of physical activity measures used in middle-aged women. Med Sci Sports Exerc. 2009;41(7):1403–12.

70. Ainsworth BE. Issues in the assessment of physical activity in women. Res Q Exerc Sport. 2000;71(2 Suppl):S37–42.

71. National Institutes of Health State-of-the-Science Conference statement: management of menopause-related symptoms. Ann Intern Med. 2005;142(12 Pt 1):1003–13.

72. Bromberger JT, Harlow S, Avis N, Kravitz HM, Cordal A. Racial/ethnic differences in the prevalence of depressive symptoms among middle-aged women: The Study of Women's Health Across the Nation (SWAN). Am J Public Health. 2004;94(8):1378–85.

18

# Impact of urinary incontinence on female sexual health in women during midlife

Christine M. Chu[*], Lily A. Arya and Uduak U. Andy

## Abstract

Sexual health is important to the self worth, emotional well being, and overall quality of life of women in midlife. However, urinary incontinence, which is prevalent in this population, has a negative impact on sexual function. The purpose of this article is to review the impact of urinary incontinence on female sexual dysfunction and discuss the impact of urinary incontinence treatment on sexual function. We carried out a literature review on the effect of stress urinary incontinence and urgency urinary incontinence on sexual health and physiological response, including coital incontinence, satisfaction, desire, orgasm, frequency, and partner relationships. We examined the literature regarding changes in sexual function related to non-surgical and surgical interventions for incontinence. Overall, though studies are lacking and of poor quality, treatment of incontinence has been shown to improve sexual function. Both pelvic muscle training and midurethral slings have been shown to improve sexual function in those with stress urinary incontinence. In urgency urinary incontinence, evidence indicates improvement in sexual function after treatment with anti-muscarinic medications. Coital incontinence commonly improves with treatment of the underlying incontinence subtype. Although problems related to sexual health are complex and involve both psychological and physical factors, it is important to consider treatment of urinary incontinence as part of management of sexual dysfunction.

**Keywords:** Sexual function, Sexual dysfunction, Urinary incontinence, Urge urinary incontinence, Stress urinary incontinence, Coital incontinence, Treatment outcome, Middle aged

## Introduction

Urinary incontinence (UI) is a common condition, with reported prevalence ranging from 28 to 47 % in women during midlife [1, 2]. The risk of incontinence increases incrementally from the age of 40 to 60, with prevalence nearly doubled by age 55 [3]. Common types of incontinence include stress incontinence (urinary leakage with activity that increase intra-abdominal pressure), urgency urinary incontinence (leakage related to urgency and irritative bladder symptoms associated with overactive bladder), and mixed incontinence (a combination of stress and urgency urinary incontinence). Stress urinary incontinence is the most common type of urinary incontinence, accounting for 52 - 65 % of urinary incontinence in women aged 30 to 60 [4]. Treatment of stress UI is primarily surgical, while urgency urinary incontinence, a common problem that

may affect 20 % of middle-aged women [5], is mainly treated with non-surgical options. In those with mixed urinary incontinence, the most bothersome and dominant incontinence type is treated first. However, coital incontinence, the leakage of urine during sexual intercourse, may have the most impact on sexual health and commonly occurs in women with any type of incontinence, with an overall prevalence from 11 to 60 % in middle-aged women with UI [6].

UI, even when not directly associated with intercourse, plays an important role in altering behaviors of human sexual function. This is concerning, as sexual health is very important in the overall quality of life and is tied to a woman's self worth, emotional well-being, and even cognitive function [7]. In a recent report, 86 % of women with urinary incontinence reported that sexual health was an important issue; however, few women with UI will discuss problems with sexual health unless directly asked [8]. Our aim is to review the impact of urinary incontinence on female sexual dysfunction and discuss the

* Correspondence: christine.chu@uphs.upenn.edu
Division of Urogynecology, Department of Obstetrics and Gynecology, University of Pennsylvania School of Medicine, 3400 Spruce St., 1000 Courtyard Building, Philadelphia, PA 19104, USA

impact of urinary incontinence treatment on sexual health of women in midlife.

Given the rarity of major, high-level evidence with regards to UI, treatment, and its relationship to sexual health, we searched for any trials related to these topics, prioritizing randomized controlled trials and prospective studies. We conducted a wide and comprehensive literature search in Pubmed (up to December 2014) on any articles examining overall changes in sexual health (overall subject-described impact). Additionally, we looked for the impact of urinary incontinence and treatment on aspects of the sexual physiologic responses (frequency, libido, desire, arousal, lubrication, orgasm, satisfaction, pain). No date or language restriction was used. Questionnaires and questionnaire subdomains used by studies to evaluate changes in sexual health are briefly described in Table 1.

## Review
### Urinary incontinence and overall impact on sexual health
Because of the proximity of the bladder and urethra to the vagina and vulva, UI may have major effects on the sexual health of affected women. In clinic settings, incontinent middle-aged women commonly report disruption of sexual health with a median percentage of 28 % [9]. Complete abstinence from sex secondary to urinary incontinence can range from 5.9 to 38 %, a wide range owing to the diversity of the populations included in these studies [10–12]. Older women with urinary incontinence report decreased self-rated health and a greater incidence of depression [5], which may also affect sexual health. Women with UI show greater dysfunction on validated

sexual function questionnaires compared to those without incontinence [13], regardless of menopausal status [14].

When examining sexual health in women with stress UI, older age, postmenopausal state, greater prolapse, and greater parity have been associated with worse sexual function scores [15]. The severity and duration of stress UI may not be associated with the level of sexual function [16, 17]. In patients with urgency UI, twenty-five percent of women with urgency UI report negative impacts on their sex life [18, 19]. Urgency UI is also significantly associated with lower self-esteem [20], which significantly influences sexual dysfunction [21].

### Impact on the female sexual response
Severe UI has been found to be significantly associated with decreased libido and vaginal dryness [22], decreased interest, and decreased satisfaction with sexual intercourse, including orgasmic dysfunction [9].

In particular, women with stress UI have been noted to have problems with desire, arousal, and lubrication [23]. Decreased desire in these women may be related to unsatisfying partner relationship, worries about coital incontinence, and unsatisfying somatic health [21]. In spite of decreased sexual desire, a majority of women with stress UI (78 %) are able to achieve orgasm [16], and may not necessarily display decreased sexual activity [24]. Women with urgency UI similarly also report significant difficulty with hypoactive sexual desire, and arousal disorder; however, achieving orgasm is also difficult in this population [25–27]. In women with urgency UI, this results in decreased sexual activity [28] and decreased sexual satisfaction associated with urgency UI [2].

**Table 1** Sexual function questionnaires and subscale domains

| Questionnaire or Subscale Name | Items | Domains/Descriptions |
|---|---|---|
| Female Sexual Function Index (FSFI) | 19 | Desire, Arousal, Satisfaction, Lubrication, Orgasm, Pain |
| Bristol Female Lower Urinary Tract Symptoms (BFLUTS): Sex Life Items | 4 | Urinary related sex life problems (2), Pain, Coital Incontinence |
| King's Health Questionnaire (KHQ): Personal Relationship Domain | 3 | Relationship with partner, Effect on sex life, Effect of family life |
| Short form Personal Experiences Questionnaire (SPEQ): 3 Domains | 3 | Libido, Arousal, Dyspareunia |
| Pelvic Organ Prolapse-Urinary Incontinence Sexual Function Questionnaire (PISQ) | 31 Short form: 12 | 31: Behavioral/Emotive (15), Physical (10), Partner-related (6) Short form: Behavioral/Emotive (4), Physical (5), Partner-related (3) |
| Beck Depression Inventory II: Question 21 | 1 | Loss of interest in sex |
| Sexual Quality of Life-Female (SQOL-F) | 19 | Desire, Lubrication, Arousal, Pain, Orgasm, Satisfaction |
| Arizona Sexual Experience Scale | 5 | Desire, Arousal, Lubrication, Orgasm, Satisfaction |
| Nine questions regarding Sexual Functioning (NSF-9) | 9 | Libido, Frequency, Lubrication, Orgasm, Time to Orgasm, Pain, Satisfaction |
| Lemack | 8 | Presence of pre-operative sexual activity, Frequency, Satisfaction with intercourse, Satisfaction with surgery, Coital incontinence, Partner pain |
| Electronic Pelvic Floor Symptoms Assessment Questionnaire (ePAQ): Urinary domain | 4 | Impact of urinary symptoms on sex life, Anxiety, Avoidance of sex, Partner avoidance of sex |

Dyspareunia, pain with intercourse, often accompanies UI and varies in prevalence from 8 to 42 % amongst middle-aged women with UI [9]. Studies have reported significantly greater rates of dyspareunia in women with UI and other lower urinary tract symptoms compared to controls [22, 25]. Dyspareunia has been noted more frequently in women with stress UI compared to those with overactive bladder [15]. However, dyspareunia does commonly accompany urgency UI [28, 29].

### Impact on partners' sexual health

UI also affects the sexual function of partners. Male partners of women with any type of UI report decreased overall sexual function, satisfaction, frequency of intercourse, and increased rates of erectile dysfunction as compared with partners of women without UI [30]. In spite of these negative effects, 42 % were unaware of the presence of coital incontinence. Of those who were aware, the majority (65 %) did not consider the UI to be the main problem affecting sexual health [21]. Negative effects on marital relationships have been correlated specifically with the presence of urgency UI [31].

### Coital incontinence and impact on sexual health

Coital incontinence deserves particular focus as it is often directly associated with sexual dysfunction. Coital incontinence is prevalent in up to 56 % of middle-aged women with incontinence [9], and peaks around the age of 50, with subsequent decrease as women enter their sixth decade of life [32]. Risk factors for coital incontinence include severity of incontinence [33], obesity [34], parity [35], and anterior and posterior vaginal wall prolapse [35]. The severity of the coital incontinence may be associated with the degree of sexual dysfunction [35, 36].

The impact of coital incontinence on sexual function is multifold. Actual leakage during coitus can affect sexual satisfaction. However, worry about leakage also contributes, and is significantly associated with decreased sexual desire and sexual satisfaction [21]. Embarrassment, guilt and anxiety about sexual activities are highly prevalent in this population [37]. Arousal can be also compromised, as patients with coital incontinence have significantly greater issues with lubrication [37]. Dyspareunia may be increased in women with coital incontinence compared to those without urinary complaints [37]. Avoidance of intercourse specifically because of coital incontinence is common [37]. Among partners of women with coital incontinence, an association with increased ejaculation before reaching full erection was noted [37].

Coital incontinence may occur at any time during intercourse, but is most commonly noted during penetration and orgasm [21, 38], although it is also frequently reported during clitoral stimulation and arousal [21]. Coital incontinence during penetration is commonly associated with stress UI [35, 39–41], while detrusor spasms have been implicated in coital incontinence during orgasm [39, 42]. Coital incontinence resulting from stress UI during penetration may be due to the alteration of the urethrovesical angle and elevation of the bladder neck by the erect penis during moments of increased intra-abdominal pressure. The mechanism of urinary incontinence during orgasm is unclear. It is postulated that penile stimulation of the nerve rich area of the bladder base and trigone may trigger detrusor overactivity in those with severe overactive bladder [42]. Alternately, stimulation of the vanilloid receptors in this area, which are reportedly increased in density in patients with urgency, may trigger detrusor contractions [43]. However, other studies have found no relationship between timing of coital incontinence and stress UI, detrusor overactivity, or mixed urinary incontinence [38, 44]; and that regardless of timing of coital incontinence, stress UI was the most frequently diagnosed type of incontinence, while detrusor overactivity was uncommon [45].

### The impact of treatment of urinary incontinence on sexual health

Treatment of incontinence includes both non-surgical and surgical modalities. Non-surgical treatment for stress UI includes pelvic muscle training (strengthening the levator ani muscles, the main support for the bladder during increased intra-abdominal pressure) [46], anti-incontinence pessaries, and transvaginal electrical stimulation. However, the treatment of stress UI is primarily surgical, and includes midurethral mesh slings, Burch colposuspension, and periurethral bulking injection (injection of bulking agents into the urethral wall to improve continence) [47]. Urgency UI is typically treated by non-surgical methods, including pelvic muscle training and biofeedback, transvaginal electrical stimulation, medication, percutaneous tibial nerve stimulation (involving stimulation of sacral plexus via the tibial nerve). Surgical therapies for urgency UI include botulinum toxin injection of the detrusor muscle and sacral neuromodulation (implantation of a device that stimulates the sacral nerve). Treatment of coital incontinence, like treatment for mixed urinary incontinence, is generally based on the treatment of the dominant incontinence type.

In the discussion below, we will address the effect of treatments for stress UI and urge UI on sexual function, the physiological female sexual response, and coital incontinence.

### Non-surgical treatment of urinary incontinence

Table 2 summarizes the effect of non-surgical treatments for stress UI and urgency UI on sexual function.

In stress UI, several high level, large trials support the idea that pelvic floor muscle training can significantly decrease urinary-related sexual problems [48] as well as

**Table 2** Effect of non-surgical treatments for urinary incontinence on sexual function

| Study | Study Design | N | Treatment | Treatment Length | Instrument | Findings | |
|---|---|---|---|---|---|---|---|
| | | | | | | Sexual Function | Coital Incontinence |
| Pelvic Floor Muscle Training (SUI) | | | | | | | |
| Bo et al [48] | Randomized controlled trial | 1. PMFT: 25 2. Control: 30 | PMFT | 6 months | B-FLUTS | • Non-significant improvement in pain, urinary-related sexual problems | • Improved |
| Zahariou et al [49] | Prospective case series | Total: 58 | PFMT | 12 months | FSFI | • Improvement in FSFI and subscale scores ($p < 0.05$) | • Improved ($p < 0.005$) |
| Pelvic Floor Muscle Training (UUI) | | | | | | | |
| Wang et al [50] | RCT | 1. PFMT: 34 2. Biofeedback-assisted PFMT: 34 3. Transvaginal electrical stimulation: 35 | 1. PFMT 2. Biofeedback-assisted PFMT 3. Transvaginal electrical stimulation | 12 weeks | KHQ: Personal Relationship Domain | • Non-significant improvement in Personal Relationship Domain in biofeedback-assisted PFMT group | N/A |
| Anti-incontinence Pessary (SUI) | | | | | | | |
| Handa et al [52] | Randomized controlled trial | 1. Continence pessary: 149 2. Behavioral therapy: 146 3. Combo: 150 | 1. Continence pessary 2. PMFT 3. Combination | 12 months | SPEQ (3 domains), PISQ-12 | Responders (vs. non-responders): • PISQ improved ($p = 0.007$) • Restriction of sex due to UI improved ($p = 0.008$) • Dyspareunia improved ($p = 0.017$) | • Improved ($p = 0.0002$) • Greater improvement • with combo therapy ($p = 0.019$) and behavioral ($p = 0.02$) vs. pessary alone |
| Transvaginal electrical stimulation (SUI and UUI) | | | | | | | |
| Giuseppe et al [51] | Prospective case series | Total: 23 SUI: 8 UUI: 10 MUI: 5 | Transvaginal electrical stimulation | 3 months | FSFI | Significant improvement in FSFI and all subscale scores ($p \leq 0.01$) except arousal, orgasm | N/A |
| Anti-cholinergic medication (UUI) | | | | | | | |
| Sand et al [53] | RCT | Total: 2878 Female: 2508 | 1. Patient education & transdermal oxybutynin 2. Transdermal oxybutynin only | 12 weeks | KHQ: Personal Relationship Domain | Significant improvement in KHQ score, bladder pain, effect of OAB on sex life, interest in sex | Improved |
| Rogers et al [54] | RCT | 1. Placebo: 189 2. Tolterodine: 188 | 1. Placebo 2. Tolterodine 4 mg ER daily | 12 weeks | PISQ | Significant improvement of PISQ and domain scores after 12 weeks  Stable but no continued improvement if used 12 additional weeks except in Physical domain | N/A |
| Danilova et al [58] | Prospective case series | 57 | Trospium 15 mg three times daily | 16 weeks | Unknown | Sexual dysfunction decreased | N/A |
| Chapple et al [56] | RCT | 1. Placebo: 283 | 1. Placebo | 12 weeks | KHQ: Personal | Patients with OAB, total | N/A |

**Table 2** Effect of non-surgical treatments for urinary incontinence on sexual function *(Continued)*

| | | | | | | | | |
|---|---|---|---|---|---|---|---|---|
| | | 2. Fesoterodine 4/8 mg: 272 | 2. Fesoterodine 4 mg | | | Relationship Domain | Statistically significant improvement in fesoterodine 8 mg (vs. placebo) (mean score change of -11.9 v -6.2, $p < 0.05$) | |
| | | 3. Tolterodine ER 4 mg: 290 | 3. Fesoterodine 8 mg | | | | Patients with both UUI & OAB: | |
| | | | 4. Tolterodine ER 4 mg | | | | Statistically significant improvement in tolterodine (vs. placebo) (-12.7 v -6.8, p < 0.05) | |
| Percutaneous tibial nerve stimulation (UUI) | | | | | | | | |
| Eftekhar et al [59] | RCT | 1. Percutaneous tibial nerve stimulation and tolterodine 4 mg daily: 25 | 1. Percutaneous tibial nerve stimulation and tolterodine 4 mg daily | 12 weeks | FSFI | Within each arm: | | N/A |
| | | 2. Tolterodine 4 mg daily: 25 | 2. Tolterodine 4 mg daily | | | Significant improvement in FSFI and subscale scores after 12 weeks ($p < 0.001$) | | |
| | | | | | | Between arms: | | |
| | | | | | | No significant difference in FSFI, subscale scores | | |
| van Balken et al [60] | Prospective case series | Total: 121 | Percutaneous tibial nerve stimulation | 12 weeks | NSF-9 | Significant improvement in Satisfaction ($p < 0.005$), Frequency ($p < 0.005$), Orgasm ($p < 0.05$) | | N/A |
| | | Female: 76 | | | | No significant change in dyspareunia, lubrication | | |

*B-FLUTS* Bristol female lower urinary tract symptoms; *FSFI* Female sexual function index; *PISQ-12* Short form pelvic organ prolapse-urinary incontinence sexual function questionnaire; *PFMT* Pelvic floor muscle training; *RCT* Randomized controlled trial; *SA* Sexual activity; *SPEQ*: Short form personal experience questionnaire

improve sexual physiological response in the areas of desire, arousal, lubrication, orgasm, and satisfaction [49]. These improvements may be correlated to increased pelvic muscle strength [49]. Coital incontinence was found to be improved with muscle training [48, 49]. Pelvic muscle training, in combination with biofeedback and occasionally transvaginal electrical stimulation, is also used to treat urgency UI. The effect on sexual function in this population has not been extensively studied, and involves mostly small case series. A small randomized controlled trial comparing traditional pelvic exercises to biofeedback-assisted exercises and transvaginal electrical stimulation found that biofeedback-assisted pelvic floor muscle training resulted in greatest improvement in the King's Health Questionnaire Personal Relationship domain [50].

Transvaginal electrical stimulation can be used to treat stress and urgency UI through strengthening of the pelvic floor muscles. One case series that included 12 women with stress UI and sexual dysfunction prior to treatment reported statistically significant improvements in overall sexual health (as indicated by improvement in Female Sexual Function Index score) and most subscale domains related to physiological response after 3 months of transvaginal electrical stimulation therapy [51]. Likewise, this modality can be used to treat urgency UI. In the same case series, which included ten women with urgency UI, transvaginal electrical stimulation also led to improved scores in the subjects with urgency UI [51]. A small randomized controlled trial found that transvaginal electrical stimulation resulted to less improvement in the King's Health Questionnaire Personal Relationship domain than pelvic muscle training [50].

Anti-incontinence pessaries are commonly used for stress UI. One randomized controlled trial comparing anti-incontinence pessaries, pelvic floor muscle training/ continence strategies, or both found no difference in the rates of incontinence, overall sexual function improvement, or sexual response achieved by pessaries compared to pelvic muscle training. Pessary users who had improvement in urinary symptoms (58.8 %) had greater improvement in overall sexual health (as indicated by higher Pelvic Organ Prolapse/Incontinence Sexual Questionnaire scores) than those who did not (2.26 ± 3.24 versus 0.48 ± 3.76, $p = 0.0007$) [50]. However, pelvic muscle training may be potentially more effective alone or in combination with anti-incontinence pessaries than with pessaries alone [50].

Anticholinergic medications are one of the first-line treatments for urgency UI. Though these medications are well studied, many large trials do not include specific assessment of changes in sexual function. Oxybutynin and tolterodine are two anti-cholinergic medications with high-quality evidence supporting improvement in sexual function with use. In the Multicentre Assessment of Transdermal Therapy in Overactive Bladder with Oxybutynin (MATRIX), which included 2878 subjects, 19.1 % of women reported improvement in sex life while 11.2 % reported worsening following 6 months of treatment with oxybutnin [52]. Similar proportions of women reported improvement in partner relationships and sexual desire [52]. Treatment with tolterodine was found to improve overall sexual health (higher sexual function questionnaire scores) compared with baseline in two studies, with particular improvement in desire, arousal, orgasm, lubrication, and satisfaction subscales [53, 54]. Fesoterodine likewise was found to improve subjects' Personal Relationship scores as compared to controls [55]. Other smaller prospective studies have reported some improvement in sexual health following treatment with solifenacin [56] and trospium [57]. Certain trials also found that antimuscarinic medication may improve coital incontinence. In the MATRIX study, oxybutynin was found to decrease the incidence of coital incontinence from 22.8 to 19.3 %, a statistically significant change [52]. In a study with tolterodine, 59 % of patients with incontinence at orgasm had improvement in response to tolterodine, though they were less likely to respond to treatment compared to those without coital incontinence (41.2 % v 17 %, $p = 0.023$) [39].

There are currently no studies evaluating the effect of a newer class of medication, beta-3 agonists, on sexual health.

Two small, poor quality trials on percutaneous tibial nerve stimulation found mixed sexual health outcomes. In two studies that included middle-aged women, one found no improvement in Female Sexual Function Index scores [58], while the other noted improvement in the Nine Questions Regarding Sexual Functioning scores, particularly in satisfaction, frequency, and orgasm [59].

Overall, there is strong evidence that pelvic muscle training can significantly improve sexual health in women with stress and urgency UI respectively. Transvaginal electrical stimulation (for both stress and urgency UI), pelvic

muscle training (urgency UI), and anti-cholinergic medication (urgency UI) may improve sexual health, but data is limited by quantity and quality. Literature on anti-incontinence pessaries (stress UI) and percutaneous tibial nerve stimulation (urgency UI) show mixed improvement in sexual health; more trials are needed.

**Surgical treatment of urinary incontinence**
Surgical treatment of stress and urgency UI differ, but both seem to result in overall improvement in sexual health. Table 3 summarizes the effect of surgical treatments of stress UI on sexual function as reported in prospective studies. Midurethral slings are the gold standard for treatment of stress UI in middle-aged women, making up the majority of incontinence procedures performed on women aged 18 to 64 [47]. The effect of midurethral slings on sexual health is supported by several large prospective trials and randomized controlled trials.

There is a trend towards improvement in sexual health after correction with a midurethral sling. A meta-analysis of 21 studies noted that the pooled chance of improvement of sexual health following sling placement was 33.9 %, with improvement ranging from 1.8 to 94 % (0.95, 95 % CI 0.34, 1.56) [44]. One study that included 133 middle-aged women reported that 40 % of non-sexually active women reestablished intercourse after surgery [60].

Several studies reported improvement in aspects of female sexual response. There was an association between midurethral sling and decreased anxiety [61], resulting in improvement in sexual spontaneity, arousal, and orgasm in certain patients [62]. However, when examining other specific subdomains, most studies found no changes in sexual desire [63, 64], orgasmic capabilities [63, 64], intercourse frequency [63, 65], or satisfaction [63, 64] following sling surgery. Zycynski et al reported improvement in dyspareunia rates in a group of 406 subjects aged 52.9 $^{+}/_{-}$ 11.0 years following sling surgery for stress UI [66].

Anti-incontinence surgeries can be very effective in treating coital incontinence. In fact, improvement after surgery was primarily attributed to decreased urinary-related sexual complaints such as coital incontinence [32, 61]. Pooled data on midurethral slings from a meta-analysis showed a significant reduction in coital incontinence with an OR 0.12 (CI 0.08-0.17) [44]. Post-operatively, patients also reported decreased fear and embarrassment of coital incontinence [67]. Women with coital incontinence and stress UI at baseline were also more likely to display improvement in frequency and enjoyment of intercourse as compared to those without coital incontinence (32.5 % v 6.8 %) [68].

Worsening of sexual function after midurethral sling placement is less common but possible, approximately 13.1 % in a meta-analysis by Jha et al [44]. This can

**Table 3** Effect of surgical treatments of stress urinary incontinence on sexual function

| Study | Design | N | Treatment | Length of Follow Up (months) | Instrument | Findings | | | | Coital Incontinence |
|---|---|---|---|---|---|---|---|---|---|---|
| | | | | | | Overall Post-Operative Sexual Function | Improved | Worsened | No Difference | |
| **Midurethral sling: Retropubic (TVT)** | | | | | | | | | | |
| Jha et al [62] | Prospective case series | 62 | TVT | 3 | ePAQ | N/A | • Impact of LUTS on sex (p < 0.001)<br>• Avoidance of sex (p < 0.001)<br>• Anxiety of UI & sex (p < 0.001) | N/A | • Partner avoidance of sex (p = 0.06) | • Improved (p < 0.001) |
| Ghezzi et al [70] | Prospective case series | 53 | TVT | 6-12 | PISQ | • Improved: 34 %<br>• Worsened: 3.8 % | N/A | N/A | • Fear of incontinence<br>• Frequency | • Improved in 87 %, with associated improvement:<br>• Frequency<br>• Fear of CI<br>• Embarrassment |
| **Midurethral sling: Retropubic (TVT) versus Transobterator (TVT-O, TOT) comparative studies** | | | | | | | | | | |
| Elzevier et al [71] | Prospective cohort | 1. TVT-O: 34<br>2. TOT: 44 | 1. TVT-O<br>2. TOT | 3-4 | Lemack | • Improved: 20.6 & 18.2 % (TVT, TVT-O respectively)<br>• Worsened: 5.9 & 18.2 % (TVT, TVT-O respectively) | N/A | • Dyspareunia from vaginal narrowing in TOT [vs TVT-O] (p = 0.026) | • Frequency<br>• Lubrication loss (p = 0.612)<br>• Clitoral lumescence reduction, sensibility (p = 0.191, p = 0.346 respectively) | • Improved |
| Jha et al [64] | Prospective cohort | 1. TVT: 43<br>2. TVT-O: 11 | 1. TVT<br>2. TVT-O | 6 | PISQ | N/A | • Total PISQ (p < 0.001)<br>• Partner, Physical subdomains (p = 0.002, p < 0.001 respectively) | N/A | • Behavior emotive subdomain (p = 0.7) | • Improved (p < 0.002) |
| Zyczynski et al [67] | RCT | 1. TVT: 298<br>2. TOT: 299 | 1. TVT<br>2. TOT | 24 | PISQ | N/A | • Total PISQ (p < 0.0001)<br>• Pain (p = 0.003)<br>• Fear of UI & sex (p < 0.0001) | • PISQ in surgical failure [vs success] (p = 0.009) | • PISQ between TVT & TOT<br>• Proportion of sexually active patients post-op | • Improved (p < 0.0001) |
| Filocamo et al [61] | Prospective cohort | 1. TVT: 28 | 1. TVT | 12 | FSFI | N/A | • Total FSFI (p < 0.002) | N/A | • FSFI between TVT & TOT | N/A |

**Table 3** Effect of surgical treatments of stress urinary incontinence on sexual function (Continued)

| Study | Design | Intervention (N) | Questionnaire | Score | Outcome | Findings |
|---|---|---|---|---|---|---|
| | | 2. TOT: 105 | 2. TOT | | | • All subdomains (p < 0.002) • Sexual dysfunction (P = 0.05) |
| Cayan et al [75] | Prospective cohort | 1. TVT or vaginal repair: 53 | 1. TVT or vaginal repair | FSFI | 1. Sling: 32.1 +/- 13.7 | • Improved: 24.5 & 12.2 % (TVT, Burch respectively) | N/A · Total FSFI (p < 0.001) · Pain (p = 0.162) N/A |
| | | 2. Burch 41 | 2. Burch | | 2. Burch: 35.7 +/- 16.7 | • Worsened: 47.2 & 63.4 % (TVT, Burch respectively) | • Desire, arousal, lubrication, orgasm, satisfaction subdomains (p ≤ 0.002) • Total FSFI, desire, arousal, lubrication, orgasm in Burch [vs TVT] (p = 0.004-0.026) |
| **Periurethral bulking injection** | | | | | | |
| Leone Roberti Maggiore et al [76] | Prospective case series | Polyacrylamide hydrogel periurethral injection 29 | 12 | PISQ, Global sexual satisfaction VAS score | N/A | • Total PISQ (p < 0.001) • Desire, orgasm frequency, excitation, satisfaction, fear of UI & sex, negative emotional reaction, orgasm intensity (p < 0.001) • Global sex satisfaction VAS score (p < 0.001) | • Global sex satisfaction in surgical failure [vs success] (p < 0.001) • Pain (p = 0.244) • Improved (p < 0.001) |

*CI* Coital incontinence; *ePAQ* Electronic Pelvic Floor Symptoms Assessment Questionnaire; *FSFI* Female sexual function index; *PISQ* Pelvic Organ Prolapse-Urinary Incontinence Sexual Function Questionnaire; *RCT* Randomized controlled trial; *SA* Sexually active; *TVT* Tension-free vaginal tape; *TVT-O* Tension-free vaginal tape - obturator; *TOT* transobturator tape; *VAS* visual analog scale manifest as new-onset dyspareunia [67], loss of libido [67], and de novo anorgasmia [64, 69]. The mechanism is not understood, but may be attributed to mesh complications such as erosion [70], changes in clitoral blood flow after dissection in the periurethral area, narrowing of the vaginal opening, or potential injury to the pudendal nerve branches [70, 71]. Removal or revision of mesh may improve sexual dysfunction; one case series showed that use of vaginal estrogen or correction of erosion after mesh slings were found to have improvement in all Female Sexual Function Index scores except orgasm [72].

Burch colposuspension is less commonly used to treat stress UI given the availability of minimally invasive techniques. Evidence on the effect of Burch colposuspension on overall sexual health is poor in quality and contradictory. One retrospective study comparing tension-free vaginal tape to Burch found no significant difference in sexual improvement post-operatively, though there was a non-significant increase in worsening of intercourse after tension-free vaginal tape [73]. Another small prospective study found decreased sexual function in both groups, but to a greater degree in patients who underwent Burch colposuspension [74].

Periurethal bulking injections are useful for management of stress UI in women who are poor candidates for general anesthesia, as these procedures can be performed with local anesthetics. Data on the effect of bulking agents on sexual function is limited in number and quality. One small

prospective study on 29 patients (mean age: 53 years old) treated with polyacrylamide hydrogel injections reported significant improvement in total Pelvic Organ Prolapse/Incontinence Sexual Questionnaire-12 scores, and 6 patients reestablished sexual activity post-operatively [75]. Sexual response (desire, excitement, and orgasm) likewise improved. Four patients who presented with coital incontinence prior to injections achieved resolution of their incontinence [75].

Table 4 shows the effect of surgical treatments of urgency UI on sexual function. Studies on onabotulinumtoxin A injection and sexual function have not been conducted, though an randomized controlled trial by Nitti et al did note a significant improvement in the King's Health Questionnaire Personal Relationships domain score following treatment with Botox in women with urgency UI [76]. Data on sacral neuromodulation is mixed. Four low quality studies showed significant improvement in sexual function questionnaire scores [77–80], while one did not [81]. Subscale improvements were noted in lubrication, pain, arousal, satisfaction, and orgasm intensity [77–80]. One case series on sacral neuromodulation indicated decreased coital incontinence in 3 patients, and cured coital incontinence in 2 patients, as well as decreased fear of coital incontinence [79].

Overall, there is high quality data to support improvement of sexual function after treatment with midurethral slings. Periurethral injection may improve sexual health, though larger studies are needed. The effect of Burch

**Table 4** Effect of surgical treatments of urge urinary incontinence on sexual function

| Author | Study Design | N | Treatment | Instrument | Findings |
|---|---|---|---|---|---|
| Obotulinumtoxin A injection | | | | | |
| Nitti et al [77] | RCT | 1. Placebo: 243<br>2. Botox: 249 | 1. Placebo<br>2. Botox 100 U follow up: 12 weeks | KHQ (Personal Relationship Domain) | • Clinically significant improvement in all KHQ scores, including Personal Relationship (-13.4 v -1.1, $p < 0.001$) |
| Sacral neuromodulation | | | | | |
| Zahibi et al [78] | Prospective case series | 36 | SNM follow up: 6 months | FSFI | • Significant ↑ FSFI total and all subscale scores except desire<br>• Pts with voiding dysfunction only: 157 % improvement in total FSFI |
| Signorello et al [79] | Prospective case series | 30 | SNM follow up: median 36.3 months | FSFI | • Significant improvement in total FSFI and most domains except orgasm<br>• 25 % showed >50 % improvement on total FSFI |
| Gill et al [80] | Prospective case series | 8 | SNM follow up: median 3.2 months | FSFI, Female Sexual Health Questionnaire | • Significant improvement in arousal, satisfaction, orgasm<br>• 50 % ↓ CI, restriction of SA due to UI |
| Pauls et al [81] | Prospective case series | 7 | SNM | FSFI | • Significant ↑ frequency, improvement of FSFI total and desire, lubrication, satisfaction, pain scores |
| Ingber et al [82] | Prospective case series | 27 | SNM follow up: 6 months | FSFI | • Non-significant improvement in FSFI in OAB patients (18.6 → 22.4, $p = 0.257$) |

*SA* Sexual activity, *FSFI* Female Sexual Function Index; *KHQ* King's Health Questionnaire; *CI* Coital incontinence; *RCT* Randomized controlled trial; *SNM* Sacral neuromodulation colposuspension on sexual function is mixed, and more evidence is required. High quality, large studies examining the effect of surgical treatments of urgency UI on sexual function are needed, though sacral neuromodulation shows promise in a few low quality studies.

## Conclusions

Urinary incontinence is a bothersome condition that is prevalent in middle age women. There is significant data to support that urinary incontinence is detrimental to sexual function, especially in women in midlife. While data on the effect of urinary incontinence treatments on sexual function is limited by the lack of large trials and high quality trials, treatment of any incontinence has been shown to improve sexual function. For stress UI, non-surgical and surgical treatments - pelvic muscle training and midurethral slings - have been shown to improve sexual function. For urgency UI, treatment with pelvic muscle training and anti-muscarinic medications has the most evidence of improvement in sexual function. Coital incontinence generally improves with treatment of the underlying incontinence subtype. Though problems with sexual health in middle-aged women with incontinence are admittedly complex, and involve both psychological and physical factors, evaluation and treatment of urinary incontinence is important in the management of this important issue.

### Abbreviations
ATLAS: Ambulatory treatments for leakage associated with stress; UI: Urinary incontinence.

### Competing interests
The authors declare that they have no competing interests.

### Authors' contributions
CC conceived and designed the aims of this review, conducted literature searches, and drafted the manuscript. LA participated in study design and critical revisions of the manuscript. UA aided in the design and coordination of the review and data acquisition, and helped to draft the manuscript. All authors read and approved the final manuscript.

### References
1. Dooley Y, Kenton K, Cao G, Luke A, Durazo-Arvizu R, Kramer H, et al. Urinary incontinence prevalence: results from the National Health and Nutrition Examination Survey. J Urol. 2008;179(2):656–61.
2. Waetjen LE, Liao S, Johnson WO, Sampselle CM, Sternfield B, Harlow SD, et al. Factors associated with prevalent and incident urinary incontinence in a cohort of midlife women: a longitudinal analysis of data: study of women's health across the nation. Am J Epidemiol. 2007;165(3):309–18.
3. Moller LA, Lose G, Jorgensen T. The prevalence and bothersomeness of lower urinary tract symptoms in women 40 ± 60 years of age. Acta Obstet Gynecol Scand. 2000;79:298–305.
4. Hannestad YS, Rortveit G, Sandvik H, Hunskaar S, Norwegian EPINCONT study. Epidemiology of Incontinence in the County of Nord-Trondelag. A community-based epidemiological survey of female urinary incontinence: The norwegian EPINCONT study. epidemiology of incontinence in the county of nord-trondelag. J Clin Epidemiol. 2000;53(11):1150–7.
5. Stewart WF, Van Rooyen JB, Cundiff GW, Abrams P, Herzog AR, Corey R, et al. Prevalence and burden of overactive bladder in the united states. World J Urol. 2003;20(6):327–36.
6. Barber MD, Dowsett SA, Mullen KJ, Viktrup L. The impact of stress urinary incontinence on sexual activity in women. Cleve Clin J Med. 2005;72(3):225–32.
7. Ratner ES, Erekson EA, Minkin MJ, Foran-Tuller KA. Sexual satisfaction in the elderly female population: A special focus on women with gynecologic pathology. Maturitas. 2011;70(3):210–5.
8. Nilsson M, Lalos O, Lindkvist H, Lalos A. How do urinary incontinence and urgency affect women's sexual life? Acta Obstet Gynecol Scand. 2011;90(6):621–8.
9. Shaw C. A systematic review of the literature on the prevalence of sexual impairment in women with urinary incontinence and the prevalence of urinary leakage during sexual activity. Eur Urol. 2002;42(5):432–40.
10. Lam GW, Foldspang A, Elving LB, Mommsen S. Social context, social abstention, and problem recognition correlated with adult female urinary incontinence. Dan Med Bull. 1992;39(6):565–70.
11. Rizk DE, Shaheen H, Thomas L, Dunn E, Hassan MY. The prevalence and determinants of health care-seeking behavior for urinary incontinence in united arab emirates women. Int Urogynecol J Pelvic Floor Dysfunct. 1999;10(3):160–5.
12. Norton PA, MacDonald LD, Sedgwick PM, Stanton SL. Distress and delay associated with urinary incontinence, frequency, and urgency in women. BMJ. 1988;297(6657):1187–9.
13. Sen I, Onaran M, Aksakal N, Acar C, Tan MO, Acar A, et al. The impact of urinary incontinence on female sexual function. Adv Ther. 2006;23(6):999–1008.
14. Aslan G, Koseoglu H, Sadik O, Gimen S, Cihan A, Esen A. Sexual function in women with urinary incontinence. Int J Impot Res. 2005;17(3):248–51.
15. Oh SJ, Ku JH, Choo MS, Yun JM, Kim DY, Park WH. Health-related quality of life and sexual function in women with stress urinary incontinence and overactive bladder. Int J Urol. 2008;15(1):62–7.
16. Liebergall-Wischnitzer M, Paltiel O, Hochner-Celnikier D, Lavy Y, Manor O, Woloski Wruble AC. Sexual function and quality of life for women with mild-to-moderate stress urinary incontinence. J Midwifery Womens Health. 2011;56(5):461–7.
17. Berglund AL, Fugl-Meyer KS. Some sexological characteristics of stress incontinent women. Scand J Urol Nephrol. 1996;30(3):207–12.
18. Sand PK, Appell R. Disruptive effects of overactive bladder and urge urinary incontinence in younger women. Am J Med. 2006;119(3 Suppl 1):16–23.
19. Heidler S, Mert C, Wehrberger C, Temml C, Ponholzer A, Rauchenwald M, et al. Impact of overactive bladder symptoms on sexuality in both sexes. Urol Int. 2010;85(4):443–6.
20. Woods NF, Mitchell ES. Consequences of incontinence for women during the menopausal transition and early postmenopause: Observations from the seattle midlife women's health study. Menopause. 2013;20(9):915–21.
21. Nilsson M, Lalos O, Lindkvist H, Lalos A. Impact of female urinary incontinence and urgency on women's and their partners' sexual life. Neurourol Urodyn. 2011;30(7):1276–80.
22. Handa VL, Harvey L, Cundiff GW, Siddique SA, Kjerulff KH. Sexual function among women with urinary incontinence and pelvic organ prolapse. Am J Obstet Gynecol. 2004;191(3):751–6.
23. Sako T, Inoue M, Watanabe T, Ishii A, Yokoyama T, Kumon H. Impact of overactive bladder and lower urinary tract symptoms on sexual health in japanese women. Int Urogynecol J. 2011;22(2):165–9.
24. Lukacz ES, Whitcomb EL, Lawrence JM, Nager CW, Contreras R, Luber KM. Are sexual activity and satisfaction affected by pelvic floor disorders? analysis of a community-based survey. Am J Obstet Gynecol. 2007;197(1):88.e1–6.
25. Salonia A, Zanni G, Nappi RE, Briganti A, Dehò F, Fabbri F, et al. Sexual dysfunction is common in women with lower urinary tract symptoms and urinary incontinence: Results of a cross-sectional study. Eur Urol. 2004;45(5):642–8. discussion 648.
26. Cohen BL, Barboglio P, Gousse A. The impact of lower urinary tract symptoms and urinary incontinence on female sexual dysfunction using a validated instrument. J Sex Med. 2008;5(6):1418–23.
27. Del Rosso A, Pace G, Di Pierro ED, Masciovecchio S, Galatioto GP, Vicentini C. Impact of overactive bladder on sexual function in women. Urologia. 2011;78(3):200–2.
28. Coyne KS, Sexton CC, Thompson C, Kopp ZS, Milsom I, Kaplan SA. The impact of OAB on sexual health in men and women: Results from EpiLUTS. J Sex Med. 2011;8(6):1603–15.

29. Zahariou A, Karamouti M, Tyligada E, Papaioannou P. Sexual function in women with overactive bladder. Female Pelvic Med Reconstr Surg. 2010;16(1):31–6.

30. Bekker MD, Beck JJ, Putter H, Van Driel MF, Pelger RC, Weijmar Schultz WC, et al. Sexual experiences of men with incontinent partners. J Sex Med. 2010;7(5):1877–82.

31. Yip SK, Chan A, Pang S, Leung P, Tang C, Shek D, et al. The impact of urodynamic stress incontinence and detrusor overactivity on marital relationship and sexual function. Am J Obstet Gynecol. 2003;188(5):1244–8.

32. Moller LA, Lose G, Jorgensen T. The prevalence and bothersomeness of lower urinary tract symptoms in women 40-60 years of age. Acta Obstet Gynecol Scand. 2000;79(4):298–305.

33. Nygaard I, Milburn A. Urinary incontinence during sexual activity: Prevalence in a gynecologic practice. J Womens Health. 1995;4(1):83–6.

34. Melin I, Falconer C, Rössner S, Altman D. Sexual function in obese women: impact of lower urinary tract dysfunction. Int J Obes (Lond). 2008;32(8):1312–8.

35. El-Azab AS, Yousef HA, Seifeldein GS. Coital incontinence: relation to detrusor overactivity and stress incontinence. Neurourol Urodyn. 2011;30(4):520–4.

36. Hayder D. The effects of urinary incontinence on sexuality: seeking an intimate partnership. J Wound Ostomy Continence Nurs. 2012;39(5):539–44.

37. Kizilkaya Beji N, Yalcin O, Ayyildiz EH, Kayir A. Effect of urinary leakage on sexual function during sexual intercourse. Urol Int. 2005;74(3):250–5.

38. Vierhout ME, Gianotten WL. Mechanisms of urine loss during sexual activity. Eur J Obstet Gynecol Reprod Biol. 1993;52(1):45–7.

39. Serati M, Salvatore S, Uccella S, Nappi RE, Bolis P. Female urinary incontinence during intercourse: a review on an understudied problem for women's sexuality. J Sex Med. 2009;6(1):40–8.

40. Hilton P. Urinary incontinence during sexual intercourse: a common, but rarely volunteered, symptom. Br J Obstet Gynaecol. 1988;95(4):377–81.

41. Emery J, Book NM, Novi JM. The association between post-void leakage and coital incontinence and intrinsic sphincter deficiency among women with urinary incontinence. Female Pelvic Med Reconstr Surg. 2010;16(6):349–52.

42. Serati M, Salvatore S, Uccella S, Cromi A, Khullar V, Cardozo L, et al. Urinary incontinence at orgasm: relation to detrusor overactivity and treatment efficacy. Eur Urol. 2008;54(4):911–5.

43. Liu L, Mansfield KJ, Kristiana I, Vaux KJ, Millard RJ, Burcher E. The molecular basis of urgency: regional difference of vanilloid receptor expression in the human urinary bladder. Neurourol Urodyn. 2007;26(3):433–8.

44. Jha S, Ammenbal M, Metwally M. Impact of incontinence surgery on sexual function: a systematic review and meta-analysis. J Sex Med. 2012;9(1):34–43.

45. Moran PA, Dwyer PL, Ziccone SP. Urinary leakage during coitus in women. J Obstet Gynaecol. 1999;19(3):286–8.

46. Kegel AH. Stress incontinence of urine in women; physiologic treatment. J Int Coll Surg. 1956;25(4 Part 1):487–99.

47. Jonsson Funk M, Levin PJ, Wu JM. Trends in the surgical management of stress urinary incontinence. Obstet Gynecol. 2012;119(4):845–51.

48. Bo K, Talseth T, Vinsnes A. Randomized controlled trial on the effect of pelvic floor muscle training on quality of life and sexual problems in genuine stress incontinent women. Acta Obstet Gynecol Scand. 2000;79(7):598–603.

49. Zahariou AG, Karamouti MV, Papaioannou PD. Pelvic floor muscle training improves sexual function of women with stress urinary incontinence. Int Urogynecol J Pelvic Floor Dysfunct. 2008;19(3):401–6.

50. Wang AC, Wang YY, Chen MC. Single-blind, randomized trial of pelvic floor muscle training, biofeedback-assisted pelvic floor muscle training, and electrical stimulation in the management of overactive bladder. Urology. 2004;63(1):61–6.

51. Giuseppe PG, Pace G, Vicentini C. Sexual function in women with urinary incontinence treated by pelvic floor transvaginal electrical stimulation. J Sex Med. 2007;4(3):702–7.

52. Sand PK, Goldberg RP, Dmochowski RR, McIlwain M, Dahl NV. The impact of the overactive bladder syndrome on sexual function: a preliminary report from the multicenter assessment of transdermal therapy in overactive bladder with oxybutynin trial. Am J Obstet Gynecol. 2006;195(6):1730–5.

53. Rogers RG, Omotosho T, Bachmann G, Sun F, Morrow JD. Continued symptom improvement in sexually active women with overactive bladder and urgency urinary incontinence treated with tolterodine ER for 6 months. Int Urogynecol J Pelvic Floor Dysfunct. 2009;20(4):381–5.

54. Hajebrahimi S, Azaripour A, Sadeghi-Bazargani H. Tolterodine immediate release improves sexual function in women with overactive bladder. J Sex Med. 2008;5(12):2880–5.

55. Chapple CR, Van Kerrebroeck PE, Junemann KP, Wang JT, Brodsky M. Comparison of fesoterodine and tolterodine in patients with overactive bladder. BJU Int. 2008;102(9):1128–32.

56. Capo Jr JP, Laramée C, Lucente V, Fakhoury A, Forero-Schwanhaeuser S. Solifenacin treatment for overactive bladder in Hispanic patients: patient-reported symptom bother and quality of life outcomes from the VESIcare Open-Label Trial. Int J Clin Pract. 2008;62(1):39–46.

57. Danilova TI, Danilov VV, Luchinskii SA, Danilov VV, Vasil'chenko AV. Sexual dysfunction in women with overactive bladder and their correction with m-cholinolytic spasmex. Urologiia. 2010;6(6):30–4.

58. Eftekhar T, Teimoory N, Miri E, Nikfallah A, Naeimi M, Ghajarzadeh M. Posterior tibial nerve stimulation for treating neurologic bladder in women: a randomized clinical trial. Acta Med Iran. 2014;52(11):816–21.

59. van Balken MR, Vergunst H, Bemelmans BL. Sexual functioning in patients with lower urinary tract dysfunction improves after percutaneous tibial nerve stimulation. Int J Impot Res. 2006;18(5):470–5.

60. Filocamo MT, Serati M, Frumenzio E, LiMarzi V, Cattoni E, Champagne A, et al. The impact of mid-urethral slings for the treatment of urodynamic stress incontinence on female sexual function: a multicenter prospective study. J Sex Med. 2011;8(7):2002–8.

61. Jha S, Radley S, Farkas A, Jones G. The impact of TVT on sexual function. Int Urogynecol J Pelvic Floor Dysfunct. 2009;20(2):165–9.

62. Roos A, Thakar R, Sultan A, de Leeuw J, Paulus A. The impact of pelvic floor surgery on female sexual function: a mixed quantitative and qualitative study. BJOG. 2013.

63. Jha S, Moran P, Greenham H, Ford C. Sexual function following surgery for urodynamic stress incontinence. Int Urogynecol J Pelvic Floor Dysfunct. 2007;18(8):845–50.

64. Yeni E, Unal D, Verit A, Kafali H, Ciftci H, Gulum M. The effect of tension-free vaginal tape (TVT) procedure on sexual function in women with stress urinary incontinence. Int Urogynecol J Pelvic Floor Dysfunct. 2003;14(6):390–4.

65. Berthier A, Sentilhes L, Taibi S, Loisel C, Grise P, Marpeau L. Sexual function in women following the transvaginal tension-free tape procedure for incontinence. Int J Gynaecol Obstet. 2008;102(2):105–9.

66. Zyczynski HM, Rickey L, Dyer KY, Wilson T, Stoddard AM, Gormley EA, et al. Sexual activity and function in women more than 2 years after midurethral sling placement. Am J Obstet Gynecol. 2012;207(5):421.e1–6.

67. Mazouni C, Karsenty G, Bretelle F, Bladou F, Gamerre M, Serment G. Urinary complications and sexual function after the tension-free vaginal tape procedure. Acta Obstet Gynecol Scand. 2004;83(10):955–61.

68. Bekker M, Beck J, Putter H, Venema P, Lycklama à Nijeholt A, Pelger R, et al. Sexual function improvement following surgery for stress incontinence: the relevance of coital incontinence. J Sex Med. 2009;6(11):3208–13.

69. Ghezzi F, Serati M, Cromi A, Uccella S, Triacca P, Bolis P. Impact of tension-free vaginal tape on sexual function: results of a prospective study. Int Urogynecol J Pelvic Floor Dysfunct. 2006;17(1):54–9.

70. Elzevier HW, Putter H, Delaere KP, Venema PL, Nijeholt AA L a, Pelger RC. Female sexual function after surgery for stress urinary incontinence: Transobturator suburethral tape vs. tension-free vaginal tape obturator. J Sex Med. 2008;5(2):400–6.

71. Mouritsen L. Pathophysiology of sexual dysfunction as related to pelvic floor disorders. Int Urogynecol J Pelvic Floor Dysfunct. 2009;20 Suppl 1:S19–25.

72. Kuhn A, Eggeman C, Burkhard F, Mueller MD. Correction of erosion after suburethral sling insertion for stress incontinence: results and related sexual function. Eur Urol. 2009;56(2):371–6.

73. Demirkesen O, Onal B, Tunc B, Alici B, Cetinele B. Does vaginal anti-incontinence surgery affect sexual satisfaction? A comparison of TVT and burch-colposuspension. Int Braz J Urol. 2008;34(2):214–9.

74. Cayan F, Dilek S, Akbay E, Cayan S. Sexual function after surgery for stress urinary incontinence: vaginal sling versus burch colposuspension. Arch Gynecol Obstet. 2008;277(1):31–6.

75. Leone Roberti Maggiore U, Alessandri F, Medica M, Gabelli M, Venturini PL, Ferrero S. Periurethral injection of polyacrylamide hydrogel for the treatment of stress urinary incontinence: the impact on female sexual function. J Sex Med. 2012;9(12):3255–63.

76. Nitti VW, Dmochowski R, Herschorn S, Sand P, Thompson C, Nardo C, et al. OnabotulinumtoxinA for the treatment of patients with overactive bladder and urinary incontinence: results of a phase 3, randomized, placebo controlled trial. J Urol. 2013;189(6):2186–93.

77. Zabihi N, Mourtzinos A, Maher MG, Raz S, Rodriguez LV. The effects of bilateral caudal epidural S2-4 neuromodulation on female sexual function. Int Urogynecol J Pelvic Floor Dysfunct. 2008;19(5):697–700.

78. Signorello D, Seitz CC, Berner L, Trenti E, Martini T, Galantini A, et al. Impact of sacral neuromodulation on female sexual function and his correlation with clinical outcome and quality of life indexes: A monocentric experience. J Sex Med. 2011;8(4):1147–55.

79. Gill BC, Swartz MA, Firoozi F, Rackley RR, Moore CK, Goldman HB, et al. Improved sexual and urinary function in women with sacral nerve stimulation. Neuromodulation. 2011;14(5):436–43. discussion 443.

80. Pauls RN, Marinkovic SP, Silva WA, Rooney CM, Kleeman SD, Karram MM. Effects of sacral neuromodulation on female sexual function. Int Urogynecol J Pelvic Floor Dysfunct. 2007;18(4):391–5.

81. Ingber MS, Ibrahim IA, Killinger KA, Diokno AC, Peters KM. Neuromodulation and female sexual function: does treatment for refractory voiding symptoms have an added benefit? Int Urogynecol J Pelvic Floor Dysfunct. 2009;20(9):1055–9.

82. Handa VL, Whitcomb E, Weidner AC, Nygaard I, Brubaker L, Bradley CS, et al. Sexual function before and after non-surgical treatment for stress urinary incontinence. Female Pelvic Med Reconstr Surg. 2011;17(1):30–5.

# 19

# Confronting the challenges of the menopausal transition

Robert L. Reid* and Bryden A. Magee

**Abstract**

Canada's Generation X is now entering the menopausal transition and pursuing effective therapy for bothersome vasomotor symptoms. They do so at a time when confusion about the safe and appropriate use of menopausal hormone therapy (MHT) has never been greater. Misplaced fears among women and their health care providers about MHT have, in many circumstances, led them to abandon this most effective therapy. This review discusses the physiology of the menopausal transition, the nature of symptoms related to withdrawal of ovarian estrogen production, and the potential benefits and risks of MHT. It is now clear that for most recently menopausal women the benefits of MHT outweigh the risks. The rationale for choosing different dosages, formulations, and regimens is reviewed.

**Keywords:** Menopause, Vasomotor symptoms, Menopausal hormone therapy

## Introduction

Those involved in the care of menopausal women when the first Women's Health Initiative (WHI) results were published in 2002 will remember that year as pivotal in the management of women entering the menopausal transition. The sensational way that negative results were fed to the media [1] triggered a cascade of events that created a fear of menopausal hormone therapy (MHT) leading women and their care providers to abandon the most effective treatment for menopausal vasomotor symptoms and substitute a variety of untested alternatives for which the risk-benefit profile was largely unknown.

In Canada for example, a reciprocal relationship in prescribing practices for prescriptions of MHT and selective serotonin reuptake inhibitors (SSRIs) was seen, beginning in 2002. As shown in Fig. 1, the number of prescriptions written for antidepressants increased while those written for MHT quickly dropped off, suggesting that "antidepressants were being prescribed for symptoms (psychological, physical) previously controlled with the use of hormone replacement therapy" [2].

The absence of effective therapies for distressing vasomotor symptoms has contributed to a burgeoning market for complementary and alternative medicines (CAMs) and the unscrupulous marketing of purportedly "safer" hormone therapy in the form of individualized compounded bio-identical hormones [3]. There is, in fact, considerable evidence that many CAMs are adulterated and fail to contain the constituents as advertised. More so, most CAMs have yet to establish any scientific evidence of efficacy beyond a placebo effect [4]. Ultimately, there is no evidence that compounded bio-identical hormones are more effective or safer than regulated pharmaceuticals that have undergone rigorous clinical trials before reaching the market [5].

A significant shortcoming of the WHI was the inclusion of women well beyond the age of menopause. Women up to age 79 were eligible to participate and ultimately, $2/3^{rds}$ of recruited subjects were over age 60 years. A 2002 editorial warned of this flaw, suggesting that if the role of exercise for cardiovascular disease prevention had been tested in the same age group as the WHI, it is likely that the number of induced cardiac events would have led to the conclusion that exercise is bad for the heart [6]. A full decade after the original WHI report, a publication from several WHI lead investigators acknowledged that "the unfortunate effects of the WHI came not from problems with the design or

* Correspondence: Robert.reid@queensu.ca
Division of Reproductive Endocrinology and Infertility, Queen's University, Kingston, Ontario K7L 4 V1, Canada

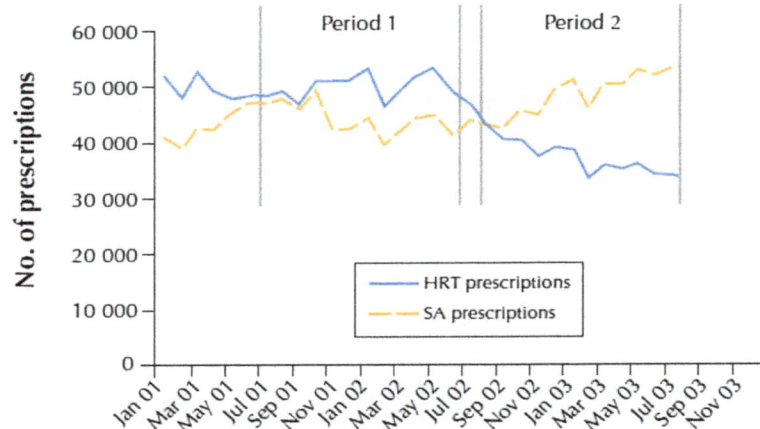

**Fig. 1** Prescriptions of MHT and Selective serotonin reuptake inhibitors in Canada showing a reciprocal trend after 2002. With permission from McIntyre RS, Konarski JZ, Grigoriadis S, Fan NC, Mancini DA, Fulton KA, Stewart DE, Kennedy SE. Hormone replacement therapy and antidepressant prescription patterns: a reciprocal relationship CMAJ 2005; 172 (1):57–59. Reproduced with permission of the Canadian Medical Association Journal

the findings; rather, they were the result of generalizing findings from a well-conducted study to a subgroup that was not adequately represented". In other words, the adverse consequences of MHT observed in older women were, in error, extrapolated to younger, newly menopausal women started on MHT. These authors further concluded: "With initiation of HT near menopause, the weight of evidence supports benefits over risks, with the potential to prevent or ameliorate downstream morbidity" [7].

Unfortunately, the damage from 10 years of adverse publicity about MHT has already been done. According to Vincent Convello from the Centre for Risk Communication at Columbia University "strong beliefs about risk, once formed, change very slowly and are extraordinarily persistent in the face of contrary evidence". This seems particularly so for MHT. Despite the recent reanalyses of the WHI, which confirm that benefits outweigh risks for most newly menopausal women, fear and confusion continue to linger. This is no doubt exacerbated by the fact that rare adverse events remain a focus for media and for lawyers looking to add additional treatments to the 1–800 BAD-DRUG list.

Leading medical societies devoted to the care of menopausal women in 2012 published a consensus document to try to bring clarity to the benefits and risks of MHT and concluded that "there is no question that hormone therapy has an important role in managing symptoms for women during the menopausal transition and in early menopause" [8].

This reassurance however, is not enough because a generation of medical graduates have now been trained in an environment where use of MHT is frowned upon. This has resulted in limited or, in some cases, non-existent exposure to prescribing MHT or addressing side effects of treatment.

This review will summarize benefits and risks of MHT based on the best available evidence today and will provide practitioners with directions to assist them in prescribing MHT appropriately to women with disruptive symptoms during the midlife transition.

## Review
### Understanding the menopausal transition
The developing follicle is the primary source of estrogen in women during the reproductive years. In general, unless perturbed by pregnancy, extremes of body weight or other hormonal disorders, the menstrual cycle throughout the reproductive years tends to have a monthly periodicity. As the pool of oocytes diminishes, women in their 40's often experience a decade of increasingly variable menstrual cycle length.

Between the ages of 40 and 45, the process of oocyte maturation accelerates, such that the follicular phase shortens to 7–8 days instead of the typical 14 days in younger women. An aberrant luteal phase elevation of estrogen (a so-called LOOP event [9]) leads to an early LH surge in the subsequent cycle and is considered one explanation for this abbreviated follicular phase. In other women, if the LOOP event does not result in ovulation, it may lead to delayed follicular development and prolongation of the subsequent cycle. Coupled with heavier and longer menses (often 8–10 days due to anatomic (adenomyosis or fibroids) or other factors (excessive prostacyclin or fibrinolytic activity), this menstrual cycle irregularity will result in many women seeking treatment for dysfunctional uterine bleeding.

Between the ages of 45 and 50, the remaining oocytes are those that have been most resistant to gonadotropin stimulation. Follicular development may halt temporarily until FSH levels rise sufficiently to force maturation. During intervals with arrested follicular development, estrogen levels fall and women experience the typical menopausal hot flashes and night sweats. Then, if and when follicular maturation resumes, estrogen levels rise and menopausal symptoms subside, only to be replaced by typical menstrual-cycle related symptoms such as breast tenderness, bloating and mood changes followed by often heavy and unpredictable menstruation.

The conventional term "perimenopause", which was originally defined by the World Health Organization, encompasses the period of time from the onset of menstrual irregularity (usually in the mid 40's) until one year after the final menstrual period when the postmenopausal phase begins [10]. More recently, the Stages of Reproductive Aging Workshop + 10 (STRAW +10), developed an updated staging system for ovarian aging in an attempt to standardize nomenclature. As such, the period of time from onset of menstrual irregularity to the final menstrual period is now defined as the "menopausal transition" [11].

It is hardly surprising that the perimenopause is a time of confusion and therapeutic frustration for women and their health care providers alike. The intermittent nature of clinical signs and symptoms of menopause leave uncertainty about whether the final menstrual period has occurred and with this variability, there may be confusion about the ongoing need for contraception, menstrual cycle regulation and/or hormone supplementation. Ultimately, most women can expect to exhaust their pool of oocytes by their mid-fifties with the average age of menopause being 51.5 years. Sustained amenorrhea with repeated elevation of FSH levels is diagnostic of menopause however therapy for distressing symptoms need not be delayed until the retrospective diagnosis of menopause has been proven.

Typical early menopausal symptoms include hot flashes and night sweats (vasomotor symptoms), and frequent night time wakenings with subsequent daytime fatigue or irritability [12]. Somatic aches and pains are the most frequent symptoms reported by women entering menopause [13, 14] but because most women assume that arthritic changes are a natural part of aging, vasomotor symptoms remain the most common reason for women to seek medical attention. In some women, mood changes may play a major role and clinical depression is a documented consequence in susceptible individuals [15]. Later on, prolonged estrogen deficiency plays a contributory role in the development of Genitourinary Syndrome of Menopause (GSM) – a condition marked by the gradual development of vaginal dryness and dyspareunia [16], increased risk for recurrent bladder or vaginal infections [17], and in some women, bladder overactivity.

Other effects of estrogen loss that lead to late clinical manifestations include accelerated bone loss (contributing to osteoporotic fractures) and certain adverse changes in cardiovascular risk factors such as lipids, obesity, diabetes, coronary artery calcium (CAC) accumulation and carotid intima-media thickness – all contributors to cardiovascular diseases [18]. Premature loss of endogenous estrogen has been shown to lead to earlier development of these menopause-associated conditions [19, 20].

**Benefits of MHT**
Although estrogen therapy has been shown to diminish somatic aches and pains and to reduce new onset of joint symptoms in menopausal women [21, 22] this seems to have remained a well-guarded secret. MHT (estrogen alone, progestin alone, or combination therapy) is best known for the dramatic relief afforded from distressing vasomotor symptoms. Systemic estrogen supplementation, even in low doses, can achieve up to an 80 percent decrease in hot flashes and night sweats with the peak effect generally evident by 4 weeks of treatment [23, 24].

Vaginal estrogen dosages recommended for treatment of GSM result in minimal systemic absorption and are therefore not effective for systemic complaints such as joint pain or vasomotor symptoms. Higher doses of vaginal estrogen do achieve systemic levels sufficient to control vasomotor symptoms [25].

The use of MHT confers the additional benefit of protecting against the accelerated bone loss of menopause and should be considered first line treatment for bone protection in symptomatic women [26]. The benefits of estrogen for prevention of further bone loss and stabilization of bone mineral density are seen even when estrogen treatment is delayed for a number of years after menopause [27] but the accelerated bone loss of menopause resumes rapidly once estrogen is discontinued [28].

Systemic MHT sometimes, and vaginal estrogen therapy almost always, provide protection of urogenital tissues from the effects of diminished estrogen exposure after menopause. Vaginal epithelium maintains healthy rugation with a more normal stratified squamous cell layer, better blood flow, and improved secretion (transudate), all of which contribute to better lubrication, less dyspareunia, increased sensation, and greater sexual satisfaction. Intravaginal but not systemic estrogen appears to improve the symptom of urgency incontinence but remains only one component of a multifaceted approach to treatment of this condition [29].

The role of hormone therapy for prevention of coronary artery disease (CAD) has been the focus of considerable confusion and debate [30, 31]. Observational studies like the Nurse Health Study, which found that MHT users were half as likely to develop CAD, are prone to certain biases due to differences in patient characteristics and behaviours between the two groups. MHT users differed in other attributes from non-MHT users, in that they were more likely to adopt other health promotion strategies like regular exercise and a healthy diet [32]. The Women's Health Initiative found that the use of MHT soon after menopause did delay the onset of coronary artery calcium (CAC) deposition [31, 33, 34] and that women with VMS had less CAC, which was attributed to prior MHT exposure [35]. In newly menopausal women MHT resulted in a small reduction in deaths due to CAD (1 fewer death per 1000 women years). However, MHT started in older women or those with pre-existing CAD increased the risk of adverse events [36–38]. This and observations from animal studies suggesting that healthy coronary arteries respond differently to estrogen than diseased vessels [39, 40] led to the "window of opportunity" theory for initiation of MHT while coronary arteries were still healthy [41].

We will probably never have the type of data needed to completely resolve this issue. It would be extremely difficult to recruit symptomatic newly menopausal women to a placebo controlled trial of sufficient duration to see outcome data for CAD. Depypere has calculated that it would be necessary to enrol over 185,000 women to detect a 10 % decrease in 10-year mortality [42].

MHT does appear to improve insulin sensitivity and reduce the incidence of new onset diabetes mellitus [43]. The WHI found 1 fewer case of new onset diabetes per 625 women years of use [44]. Recent evidence indicates that MHT has little impact on centripetal obesity, weight gain or blood pressure [45–47].

## Risks of MHT
### Keeping perspective
As discussed above, the true risks of MHT have been inflated in the media, creating fear among many women and health care providers [48]. The persistence of this fear stems from a distorted perception of the apparent risks, and this distortion that has been demonstrated by a large Australian population survey [49]. Breast cancer was perceived as a major health risk by 27 % of women compared to only 11 % who cited heart disease as a concern. In contrast to perceived risk, actual female mortality figures show that these conditions account for 3 % and 41 % of mortality respectively.

## What are the risks of MHT in the perimenopausal or recently menopausal woman?
### Cardiovascular diseases
#### Venous Thromboembolism (VTE)
Venous thromboembolism includes deep vein thrombosis and pulmonary embolism. Advancing age and obesity are important contributors to VTE risk in women on MHT [50].

In the Women's Health Initiative, women using MHT between the ages of 50–59 experienced 1 more case of VTE for every 1000 women per year [51]. This doubled for women 60–69 and tripled for women 70–79. Women with a body mass index (BMI) 25–30 kg/m$^2$ had double the risk of women with BMI <25 kg/m$^2$ and in those with BMI >30 kg/m$^2$ the risk was tripled. Cigarette smoking does not appear to be a risk for VTE though it is clearly a risk factor for coronary artery disease and stroke [52].

Risk of VTE is greatest in the first year after initiation of MHT, just as is seen with combined hormonal contraception. Hence, the actual risk to women who have safely used MHT for several years is probably lower than short-term studies indicate.

Air travel has also been identified as an important contributor to VTE, likely due to cramped seating, immobility, hypoxia and dehydration. Recent research indicates that risk of symptomatic events is 1/600 for flights over 4 h and 1/500 for flights over 12 h in travellers over 50 years of age and that this risk may be doubled in women on MHT [53].

Observational data suggest that the risk of VTE can be reduced by using lower dose MHT or transdermal formulations [54]. Findings from the large prospective Million Women cohort study in the UK suggest that estrogen-only MHT or combined estrogen/progestin therapy (EPT) containing norgestrel/norethisterone progestins instead of medroxprogesterone actetate are also associated with lower VTE risk [55].

### Stroke
Stroke remains a leading cause of morbidity and mortality in women, so any effect of MHT on stroke risk could be important. Results of past studies have been contradictory with some showing protection from ischemic stroke and others demonstrating small increases in risk. In the WHI study, hemorrhagic stroke risk was not influenced by MHT.

The attributable risk for ischemic stroke in the combined estrogen/progestin trial for all age groups was 0.9/1000 women years. For women ages 50–59 years the attributable risk of stroke was approximately 1/2500 women years of hormonal exposure [44, 56]. The attributable risk for all women enrolled in the estrogen alone arm of the trial was 1.1/1000 women years. Women aged 50–59 receiving estrogen alone showed no increase in the risk of stroke compared to placebo users [44, 57]. The impact of MHT on ischemic stroke seems to be related to hormone dosage and possibly also the route of delivery [58]. Although transdermal delivery has been suggested as a safer delivery route for MHT there is evidence that higher doses delivered transdermally may still increase the risk of stroke [59].

### Coronary Artery Disease (CAD)
As per the discussion above, MHT may carry a small risk of a coronary event when started in women beyond age 60 or more than 10 years after menopause because coronary arteries may already be diseased by this time. The absolute increase in mortality in older MHT users in the WHI was small, at 1.6 per 1000 women years. Nevertheless it is clear that co-morbidities (diabetes, obesity, hypertension dyslipidemia, smoking, inactivity) should be addressed before initiating MHT in older women. The low absolute risk of adverse outcomes should not preclude a clinical trial of MHT for distressing VMS in women beyond age 60 or more than 10 years after menopause.

### Cancers
#### Endometrial cancer
Unopposed estrogen in women with a uterus may lead to endometrial neoplasia and in some cases this may become apparent years after MHT treatment has been stopped. The risk of progression from endometrial hyperplasia to cancer depends on the type of hyperplasia identified. When atypical features exist the risk of progression to adenocarcinoma may be as high as 30 % [60].

Progestin co-therapy of sufficient dosage and duration will generally protect against the risk of endometrial neoplasia associated with unopposed estrogens [61]. For many women, progestin co-therapy results in unwanted side effects (spotting, mood changes and bloating) so alternative approaches have been explored including systemic estrogen combined with a progestin releasing intrauterine system [62] or a combination of estrogen and a selective estrogen receptor modulator [63].

#### Breast cancer
Breast cancer remains the greatest fear of most women considering MHT. Much of the breast cancer anxiety can be attributed to the enormous success of breast cancer awareness campaigns and the accompanying "pink ribbon" merchandising of everything from Kentucky Fried Chicken and Campbell's soup to jewelry and perfume [64]. The challenge for health care providers is to dispel distorted concepts about risk and to put true "absolute" or "attributable" risks into perspective [65, 66].

Table1 shows the actual risks of breast cancer for a hypothetical cohort of 1000 women over successive 10-year intervals compared to other (mostly cardiovascular) causes of mortality [67].

The WHI reported a hazard ratio for breast cancer among women using combined estrogen/progestin therapy of 1.3 with an attributable risk of 8/10,000 users per

year [68, 69]. In women randomized to estrogen-alone the hazard ratio for breast cancer was 0.77 indicating an attributable benefit of 7/10,000 fewer invasive breast cancers per year [70, 71]. While other data on the effects of estrogen on breast cancer are contradictory [72–74], the weight of evidence suggests that the breast cancer risk is lower with estrogen alone than with combined estrogen/progestin therapy and that cancers may not appear without longer term use [75].

The level of risk attributable to use of combined EPT for more than 5 years is equivalent to the risk associated with other biological determinants (early menarche, late menopause, first birth after age 30, failure to breast feed, postmenopausal obesity) or lifestyle choices (regular use of alcohol, failure to exercise etc.) [76, 77].

Based on the level of risk "attributable " to MHT Collins has concluded that "When menopausal women present with distressing vasomotor symptoms, they can be reassured that short term (less than 5 years) use of either combined EPT or E alone will have little appreciable effect on their personal breast cancer risk. Longer term use increases risk to a level similar to risks that many women accept through lifestyles that expose them to daily alcohol ingestion, lack of regular exercise and postmenopausal obesity" [66].

For women who need MHT for control of distressing VMS and those at high risk for osteoporosis where other therapies may be poorly tolerated continued use beyond 5 years is appropriate after an individualized discussion of benefits and risks [78].

#### Colorectal cancer
Several studies have demonstrated a reduction in colorectal cancer incidence [79, 80] and mortality [81] in current users, but not former users of MHT. In the WHI, although the incidence of newly diagnosed colorectal cancers was lower in women on combined estrogen and progestin therapy, there was no survival difference due to more advanced stages of cancer in MHT users [82]. The weight of evidence does not support the use of MHT for colorectal cancer prevention.

#### Ovarian cancer
Several past studies have demonstrated a slight increase in the incidence of serous and endometrioid ovarian cancers and a decrease in mucinous ovarian cancers among women using hormone therapy [83, 84]. This risk disappeared within 2 years of cessation of MHT. The attributable risk was very small with an extra ovarian cancer occurring in 1/8,300 hormone users per year. The WHI did not find an increase in ovarian cancer incidence or mortality among MHT users [85].

**Table 1** Chances of the development of, and death from, breast cancer within the next 10 years for a cohort of 1000 women. With permission from Fletcher SW, Elmore JG. Clinical practice: Mammographic screening for breast cancer. NEJM 2003; 348(17):1672–1680 Reproduced with permission of Massachusetts Medical Society

| Age | Cases of invasive breast cancer | Death from breast cancer (per 1000 women) | Death from any cause |
|---|---|---|---|
| 40 yrs | 15 | 2 | 21 |
| 50 yrs | 28 | 5 | 55 |
| 60 yrs | 37 | 7 | 126 |
| 70 yrs | 43 | 9 | 309 |
| 80 yrs | 35 | 11 | 670 |

### Lung cancer

Reassuring data indicating that MHT has no effect on the incidence of lung cancer has come from several long-term observational studies [86]. A pooled analysis of 6 case control series involving close to 2000 lung cancer patients and a similar number of controls reported by the International Lung Cancer Consortium even suggested that MHT might reduce the risk of lung cancer by 25-30 % [87]. Nevertheless, combined estrogen/progestin therapy has been suggested as a modifying factor in the progression of lung cancer [88]. In the WHI, although MHT did not significantly alter the incidence of lung cancer, mortality from lung cancer was increased in women using combined estrogen/progestin therapy [85].

### Gall bladder disease

Published data have consistently shown that gallbladder disease (gallstones and cholecystectomy rates) are increased in current and former users of MHT (estrogen alone more than combined estrogen/ progestin, and, oral MHT more than transdermal MHT) [89, 90]. In the WHI, there was one additional case of gallbladder disease per 200 women years of MHT use [44]. Estimates suggest that transdermal MHT would avoid 1 cholecystectomy for every 600 women years of use [91].

### Addressing the needs of the perimenopausal and menopausal woman

#### The symptomatic perimenopausal woman

Therapy for intermittent menopausal symptoms (hot flashes and night sweats) of the perimenopause need not be delayed until menopause is confirmed. Rather it is appropriate to begin treatment as soon as distressing symptoms appear. Standard MHT may offer a dosage that is too low to override the intermittent ovarian activity that characterizes the perimenopause. In this case a low dose combined hormonal contraceptive may be ideal for low risk non-smokers since it provides menstrual cycle regulation, suppression of vasomotor symptoms,

and contraception. For smokers or individuals at higher risk for cardiovascular complications (obesity, immobility or diabetes) an alternative would be to combine a progestin releasing intrauterine system with systemic transdermal estrogen. The device will suppress bleeding and afford contraception while the transdermal estrogen alleviates vasomotor symptoms.

#### The symptomatic menopausal woman

For women who present after menopause is clearly established it is first important to elucidate the nature and severity of symptoms, risk factors for CVD, osteoporosis and cancer, and the extent of any co-morbidities. Ideally co-morbidities like diabetes, hypertension or dyslipidemia should be addressed before MHT is commenced. Before MHT is started a physical examination is generally wise to evaluate for hypertension or any preexisting breast or pelvic abnormalities. An endometrial biopsy or ultrasound to assess the endometrium should be considered if any abnormal uterine bleeding has occurred in the preceding months.

After a review of anticipated benefits and possible risks, a joint decision between patient and practitioner should be reached about the initial dosage, route of delivery, type of estrogen and progestin and regimen. Estrogen, either by itself or with progestins, is the most consistently effective therapy for hot flashes and night sweats.

Low-dose estrogen (doses of 0.3 mg of conjugated equine estrogen, 0.5 mg of oral micronized estradiol, 25 ug of transdermal estradiol, or 2.5 mg of ethinyl estradiol) has been shown to be effective for many women, although some women require a higher dose for relief of hot flashes [92, 93]. No convincing clinical evidence suggests that one product is safer or more efficacious than the other. Initial relief from hot flashes is generally rapid (within 1 week) but may take longer when treatment is initiated with these very low doses [24].

In the absence of specific risk factors, route of delivery can often be decided by the woman who will know best how she can maintain therapy. Observational studies suggest that transdermal delivery may be associated with a reduced risk of VTE and possibly stroke [94]. Therefore when specific risk factors for these conditions exist (smoking, obesity, immobility, or a known personal/family history of thrombophilia) a transdermal approach should be recommended.

Which progestin to use in women with a uterus has been the subject of considerable debate. Medroxyprogesterone acetate (MPA) has been widely employed in MHT throughout North America for several decades. It was chosen for the WHI investigation because of its popularity and widespread use at the time. Since then questions have surfaced about the relative safety of different progestins with some arguing for a switch to natural progesterone

[92] and others arguing that experimental data on MPA have not translated to clinical outcomes and that continued short term use of MPA is safe [95]. Used cyclically the progestin dosage is MPA 5 mg or progesterone 200 mg for 10–12 days per month. With very low doses of estrogen, especially if progestin causes side effects, progestin treatment may be administered less frequently (every two or three months). For continuous combined therapy the usual progestin dosage is MPA is 2.5 mg or progesterone is 100 mg daily. Other specific combined formulations offer a fixed dose of estrogen and progestin in a single tablet.

Traditionally, MHT employed a regimen that allowed a one week hormone-free interval per month during which time a small amount of scheduled bleeding might occur. At these very low doses there is often minimal endometrial growth and little, if any, withdrawal bleeding. On the other hand, the hormone free week is often punctuated by return of distressing vasomotor symptoms. This has led to a variety of continuous regimens employing a daily combination of estrogen and progestin in women with a uterus or estrogen alone for women after hysterectomy. Personal tolerance to spotting or preferences for scheduled cyclic bleeding may help determine whether a continuous combined MHT regimen would be preferred to a cyclic regimen with monthly withdrawal bleeding.

Counselling should include what initial side effects to anticipate (breast tenderness, spotting, discharge etc.) and when a follow-up evaluation is warranted (unscheduled bleeding after 6 months). Generally, since the peak benefit for vasomotor symptoms occurs at 1 month after initiation, a follow-up appointment in two months works well for a review. Remember to enquire about whether the systemic therapy is adequately correcting any vaginal dryness and dyspareunia – if not, add a prescription for vaginal estrogen. If symptom control is good, and the woman is satisfied, a one-year prescription and annual review is appropriate.

Regular monitoring of bone mineral density is not required while on MHT as long as there are no other significant risk factors for osteoporosis [19]. MHT may be continued for as long as the distressing symptoms persist for which the treatment was started. A brief (eg. 2 week) break from MHT will allow women to rapidly discern whether continued treatment is necessary for relief of symptoms. Among women who stopped MHT after the publication of the WHI, 25 % resumed therapy, presumably due to severity of symptoms [93, 96]. Periodic review of the need for treatment and an individualized discussion of benefits and risks is appropriate when the prescription is renewed. Often women will realize when therapy is no longer needed for control of vasomotor symptoms and this would be an appropriate time to discontinue systemic therapy. When systemic treatment is stopped it is important for the health care provider to counsel about the possible development of Genitourinary Syndrome of Menopause and therapeutic options available to prevent this. As well, in anticipation of accelerated bone loss in the next few years, a baseline BMD with follow-up in 1.5 - 2 years is appropriate.

## Conclusions

The perimenopause and menopause are periods of life that can disrupt the quality of life for many women, so an understanding of the pathophysiology and the potential consequences of waning ovarian estrogen production can inform accurate counselling and management. Most women considering MHT at this time of life can be informed that risks are few and that in fact, the benefits extend well beyond the control of vasomotor symptoms that precipitated the visit. Regular follow-up with attention to co-morbidities and periodic review of individual benefits and risks will allow for optimal duration of treatment.

**Abbreviations**
CAC: Coronary artery calcification; CAD: Coronary artery disease; CAM: Complementary and alternative medicine; CVD: Cardiovascular disease; EPT: Estrogen and progestin therapy; GSM: Genitourinary syndrome of menopause; MHT: Menopausal hormone therapy; MPA: Medroxyprogesterone acetate; SSRI: Selective serotonin reuptake inhibitors; VSM: Vasomotor symptoms; WHI: Women's health initiative.

**Competing interests**
Dr. Robert Reid has worked as a consultant and on advisory boards for the following companies:
Bayer Canada Inc
Pfizer Canada Inc
Searchlight Inc
Actavis Canada
Aspen Pharma
He sits on a Data and Safety Monitoring Board for a number of ongoing Merck clinical research trials.
He has received grants in aid of research from Ferring Canada Inc.
Dr. Bryden Magee has worked on an advisory board for Pfizer Canada Inc.
The authors declare that they have no competing interests.

**Authors' contributions**
RLR carried out the extensive literature review and initial manuscript development. BAM assisted in manuscript development, editorial review prior to submission and revisions in response to reviewers/editor feedback. All authors read and approved the final manuscript.

**References**
1. Brown S. Shock, terror and controversy: how the media reacted to the Women's Health Initiative. Climacteric. 2012;15:275–80.
2. McIntyre RS, Konarski JZ, Grigoriadis S, Fan NC, Mancini DA, Fulton KA, et al. Hormone replacement therapy and antidepressant prescription patterns: a reciprocal relationship. CMAJ. 2005;172(1):57–9.
3. Utian WH. Feminine Forever, Round 2: The Bioidentical Cult. Menopause Management. 2007;16:6–10.
4. Anonymous. Drugs for menopausal symptoms. Med Lett Drugs Ther. 2012;54(1391):41–3.
5. Pinkerton JV. Think Twice Before Prescribing Custom-Compounded Bioidentical Hormone Therapy. J Women's Health. 2014;23(8):631–3.

6. Reid RL. Translating the latest scientific advances into clinical practice. JOGC. 2002;24(10):771–4. 776–779.

7. Langer RD, Manson JA, Allison MA. Have we come full circle or moved on? The Women's Health Initiative 10 yrs on. Climacteric. 2012;15:206–12.

8. Stuenkel CA, Gass MLS, Manson JE, Lobo RA, Pal L, Rebar RW, et al. A decade after the Women's Health Initiative- the experts do agree. Fertil Steril. 2012;98(2):313–4.

9. Hale GE, Hughes CL, Burger HG, Robertson DM, Fraser IS. Atypical estradiol secretion and ovulation patterns caused by luteal out-of-phase (LOOP) events underlying irregular ovulatory menstrual cycles in the menopausal transition. Menopause. 2009;16(1):50–9.

10. WHO Scientific Group. Research on Menopause in the 1990s. Report of a WHO Scientific Group. WHO Technical Report Series. 1996;866:1–107.

11. Harlow SD, Gass M, Hall JE, Lobo R, Maki P, Rebar RW et al. Executive summary of the Stages of Reproductive Aging +10: Adressing the unfinished agenda of staging reproductive aging. Menopause. 2012;19(4):387–95.

12. Gold EB, Block G, Crawford S, Lachance L, FitzGerald G, Miracle H, et al. Lifestyle and demographic factors in relation to vasomotor symptoms: baseline results from the Study of Women's Health Across the Nation. SWAN study. Am J Epidemiol. 2004;159:1189.

13. Guthrie JR, Dennerstein L, Taffe JR, Lehert P, Burger HG. The menopausal transition: a 9-year prospective population-based study. The Melbourne Women's Midlife Health Project. Climacteric. 2004;7(4):375–89.

14. Szoeke CE, Cicuttini F, Guthrie J, Dennerstein L. Self-reported arthritis and the menopause. Climacteric. 2005;8(1):49–55.

15. Toffol E, Heikinheimo O, Partonen T. Hormone therapy and mood in perimenopausal and postmenopausal women: a narrative review. Menopause. 2015;22(5):564–78.

16. Levine KB, Williams RE, Hartmann KE. Vulvovaginal atrophy is strongly associated with female sexual dysfunction among sexually active postmenopausal women. Menopause. 2008;15:661–7.

17. Raz R, Stamm W. A controlled trial of intravaginal estriol in postmenopausal women with recurrent urinary tract infections. N Engl J Med. 1993;329:753–6.

18. El Khoudray SR, Wildman RP, Matthews K, Thurston RC, Bromberg JT, Sutton-Tyrrell K. Endogenous sex hormones impact the progression of subclinical atherosclerosis in women during the menopausal transition. Atherosclerosis. 2012;225:180–6.

19. Khan A, Fortier M. SOGC Menopause and Osteoporosis Working Group. Osteoporosis in Menopause. SOGC Clinical Practice Guideline 312. JOGC. 2014;36(9):S1–S15.

20. Wellons M, Ouyang P, Schreiner P, Herrington DM, Vaidya D. Early menopause predicts future coronary heart disease and stroke: the Multi-Ethnic Study of Atherosclerosis. Menopause. 2012;19(10):1081–7.

21. Magliano M. Menopausal arthralgia: Fact or fiction. Maturitas. 2010;76:29–33.

22. Chlebowski RT, Cirillo DJ, Eaton CB, Stefanick ML, Pettinger M, Carbone LD, et al. Estrogen alone and joint symptoms in the Women's Health Initiative randomized trial. Menopause. 2013;20(6):600–8.

23. Maclennan A, Broadbent JL, Lester S, Moore V. Oral oestrogen and combined oestrogen/progestogen therapy versus placebo for hot flushes. Cochrane Database Syst Rev. 2004;4:CD002978.

24. ACOG Committee opinion. Vasomotor Symptoms. Obstet Gynecol. 2004;4:106S–17S.

25. Rigg LA, Hermann H, Yen SS. Absorption of estrogen from vaginal creams. N Engl J Med. 1978;298(4):195–7.

26. Gallagher JC, Levine JP. Preventing osteoporosis in symptomatic postmenopausal women. Menopause. 2011;18(1):109–18.

27. Lindsay R, Hart DM, Aitken JM, MacDonald EB, Anderson JB, Clarke AC. Long-term prevention of postmenopausal osteoporosis by oestrogen. Evidence for an increased bone mass after delayed onset of oestrogen treatment. Lancet. 1976;1(7968):1038–41.

28. Gallagher JC, Rapuri PB, Haynatzki G, Detter JR. Effect of discontinuation of estrogen, calcitriol, and the combination of both on bone density and bone markers. JCEM. 2002;87(11):4914–23.

29. Reid RL, Abramson BL, Blake J, Desindes S, Dobin S, Johnston S, et al; SOGC Menopause and Osteoporosis Working Group. Managing menopause: SOGC Clinical Practice Guideline 312. JOGC. 2014;36(9):S1–S80.

30. Allison MA, Manson JE. Observational studies and clinical trials of menopausal hormone therapy: can they both be right? Menopause. 2006;13(1):1–3.

31. Hodis HN, Mack WJ. Hormone therapy and coronary artery calcification. N Engl J Med. 2007;357(12):1252–3.

32. Grodstein F, Manson JE, Colditz GA, Willett WC, Speizer FE, Stampfer MJ. A prospective, observational study of postmenopausal hormone therapy and primary prevention of cardiovascular disease. Ann Intern Med. 2000;133(12):933–41.

33. Allison MA, Manson JE, Langer RD, Carr JJ, Rossouw JE, Pettinger MB, et al. Oophorectomy, hormone therapy, and subclinical coronary artery disease in women with hysterectomy: the Women's Health Initiative coronary artery calcium study. Menopause. 2008;15(4):639–47.

34. Manson JE, Allison MA, Rossouw JE, Carr JJ, Langer RD, Hsia J, et al. Estrogen Therapy and Coronary-Artery Calcification. N Engl J Med. 2007;356:2591–602.

35. Allison MA, Manson JE, Aragaki A, Langer RD, Rossouw J, Curb D, et al. Vasomotor symptoms and coronary artery calcium in postmenopausal women. Menopause. 2010;17(6):1136–45.

36. Hulley S, Grady D, Bush T, Furberg C, Herrington D, Riggs B, et al. For the Heart and Estrogen/ progestin replacement study (HERS) Research Group. Randomized trial of estrogen plus progestin for secondary prevention of coronary heart disease in postmenopausal women. JAMA. 1998;280(7):605–13.

37. Salpeter SR, Walsh JME, Greyber E, Salpeter EE. Coronary heart disease events associated with hormone therapy in younger and older women: a meta-analysis. J Gen Intern Med. 2006;21:363–6.

38. Rossouw JE, Prentice RL, Manson JE, Wu L, Barad D, Barnabei VM, et al. Postmenopausal hormone therapy and risk of cardiovascular disease by age and years since menopause. JAMA. 2007;297(13):1465–77.

39. Holm P, Andersen HL, Andersen MR, Erhardtsen E, Steen S. The direct antiatherogenic effect of estrogen is present, absent or reversed, depending on the state of the arterial endothelium: A time course study in cholesterol-clamped rabbits. Circulation. 1999;100:1727.

40. Grodstein F, Manson JA, Stampfer MJ. Hormone therapy and coronary heart disease: The role of time since menopause and age at hormone initiation. J Women's Health. 2006;15(1):35–44.

41. Clarkson TB. Estrogen effects on arteries vary with stage of reproductive life and extent of subclinical atherosclerosis progression. Menopause. 2007;14(3):373–84.

42. Depypere HT, Tummers P, De Bacquer D, De Backer G, Do M, Dhont M. Number of women needed in a prospective trial to prove potential cardiovascular benefit of hormone replacement therapy. Climacteric. 2007;10:238–43.

43. Margolis KL, Bonds DE, Rodabough RJ, Tinker L, Phillips LS, Allen C, et al. Effect of oestrogen plus progestin on the incidence of diabetes in postmenopausal women: results from the Women's Health Initiative Hormone Trial. Diabetologia. 2004;47:1175–87.

44. Manson JE, Chlebowski RT, Stefanick ML, Aragaki Ak, Rossouw JE, Prentice RL, et al. Menopausal hormone therapy and health outcomes during the intervention and extended post stopping phases of the Women's Health Initiative randomized trials. JAMA. 2013;310(13):1353–68.

45. Sites CK, L'Hommedieu GD, Toth MJ, Brochu M, Cooper BC, Fairhurst PA. The effect of hormone replacement therapy on body composition, body fat distribution, and insulin sensitivity in menopausal women: a randomized double blind, placebo controlled trial. J Clin Endocrinol Metab. 2005;90:2701–7.

46. Norman RJ, Flight IH, Rees MC. Oestrogen and progestogen hormone replacement therapy for peri-menopause and post-menopausal women: Weight and body fat distribution. Cochrane Database Syst Rev. 2000;2011(4):CD001018.

47. Kim C, Golden SH, Kong S, Nan B, Mather KJ, Barrett-Connor E. Diabetes Prevention Program Research Group. Does hormone therapy affect blood pressure in the Diabetes Prevention Program? Menopause. 2014;21(5):477–83.

48. Atkin CK, Smith SW, McFeters C, Ferguson V. A comprehensive analysis of breast cancer news coverage in leading media outlets focusing on environmental risks and prevention. J Health Commun. 2008;13(1):3–19.

49. Deeks A, Zoungas S, Teede H. Risk perception in women: a focus on menopause. Menopause. 2008;15(2):304–9.

50. Silverstein MD, Heit JA, Mohr DN, Petterson TM, O'Fallon WM, Melton LJ 3rd. Trends in the incidence of deep vein thrombosis and pulmonary embolism. Arch Intern Med. 1998;158:585–93.

51. Cushman M, Kuller LH, Prentice R, Rodabough RJ, Psaty BM, Stafford RS, et al. Women's Health Initiative Investigators. Estrogen plus progestin and the risk of venous thromboembolism. JAMA. 2004;292:1573–80.

52. Blondon M, Wiggins KL, McKnight B, Psaty BM, Rice KM, Heckbert SR, et al. The association of smoking with venous thrombosis in women. A population-based, case–control study. Thromb Haemost. 2013;109:891–6.

53. Gavish I, Brenner B. Air travel and risk of thromboembolism. Intern Emerg Med. 2011;6:113–6.

54. Laliberte F, Dea K, Duh MS, Kahler KH, Rolli M, Lefebvre P. Does the route of administration for estrogen hormone therapy impact the risk of venous thromboembolism? Estradiol transdermal system versus oral estrogen-only hormone therapy. Menopause. 2011;18(10):1052–9.

55. Sweetland S, Beral V, Balkwill A, Liu B, Benson VS, Canonico M, et al. Venous thromboembolism risk in relation to use of different types of postmenopausal hormone therapy in a large prospective study. J Thromb Haemost. 2012;10(11):2277–86.

56. Wassertheil-Smoller S, Hendrix SL, Limacher M, Heiss G, Kooperberg C, Baird A, et al. The effect of estrogen and progestin on stroke in postmenopausal women. The Women's Health Initiative: a randomized trial. JAMA. 2003;289:2673–84.

57. Hendrix SL, Wassertheil-Smoller S, Johnson KC, Howard BV, Kooperberg C, Rossouw JE, et al. WHI Investigators. Effects of conjugated equine estrogen on stroke in the Women's Health Initiative. Circulation. 2006;113:2425–34.

58. Birge SS. Estrogen and stroke: a case for low-dose estrogen. Menopause. 2006;13(5):719–20.

59. Renoux C, Dell'Aniello S, Garbe E, Suissa S. Transdermal and oral hormone replacement therapy and the risk of stroke: a nested case–control study. BMJ. 2010;340:c2519.

60. Kurman RJ, Kaminski PF, Norris HJ. The behavior of endometrial hyperplasia: a long-term study of "untreated" hyperplasia in 170 patients. Cancer. 1985;56:403–12.

61. Pickar JH, Thorneycroft I, Whitehead M. Effects of hormone replacement therapy on the endometrium and lipid parameters: a review of randomized trials, 1985–1995. Am J Obstet Gynecol. 1998;178(5):1087–99.

62. Somboonporn W, Panna S, Temtanakitpaisan T, Kaewrudee S, Soontrapa S. Effects of the levonorgestrel-releasing intrauterine system plus estrogen therapy in perimenopausal and postmenopausal women: systematic review and meta-analysis. Menopause. 2011;18:1060–6.

63. Santen RJ, Kagan R, Altomare CJ, Komm B, Mirkin S, Taylor HS. Current and evolving approaches to individualizing estrogen receptor-based therapy for menopausal women. J Clin Endocrinol Metab. 2014;99:733–47.

64. King S, Pink Ribbons Inc. Breast Cancer and the Politics of Philanthropy. Minneapolis, Minn: University of Minnesota Press; 2008.

65. Kaunitz AM. Hormone therapy and breast cancer risk: Trumping fear with facts. Menopause. 2006;13(2):160–3.

66. Collins JA. Hormones and breast cancer. Should practice be changed? Obstet Gynecol. 2006;108(6):1352.

67. Fletcher SW, Elmore JG. Clinical practice: Mammographic screening for breast cancer. NEJM. 2003;348(17):1672–80.

68. The Writing Group for the WHI Investigators. Risks and benefits of estrogen plus progestin in healthy post-menopausal women: principal results of the Women's Health Initiative randomized controlled trial. JAMA. 2002;288:321–33.

69. Anderson GL, Chlebowski RT, Aragaki AK, Kuller LH, Manson JE, Gass M, et al. Conjugated equine oestrogen and breast cancer incidence and mortality in postmenopausal women with hysterectomy: extended follow-up of the Women's Health Initiative randomized placebo-controlled trial. Lancet Oncol. 2012;13:476–86.

70. The Writing Group for the WHI Investigators. Effects of Conjugated Equine Estrogen in Postmenopausal Women With Hysterectomy The Women's Health Initiative Randomized Controlled Trial. JAMA. 2004;291(14):1701–12.

71. LaCroix AZ, Chlebowski RT, Manson JE, Aragaki AK, Johnson KC, Martin L, et al. WHI Investigators. Health Outcomes After Stopping Conjugated Equine Estrogens Among Postmenopausal Women With Prior Hysterectomy A Randomized Controlled Trial. JAMA. 2011;305(13):1305–14.

72. Jick SS, Hagberg KW, Kaye JA, Jick H. Postmenopausal estrogen-containing hormone therapy and risk of breast cancer. Obstet Gynecol. 2009;113:74–80.

73. Collaborative Group on Hormonal Factors in Breast Cancer. Breast cancer and hormone replacement therapy: collaborative reanalysis of data from 51 epidemiological studies of 52,705 women with breast cancer and 108,411 women without breast cancer. Lancet. 1997;350(9084):1047–59.

74. Colditz GA, Hankinson SE, Hunter DJ, Willett WC, Manson JE, Stampfer MJ, et al. The use of estrogens and progestins and the risk of breast cancer in postmenopausal women. N Engl J Med. 1995;32(24):1589–93.

75. Li CI, Malone KE, Porter PL, Weiss NS, Tang MT, Cushing-Haugen KL, et al. Relationship between long durations and different regimens of hormone therapy and breast cancer risk. JAMA. 2003;289:3254–63.

76. Sprague BL, Trentham-Dietz A, Egan KM, Titus-Ernstoff L, Hamptom JM, Newcomb PA. Proportion of invasive breast cancer attributable to risk factors modifiable after menopause. Am J Epidemiol. 2008;168(4):404–11.

77. Singletary SE. Rating the risk factors for breast cancer. Ann Surg. 2003;237(4):474–82.

78. Reid RL. STOP enforcing a 5-year rule for menopausal hormone therapy - START individualizing therapy to optimize health and quality of life. OBG Management. 2013;25(12):24–8.

79. Grodstein F, Newcomb PA, Stampfer MJ. Postmenopausal hormone therapy and the risk of colorectal cancer: a review and meta-analysis. Am J Med. 1999;106:574–82.

80. Lin KJ, Cheung WY, Giovannucci EL. The effect of estrogen vs combined estrogen-progestogen therapy on the risk of colorectal cancer. Intern J Cancer. 2012;130(2):419–30.

81. Chan JA, Meyerhard JA, Chan AT, Giovannucci EL, Coldit GA, Fuchs CS. Hormone replacement therapy and survival after colorectal cancer diagnosis. J Clin Oncol. 2006;24:5680–6.

82. Simon MS, Chlebowski RT, Wactawski-Wende J, Johnson KC, Muckovitz A, Kato I, et al. Estrogen plus progestin and colorectal cancer incidence and mortality. J Clin Oncol. 2012;30(32):3983–90.

83. Morch LS, Lokkegaard E, Andreasen AH, Kjaer SK, Lidegaard O. Hormone therapy and different ovarian cancers: a national cohort study. Amer J Epidemiol. 2012;175(12):1234–42.

84. Koskela-Niska V, Lyytinen H, Riska A, Pukkala E, Ylikorkala O. Ovarian cancer risk in Ovarian cancer risk in postmenopausal women using estradiol-progestin therapy - a nationwide study. Climacteric. 2013;16(1):48–53.

85. Taylor HS, Manson JE. Update in hormone therapy use in menopause. JCEM. 2011;96(2):255–64.

86. Clague J, Reynolds P, Sullivan-Halley J, Ma H, Lacey JV Jr, Henderson KD, et al. Menopausal hormone therapy does not influence lung cancer risk: results from the California Teachers Study. Cancer Epidemiol Biomarkers Prev. 2011;20(3):560–4.

87. Pesatori AC, Carugno M, Consonni D, Hung RJ, Papadoupolos A, Landi MT, et al. Hormone use and risk for lung cancer: a pooled analysis from the International Lung Cancer Consortium. Brit J Cancer. 2013;109(7):1954–64.

88. Pines A. Postmenopausal hormone therapy and lung cancer. Climacteric. 2011;14(2):212–4.

89. Simonsen MH, Erichsen R, Froslev T, Rungby J, Sorensen HT. Postmenopausal estrogen therapy and risk of gallstone disease: a population-based case–control study. Drug Saf. 2013;36(12):1189–97.

90. Nordenvall C, Oskarsson V, Sadr-Azodi O, Orsini N, Wolk A. Postmenopausal hormone replacement therapy and the risk of cholecystectomy: a prospective cohort study. Scand J Gastroenterology. 2014;49(1):109–13.

91. Liu B, Beral V, Balkwill A, Green J, Sweetland S, Reeves G; Million Women Study Collaborators. Gallbladder disease and use of transdermal versus oral hormone replacement therapy in postmenopausal women: prospective cohort study. BMJ. 2008;337:a386.

92. Notelovitz M, Lenihan JP, McDermott M, Kerber IJ, Nanavati N, Arce J. Initial 17beta-estradiol dose for treating vasomotor symptoms. Obstet Gynecol. 2000;95:726–31.

93. National Institutes of Health State-of-the-Science Conference Statement. Management of Menopause-Related Symptoms. Ann Intern Med. 2005;142:1003–13.

94. Simon JA. What if the Women's Health Initiative had used transdermal estradiol and oral progesterone instead? Menopause. 2014;21(7):769–83.

95. Stanczyk FZ, Bhavnani BR. Use of medroxyprogesterone acetate for hormone therapy in postmenopausal women: is it safe? J Steroid Biochem Mol Biol. 2014;142:30–8.

96. Grady D, Ettinger B, Tosteson A, Pressman A, Macer J. Discontinuing postmenopausal hormone therapy: predictors of difficulty stopping. Obstet Gynecol. 2003;102:1233–9.

# 20

# The course of depressive symptoms during the postmenopause

Katherine E Campbell[1]*†, Cassandra E. Szoeke[2]† and Lorraine Dennerstein[1]†

## Abstract

As the Australian population ages, significantly more women are entering the postmenopausal stage of the climacteric, yet research focusing on the prevalence of depressive symptoms in this stage of ovarian ageing is scarce. This review will examine the information provided by studies that have a cohort with data of adequate duration to explore depressive symptom prevalence in the early and late postmenopause. Longitudinal epidemiological studies of women transitioning through the postmenopause that included measures of mood and/or depressive symptoms were identified through searches of MEDLINE (1980-2014) and PsycINFO (1980-2014) databases. Population based studies with at least two time points of assessment were included. Longitudinal studies of ageing that did not categorise women as postmenopausal were not included, as this was outside the scope of this review.

Prevalence estimates of depressive symptoms varied between studies and ranged from 8.5 % to 25.7 % with percentages between 22 and 25 % being most consistently reported. Surgical postmenopause groups reported higher ratings of depressive symptoms at 18-42 % and higher incidence of major depressive disorder in all but one study. The prevalence of Major Depressive Disorder also varied with ranges from <1 % to 42 % reported. Wide ranges in prevalence were reported in the literature. Differences in definitions, inconsistent sample sizes and varying measures make it difficult to compare results across studies. The specific inclusions and exclusions of sub-samples of larger cohorts are at times inconsistent with epidemiological acquisition and, as such, impact upon generalizability of results to a healthy population.

**Keywords:** Postmenopause, Depressive symptoms, Centre for Epidemiological Studies Depression Scale (CESD)

## Background

Research consistently demonstrates a higher occurrence of depressive disorders and depressive symptoms in women compared to men [1, 2]. This difference has been demonstrated in a variety of contexts including population studies, hospital admissions, suicide attempts and the prescription of anti-depressant medication [3]. The gender difference begins during adolescence and continues into old age, corresponding roughly with a woman's reproductive years [4]. It has been proposed that changes in ovarian sex steroids may be a contributing factor in the higher vulnerability for women to develop a depressive disorder [5]. For this reason it has been suggested that there are certain windows of

vulnerability for the development of depression across the lifespan and there has been significant research conducted into the characteristics of depression in women in specific age ranges or during biological transitions such as adolescence, the postpartum period and late-life [6].

There are a number of studies which have examined mood in the menopausal transition, a time representing significant changes in physiology associated with ovarian ageing [7, 8]. However, there is limited literature examining the period of time directly following the final menstrual period, a physiological marker corresponding to the onset of early postmenopause. With the recent updates to the staging system used to characterise menopausal status [9], the consistent definition of the postmenopausal stages will allow for a greater understanding of depressive symptoms in this particular stage of reproductive ageing.

Unique hormonal changes take place in the first two years following the final menstrual period and coincide

---

* Correspondence: katherine.campbell.psy@gmail.com
†Equal contributors
[1]Department of Psychiatry, University of Melbourne, Victoria, Australia
Full list of author information is available at the end of the article

with the early postmenopausal stage of reproductive ageing as outlined in the new staging system used to characterise the menopausal transition [9]. While the final menstrual period (FMP) is a distinct and measurable physiological event in the reproductive aging cycle, it is not commonly used as a reference point for understanding the temporal characteristics of depressive symptoms across the postmenopausal period. Given the variability of length of certain menopausal stages, the FMP could serve as a consistent marker for future research examining mood in the menopause. If uniformly included in future publications, calculating years preceding or following FMP would allow for comparability across studies regardless of the definition used to categorize the menopausal stage. As our understanding of ovarian ageing advances, this physiological marker would remain a stable frame of reference regardless of amendments to the broader reproductive ageing stages.

Several longitudinal epidemiological studies were initiated to specifically examine the association between mood and menopause [10–12]. As these studies have matured those remaining now have data available on women who have entered the postmenopausal period and in some cases transitioned from early postmenopause into late postmenopause [12, 13]. The data provided in these longitudinal studies will improve our understanding of the characteristics of depressive symptoms in the postmenopausal period.

It has been estimated that by 2030, 1.2 billion women will be postmenopausal, compared to 470 million in 1990 [14]. The onset of postmenopause is variable due to the individual discrepancy in the occurrence of the final menstrual period. As the average age of postmenopause onset is between 50 and 52 years and the current life expectancy of a female in high-income countries is 82 years [15], the length of postmenopause is, on average, approximately thirty years in developed countries. As the female population ages, an increasing number of women will be experiencing postmenopause and an understanding of the risk factors associated with this period will become increasingly important.

The postmenopausal period can encompass up to a third of a woman's life, yet the distinction between the early and late stages of the postmenopause are rarely focused upon. Recent research examining the ongoing changes in estradiol and follicle stimulating hormone (FSH) levels demonstrate that distinct and observable changes in hormone levels continue for several years after the perimenopause and into the postmenopause [16]. Consistent endocrinological patterns were used to determine the reproductive stages of ageing staging system [9]. Randolph and colleagues demonstrated that the most rapid changes in FSH and estradiol occur in the two years preceding and two years following the final

menstrual period, regardless of the age at which FMP occurs [17]. This finding highlights the need to distinguish between ovarian ageing and chronological ageing when exploring the impact of menopausal status on depressive symptoms. The experience of the final menstrual period is an essential reference point in determining if changes in sexual hormones affect the risk of experiencing depressive symptoms independent of age. The recent changes in the understanding of the early postmenopause, and in turn the classification system used to describe it, emphasises the need for further study of this specific stage of the menopausal transition. Despite this, few studies identify the early postmenopause substages as periods of ovarian ageing with distinct physiological profiles. Rather the early postmenopause is often defined with arbitrary time frames or not defined at all [18]. Research examining depressive symptoms and mood across the early postmenopause, using the updated criteria, is needed.

Reproductive endocrine function has stabilised by late postmenopause [9]. Few studies of the menopausal transition have continued to follow women into late postmenopause. Women experiencing the postmenopause are entering late-life and research on depressive symptoms in this population focuses on somatic concerns and other physiological factors associated with ageing [19]. As data from longitudinal studies becomes available the impact of ovarian ageing on mood from midlife to late-life can be studied specifically.

Midlife transitions can have both a positive and negative impact on mental health issues [20]. Caregiving, changes in marital status and perceived health decline are examples of life transitions that have been shown to increase depressive symptom development in midlife women [20]. Similarly, changes in lifestyle factors and social circumstances that occur between the early stages and late stages of postmenopause may also impact the development of depressive symptoms.

## Postmenopause classification

The most commonly used menopausal status classification systems are the World Health Organisation (WHO) criteria [21] and that developed at the original Stages of Ageing Reproductive Workshop (STRAW) [22]. Both systems define 'postmenopause' as beginning after the final menstrual period (FMP) and continuing for the remainder of a woman's life [9]. The STRAW criteria, and the updated 2011 criteria (STRAW + 10), offer a further breakdown of the postmenopausal transition due to the length of the postmenopausal period. The categories outlined in the STRAW + 10 staging system are illustrated in Fig. 1 [9]. Despite this distinction few epidemiological studies distinguish between early and late

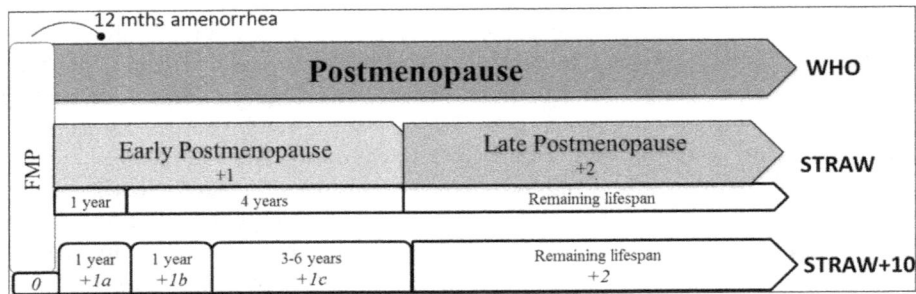

**Fig. 1** Stages of postmenopause with corresponding WHO, STRAW and STRAW + 10 criteria as described in text

postmenopause when reporting on prevalence of depressive symptoms during this period [18, 23, 24].

The early postmenopause stage has been organised into three substages: the first two of one year duration and the third stage varying between three and six years. The first stage is determined retrospectively and represents the twelve months of amenorrhea following the final menstrual period (FMP). Early postmenopause includes a period in which the FSH levels increase and estradiol levels rapidly decrease and move toward stabilisation. Vasomotor symptoms are most likely to occur during this time due to the radical fluctuation in hormones [9].

The third substage of the early postmenopause represents the period of stabilisation of low levels of estradiol and high levels of FSH. Further research is needed to determine the average timing and specific trajectories of change at which stabilisation occurs, however it is thought to be between three and six years. Due to the varied length of the third substage, the overall length of early postmenopause ranges between five and eight years [9].

Late postmenopause follows the early postmenopause stage and continues for the remainder of a woman's life. In this stage reproductive endocrine function has stabilised and further changes in sex steroids are limited [9]. It has been suggested that further research may be required to determine if further declines in FSH occur in very old women [9].

### Defining the postmenopause in examining depression

Despite the clear distinction in physiological profile between the early postmenopausal substages and late postmenopause the majority of studies examining the occurrence of depressive symptoms during postmenopause have not distinguished between these periods and include only a general distinction between early and late postmenopause [13] or no distinction at all [18, 25].

In order to better understand the trajectories of depressive symptom ratings across the postmenopause each of the unique substages of the early and late postmenopause need to be considered. Using the general term 'postmenopause' to compare longitudinal data will

not adequately capture the potential risks associated with the distinct substages of the transition.

Similarly a clear distinction needs to be made between women who experience surgical menopause and those that have a natural menopause [10, 25, 26]. Surgically postmenopausal women have been shown to demonstrate higher scores on measures of depressive symptomology [10, 25, 26]. For this reason any reports of prevalence of depressive symptoms in postmenopausal women needs to consider women who entered the postmenopause due to oophorectomy or hysterectomy as a separate group.

The goal of the following review is to examine the current information available regarding the occurrence of depressive symptoms across the postmenopausal period and to determine research questions where gaps exist in the literature.

### Methods

PsychINFO (1970-2014) and MEDLINE (1975-2014) databases were searched using the following key terms: 'depression', 'depressive disorder', 'depressive symptom', 'negative mood', 'negative affect', 'postmenopause', 'postmenopausal', 'menopausal transition' and 'menopause'. Search results of 648 (PsycINFO) and 9,780 (MEDLINE) articles were initially identified through searches using various combinations of the key terms. These were limited to articles published in English and screened for studies describing longitudinal epidemiological studies of women that had data of adequate duration to report on prevalence of depressive symptoms or depressive disorder during the postmenopause. Studies that included information on risk of experiencing depressive symptoms or depression during postmenopause were also included. Studies exploring major depressive disorder, major depressive episode, mood disorders and depressive symptoms were all reviewed to capture any potential studies for inclusion. Broad search terms were used due to the inconsistency in the definitions and measures being used between, and even within the longitudinal studies. A manual search of journal articles and bibliographies was also conducted to ensure that all relevant materials were examined. This search yielded an additional 200 articles. All abstracts were reviewed for content relevant to prevalence of depressive symptoms in the postmenopausal period.

Longitudinal population based studies of mood and menopause were included if they had at least two time points of assessment with the same cohort, if they specifically defined a postmenopausal group independent of other menopausal status groups, and if they included a standardised measure of self-reported depressive symptoms or a clinically recognised diagnostic tool for assessing Major Depressive Disorder. The following studies were included: the Women's Healthy Ageing Study (WHAP); the Seattle Midlife Women's Health Study (SWMHS); the Study of Women's Health Across the Nation (SWAN); the Manitoba Project; the Penn Ovarian Ageing Study (POAS); and the Eindhoven Perimenopausal Osteoporosis Study (EPOS). Only articles with data pertaining specifically to prevalence or standardised reports of increased risk of depressive symptoms or depressive disorder in the postmenopause are described in this review. Inconsistency in methodology, sample sizes, and analysis techniques made it unreasonable to conduct a meta-analysis without excluding important studies reporting on prevalence.

A number of different measures of depression and depressive symptoms were used by the different longitudinal studies. The most consistently used measure to assess depressive symptom severity was the Centre for Epidemiological Studies Depression Scale (CESD). The CES-D is a self-report scale specifically designed to be used in epidemiological studies to assess the presence of clinical and non-clinical symptoms of depression in the general population. It is one of the most commonly used depression measure in studies of healthy populations [27]. Items assess four areas related to depression: depressed affect, positive affect, somatic activity and interpersonal aspects [28]. The cut off ranges used to categorise normal versus mild to moderate symptoms of depression for the short and full versions are ≥10 and ≥16 respectively [27, 29]. The only other depressive symptom measure used was the Edinburgh Depression Scale, originally developed for use with post-natal women but validated for use with menopausal women [30]. Cut offs of 12 or more are used to determine risk of depression [18].

The Structured Clinical Interview for DSM-IV Axis 1 Disorders (SCID) [31], and Primary Care Evaluation of Mental Disorders (PRIME-MD) [32] were used to assess presence of depressive disorders. The SCID is a clinician administered diagnostic tool used to assess for the presence of past or current major depressive disorders based on DSM criteria. The PRIME-MD is a standardised, validated diagnostic assessment used to diagnose mood,

anxiety, alcohol and eating disorders, also using DSM criteria.

## Results

A summary of sample sizes, participant exclusion criteria, definition of postmenopausal stage and the measurements used varied between, and at times within, the larger cohort studies and have been outlined in Table 1.

### The Penn Ovarian Ageing Study

The Penn Ovarian Ageing Study (POAS) began recruitment in 1996. A baseline cross sectional sample of 436 women aged between 35 and 47 years from Pennsylvania were recruited [33]. The findings from the Penn study include results from the assessment of both depressive symptom scores and clinical diagnosis of Major Depressive Disorder. Symptoms scores were based on the CESD with cut off of at or above 16. Clinical diagnosis was made using the Primary Care Evaluation of Mental Disorders (PRIME-MD) assessment tool which determined a diagnosis of current mood disorder at each period of assessment. Six assessments were conducted at eight month intervals across approximately four years. As postmenopausal women were excluded at baseline, the maximum length of time since final menstrual period was approximately four years. The age of the postmenopausal group ranged from 44 to 51 years. The mean CESD scores for the postmenopausal group as they transitioned through the third, fourth and fifth assessment periods were: 1.0 ($n = 2$); 6.0 ($n = 4$); and 13.8 ($n = 9$). Participants did not meet criteria for Major Depressive Disorder based on the PRIME-MD at any of these time points. The mean CESD score for the group at the sixth assessment period was 10.6 (normal range) and less than 1 % met criteria for diagnosis of Major Depressive Disorder. Participants were considered as having a history of depression if they met criteria for MDD based on the PRIME-MD at any assessment point in the study. Results of the 2004 study need to be interpreted with caution due to the small sample size, with only 11 women meeting STRAW criteria for postmenopause classification [33].

A much larger sample size was included in the 2014 POAS study, with 203 postmenopausal women included in the analysis [34]. The sample was divided into groups, with CESD scores being reported separately for women with a history of depression ($n = 90$) and women with no history ($n = 113$). History of depression was determined at baseline based on self reported medical history or as determined by the PRIME-MD. The mean age at baseline was 42.8 years. The mean age at FMP was 51.1 years and ranged from 42-58 years. In this study, time since the final menstrual period was used as a marker to determine changing symptom prevalence scores across the

**Table 1** Longitudinal cohort summary of depressive symptom incidence

| Cohort Details | SubSample characteristics | Follow-Up Type and Duration | Sample and Assessment of Depression | Definition of Postmenopause/ PoM Range | Results |
|---|---|---|---|---|---|
| Penn Ovarian Ageing Study (POAS)—Baseline cross section 436 women 35-47 yrs, from Pennsylvania USA, recruited 1996. | Freeman et al., 2004 [33]. PoM $n = 11$ | Six assessments at eight month intervals over four years. | Depressive symptoms: CESD < 16 vs ≥16. Depressive Disorder: Primary Care Evaluation of Mental Disorders (PRIME-MD). | STRAW PoM Maximum Duration: 11 years | CESD mean score 10.6 (pre 12.7, early transition 14.6, late transition 13.1). Diagnosis of MDD <1 % |
| | Freeman et al., 2014 [34]. PoM $n = 203$ | Longitudinal; 14 year FU | Depressive symptoms: CESD < 16; ≥16;≥25. Depressive Disorder: Primary Care Evaluation of Mental Disorders (PRIME-MD). | STRAW + 10; PoM Maximum Duration: 14 years. Also included analysis using years since FMP as reference. | CESD of 16 or greater decreased approximately 15 % each year following FMP. OR for risk of depressive symptoms highest for first two years following FMP. ~35 % of women with a history of depression reported high scores in each postmenopausal year compared to 0-15 % of women with no history. |
| Study of Women's Health Across the Nation (SWAN)—Baseline cross section 16,065 women 40-55 yrs, from 7 geographic regions across the USA, recruited 1995-1997. | Bromberger, et al., 2007 [35]. $n = 2885$ (25 % PoM) PoM $n = $ ~721 | Longitudinal; 5 yr FU | Depressive symptoms: CESD < 16 vs ≥16 | WHO PoM Maximum Duration: 6 years | OR of having CESD score ≥16 in postmenopause (1.57) → significantly higher than premenopause. |
| | Bromberger et al., 2010 [11]. $n = 3296$ (66 % PoM) PoM $n = $ ~2175 | Longitudinal; 8 yr FU | Depressive symptoms: CESD < 16 vs ≥16 | WHO; STRAW PoM Maximum Duration: 9 years | OR of having CESD score ≥16 in postmenopause (1.79) → significantly higher than premenopause. |
| | Bromberger et al., 2011 [13]. $n = 221$ Ancillary SWAN study – Mental Health Study (MHS) – Pittsburgh site. PoM $n = 131$ | Longitudinal; 10 yr FU | Major Depressive Episode: SCID | Early PoM: (≤2 yrs amenorrheic) Late PoM: (≥2 yrs amenorrheic) PoM Maximum Duration: 11 years | PoM 9.8 %. Early PoM significantly greater risk for MDE than premenopause. |
| | Joffe et al., 2012 [26]. $n = 425$ Ancillary SWAN study (MHS) Pittsburgh site. PoM $n = 151$ Surgical PoM $n = 38$ | Longitudinal; 6 yr FU | Past or current Depressive Disorder: SCID | WHO PoM Maximum Duration: 7 years | PoM: 64/151 (42.4 %) met criteria Surgical PoM: 12/38 (31.6 %) met criteria |

**Table 1** Longitudinal cohort summary of depressive symptom incidence (*Continued*)

| | | | | | | |
|---|---|---|---|---|---|---|
| Melbourne Women's Midlife Health Project (MWMHP)/Women's Healthy Ageing Study (WHAP) Baseline cross-section 2001 | Dennerstein et al., 2004 [10]. | 314 women PoM = 207 Surgical PoM = 39 | Longitudinal; initial year of CESD assessment 1991. FU 11 years. | Depressive symptoms: CESD(Brief) < 10 vs ≥10 | STRAW PoM Maximum Duration: 11 years | CESD ≥ 10 PoM: 22 % Surgical PoM: 42 % Mean CESD Score: PoM: 6.7 Surgical PoM: 8.7 |
| women aged 45-55 yrs, from Melbourne Australia, recruited 1990-1991. | Ryan et al., 2009 [5]. | PoM=138 | Longitudinal; 2 yr FU 2002 compared to 2004. | Depressive symptoms: CESD(Brief) < 10 vs ≥10 | STRAW PoM Maximum Duration: 13 years | CESD ≥ 10 PoM: 25.4 % |
| Seattle Midlife Women's Health Study (SMWHS) Baseline cross section 508 (35-55 yrs mean age 41 yrs), from Seattle USA, recruited 1990-1992. | Woods et al., 2008 [39]. | PoM n = 87 | Baseline and 15 year FU. | Depressive symptoms: CESD < 16 vs ≥16 | STRAW Early PoM: 5 yrs from FMP PoM Maximum Duration: 5 years | No significant difference in CESD score between menopausal stages. Small but significant decrease of 0.10 in CESD score each year. |
| Eindhoven Perimenopausal Osteoporosis Study (EPOS) Baseline recruitment 1994-1995. Women born between 1941 and 1947 from Eindhoven, Netherlands. | Maartens et al., 2002 [18]. | T1: 1995 PoM: n = 646 T2: 1998 PoM n = 1379 | Assessment in 1995 and 1998, approximately 3.5 years apart. | Depressive symptoms: Edinburgh Depression Scale (EDS) < 12 vs ≥12 | Amenorrhea for at least one year. PoM Maximum Duration: unknown | T1 N = 646 - Mean EDS: 7.8 EDS > 12 – > 24.2 % T2 N = 1379 - Mean EDS 7.7 EDS >12 – > 25.7 % |
| The Manitoba Project— Baseline cross section 2500 (40-59 yrs),from Manitoba Canada, recruited 1982-1985. | Kaufert, Gilbert & Hassard, 1988 [41]. | T1-T6 PoM. n = 5, 5, 18, 24, 29, 35 | Baseline and 3 years FU with 6 monthly contact. 6 time points. | Depressive symptoms: CESD < 16 vs ≥16 | 12 months without menstruation. PoM Maximum Duration: 3 years | No significant difference in CESD score between menopausal stages. |
| | Kaufert, Gilbert & Tate, 1992 [42]. | T1-T5 PoM. n = 5, 5, 18, 24, 29 | First five time points. | Depressive symptoms: CESD < 16 vs ≥16 | 12 months without menstruation. PoM Maximum Duration: 2.5 years | Relative odds of depression (compared to pre and peri): Non-depressed PoM: 0.87 Depressive history PoM: 0.84 Hysterectomised non-depressed PoM: 1.7 Hysterectomised depressive history PoM: 0.84 |

Prevalence ratings of depressive symptoms or major depressive disorder by cohort. Original cohort baseline details provided furthest left. Details of subsample of cohort used for each article reported separately for purposes of clarity

PoM – postmenopause; ~ - approximately; SurPoM – surgical postmenopause; FU – Follow-up; T - Time point; CESD – Centre for Epidemiological Studies Depression Scale; SCID - Structured Clinical Interview for DSM Disorders; OR – odds ratio years of the postmenopause, with data reported annually up to 7 years post FMP then grouped as 'greater than 8 years'. Overall the number of scores on the CESD of 16 or greater (high scores) decreased approximately 15 % each year, suggesting a gradual decline of depressive symptoms. Approximately 35 % of women with a history of depression reported high scores in each post-menopausal year compared to 0-15 % of women with no history. Women with a history of depression had more than 13 times the risk of experiencing depressive symptoms compared to women with no history.

The odds ratio for risk of depressive symptoms following FMP were highest for the first two stages of the early postmenopause, and decreased steadily across the third substage of early postmenopause for women with a history of depression. Participants in the late postmenopausal stage (grouped as ≥8 years since FMP), were more likely to report depressive symptoms than women in the third sub-stage, but not the first two substages, of early postmenopause. For women with no history of depression 1030 % reported a higher CESD before the FMP and experienced a significant decrease after the second year following menopause with prevalence of 0 % to 15 % reported. The 2014 Penn study is the first to use STRAW + 10 criteria and makes use of the final menstrual period as a means of tracking patterns of individual annual scores across the postmenopause.

**The Study of Women's Health Across the Nation**
Of all the longitudinal studies reporting depressive symptom data the SWAN study has the most robust sample size and has distinguished between early and late postmenopause in at least one of their studies [35]. In the SWAN cohort women were recruited between 1995 and 1997 across seven geographic regions of the United States. The SWAN study also includes large samples from multiple ethnicities including Caucasians, African Americans and Americans with Chinese, Japanese and Hispanic backgrounds.

In the earliest SWAN study reporting depressive symptom prevalence, Bromberger and colleagues used CESD cutoffs of <16 and ≥16 and found that of the 721 postmenopausal women the odds ratio of having mild or moderate levels of depressive symptoms was significantly higher in postmenopause compared to premenopause [35]. In this publication, there was no distinction made between early and late postmenopause. The definition of postmenopause was in keeping with the WHO criteria (no menses in the past 12 months) [35]. The baseline age for the entire cohort was 46.5 years (SD 2.7 years) and included an age range between 42 and 52 years. The mean age for the postmenopause group was not provided separately. Eligibility into the study required no surgical menopause and menses within the last three

months. As the study included a baseline visit and five subsequent annual visits the maximum length of post-menopause was six years.

Higher odds ratio for postmenopause (1.79) compared to premenopause was demonstrated again in their follow up study where this result was confirmed with a larger sample size of 2175 postmenopausal women [36]. The maximum postmenopausal range increased to nine years in this study which reported on the 8th year of follow-up. In 2011, Bromberger and colleagues presented findings from a 10-year follow-up of a subsample of their larger SWAN cohort and specifically examined whether risk factors and prevalence of Major Depressive Disorder were different during the postmenopausal phase. Of the 221 women in this analysis (all of whom were premeno-pausal at study entry), 131 had experienced at least one interview in which they were postmenopausal based on WHO criteria [13]. Those women classified as postmen-opausal were further categorised as early (≤2 years amenorrheic) or late postmenopausal (>2 years amenor-rheic) [30]. Based on the new STRAW + 10 criteria many of these 'late postmenopause' participants would remain in the early postmenopause category which lasts up to 8 years since onset of amenorrhea [9]. The average age at baseline, for the women with no depressive history ($n$ = 152), was 45.7 years, and with depressive history ($n$ = 69) was 45.1 years. The maximum duration of postmen-opause observed during the study was eleven years. They found that women who were in the early postmeno-pausal phase were at greater risk of experiencing a major depressive episode compared to when the women were premenopausal. There was no significant difference for women in the late postmenopausal stage compared to when the women were premenopausal. These findings were based on SCID assessments identifying current or recent major depressive episode measured annually over a ten year period using data from an ancillary SWAN study called the Mental Health Study in which a subset of 221 participants from the Pittsburgh site were in-cluded in the analysis [13].

In a more recent study, the SWAN team looked at the relationship between history of depression and quality of life, again using data from the Pittsburgh cohort of the Mental Health Study [26]. In this study 425 women from the Pittsburgh site underwent annual SCID assessments. The data provided lifetime prevalence of depressive dis-order as well as menopausal status. The mean age at study entry was 46 years for the entire cohort. The mean age of the postmenopausal women was not provided. Of the 425 women, 151 (35 %) were categorised as naturally postmenopausal (as per WHO categorisations). Of these women 64 (42.4 %) met criteria for having ever had de-pressive disorder. This high number may reflect the fact that the definition of depressive disorder was broader than with other studies that considered only a diagnosis of Major Depressive Disorder. The SWAN project defined history of depression as including "an episode of major or minor depression that occurred before the current visit and resolved in the past month" and, current depression defined as: "major or minor depressive episode occurring within the past month, were in partial remission of a major depressive episode that began earlier,…. or had a current episode of dysthymia" [26].

While depressive symptom scales are able to provide a spectrum of scores from normal to severe, a diagnostic classification, such as that used in this SWAN analysis, separates participants into either having a lifetime occurrence of depressive disorder or not. The broad definition of what constituted depressive history must be taken into consideration when looking at the prevalence of depressive disorder in postmenopausal women in this cohort.

The use of specific subsamples and changing definitions for diagnostic classification used by SWAN, highlights the need for caution when generalising across studies, or as seen in this case even when generalising within large epidemiological studies that report findings using different subsamples of the original cohort.

### The Women's Healthy Ageing Project

The Women's Healthy Ageing Project, initiated as the Melbourne Women's Midlife Health Project, is a longitudinal prospective epidemiological study that draws upon a cohort of over 400 Melbourne women who were identified through random digit dialling and contacted by phone in 1991 and commenced involvement in a longitudinal study. Assessments were conducted annually between 1991 and 1999 and were readministered in 2002, 2004 and in 2012. The Affectometer, a measure of negative mood was administered at each time point with a specific measure of depressive symptoms introduced in 2002, and readministered in 2004 and 2012. WHAP is one of the longer prospective studies on mood in women and has consistently demonstrated that negative or depressed moods, as measured by the Affectometer and the CESD, decline as women age and become postmenopausal [37].

In the WHAP cohort depressive symptoms were assessed in 2002, 2004 and 2012 with the Centre for Epidemiological Studies Depression Scale (CESD), 10 item version [38]. A cut-off of 10 was used to distinguish presence of mild or moderate depressive symptoms from normal levels. The criteria used to determine postmenopausal status were based on the STRAW criteria [22]. In 2002, in the 11th year of follow-up, a total of 314 women completed the CESD 10 items. The mean age of the overall cohort was 59.9 years (range 56-67years). Of the 314 women 207 of the cohort had experienced natural menopause and 39 had undergone surgical menopause.

CESD scores indicating mild or moderate symptoms of depression were present in 22 % for the postmenopausal women and 42 % of the surgical postmenopause group with mean scores of 6.7 and 8.7 respectively [10].

In 2004, a subsample of 138 postmenopausal women were included in an analysis of endogenous hormones and depressive symptoms [5]. Surgically postmenopausal women were excluded from analysis. The mean age for the women at the 11th year of follow-up was 60.1 years, ranging from 55.9 to 66.8 years. In the 13th year of follow up, the mean age for the cohort with CESD scores less than 10 ($n = 103$) was 60.3 years and mean years since FMP was 7.0 (SD, 2.3). For those with scores greater than 10 ($n = 35$) mean age was 59.2 with mean years since FMP being 5.9 years (SD 2.5). Of the total postmenopausal sample 25.4 % scored at or above 10 on the CESD [5]. In this sample increased risk of depression symptoms was associated with a decline in total serum estradiol (OR: 3.5; 95 % CI: 1.2-9.9) and with a large increase in FSH levels (OR: 2.6; 95 % CI: 1.0-6.7).

### The Seattle Midlife Women's Health Study

The Seattle Midlife Women's Health Study initially recruited 508 participants between 1990 and 1992 [39]. A subset of 390 women from the original cohort continued to provide data across a 15 year period. In 2008, Woods and colleagues summarised the findings exploring depressed mood across the menopausal transition and into early postmenopause [36]. The overall sample size described in this article was 302, with 87 women assessed as being in early postmenopause, defined by the original STRAW criteria as the first five years since FMP.

This study was the only one to report findings for early postmenopause specifically using the original STRAW criteria. The age range at baseline was 35–55 years with a mean age of 41.4 years. The mean age score for the early postmenopause group was not provided. Woods and colleagues found that age was modestly and negatively related to depressed mood with scores of CES-D decreasing with each year of age. While age was a significant predictor of CES-D score and menopausal stage was not, in models that included stress and family history of depression, age ceased to be a significant predictor. The data indicated a rise in depressive symptom scores in the late menopausal transition stage with a slight trend toward lower CESD scores in the early postmenopause compared with the late reproductive stage. The early postmenopausal stage was not found to be significantly different from other stages of the menopausal transition in relation to higher CESD score.

### The Eindhoven Perimenopausal Osteoporosis Study

The Eindhoven Perimenopausal Osteoporosis Study (EPOS) originally recruited 6648 women born between

1941 and 1947 living in Eindhoven in the Netherlands. The longitudinal phase of the study included 2748 women from this cohort. The baseline assessment was conducted in 1995 with follow-up taking place in 1998, approximately 3.5 years after the initial assessment [18]. In the EPOS study depressive symptomatology was assessed using the Edinburgh Depression Scale (EDS) which commonly uses a cut-off of 12 to identify those at risk for depression [40]. Women were categorised into menopausal status with postmenopause women being those who had amenorrhea for at least a year. Women using hormone therapy (HT) or who had undergone surgical menopause were excluded from analysis. At the first time point of assessment in 1995, 646 postmenopausal women with an average age of 51.3 years completed the EDS. The mean score was 7.8 (SD 6.3) and 24.2 % scored at or above 12 [18].

At the second assessment carried out in 1998, 1379 women were postmenopausal with a mean age of 55.5 years. The mean score on the EDS was 7.7 (SD 6.3) and 25.7 % scores were 12 or above. While the mean score for the EDS was slightly lower at the second time point a higher percentage of women scored 12 or above. An estimation of the range of years since final menstrual period could not be determined as postmenopausal women were included at baseline and no reference was made as to how long they had been postmenopausal.

### The Manitoba Project

The Manitoba Project on Women and Their Health initially began as a cross-sectional mail survey of 2500 women aged 40-59 living in Manitoba, Canada [41]. Of the original cross-sectional cohort, 505 women were asked and agreed to continue in the longitudinal phase of the study. The cohort was assessed via phone interview at six time points spaced six months apart over three years between 1982 and 1985. The CESD was used to determine depressive symptom level and postmenopause was defined as 12 months or more without menstruation.

In analysing 330 women in the cohort who were not hysterectomised at baseline and who had completed CESD at all time-points, no association was shown between higher CESD scores and postmenopause status [41]. As would be expected the sample size for postmenopausal women varied over the study, ranging from 17 (5 %) at the first time point to 116 (35 %) at the sixth time point. When examining the entire cohort (pre, peri and postmenopausal women) the percentage of women scoring ≥16 remained relatively stable across all time points, ranging from 9–11 %. Of those women scoring ≥16 at one interview, 25 % had high scores at two or more other time points. Of all the women taking part in

the study 29 % had a score of ≥16 at least once across the assessment period.

In a re-examination of the data, Kaufert and colleagues compared the risk of developing depressive symptoms during the menopausal transition using data from 469 women who had been involved in the initial five interviews conducted as part of the Manitoba Project [42]. The age range of the cohort at baseline was 45–55 with a mean age of 48.4 years. They found that menopausal status did not significantly alter the likelihood of a woman becoming, or staying depressed. Classification into depressed versus non-depressed groups was based on CESD scores, with those scoring higher than 16 at any point of assessment being considered as depressed (or having a history of depression at following time points). For postmenopausal women who had no history of depression the relative odds of developing depression compared to premenopause and perimenopause was 0.87 and for those with a history the relative odds were 0.84 [42]. According to this study menopausal status did not have any impact on the likelihood of developing depression, however women who had undergone surgical menopause were more vulnerable to developing depression. Non-depressed women having undergone hysterectomy had relative odds of 1.7 while those with a history of depression had odds of 0.84.

A comparison of the maximum duration of the postmenopause reported for each of the subsamples is presented in a standardised format in Fig. 2. An estimation of the maximum years of data available for the postmenopause for each cohort was overlaid on the STRAW +10 staging system for reproductive ageing. The figure highlights the variation in sample sizes used within and between the larger studies. It also shows that the definition of postmenopause used by the studies varies considerably, with some studies describing a period of 2–3 years and others a period of over 15 years [25, 39]. In order to compare findings across studies a more precise indication of years since the final menstrual period should be included.

### Discussion

Standardised depressive symptom measures were used by all of the studies examined in this review. However, not all studies reported on percentage of participants having normal versus mild or moderate symptoms. The SWAN and POAS studies used the CESD full version and the WHAP used the brief version. The Eindhoven study used the EDS. The prevalence scores above the relevant cut offs to determine the presence of mild or moderate depressive symptoms was: 22 % and 25.4 % in WHAP; 24.2 % and 25.7 % in the Eindhoven study. The SWAN study reported higher odds ratio of having depressive symptoms in postmenopause compared to

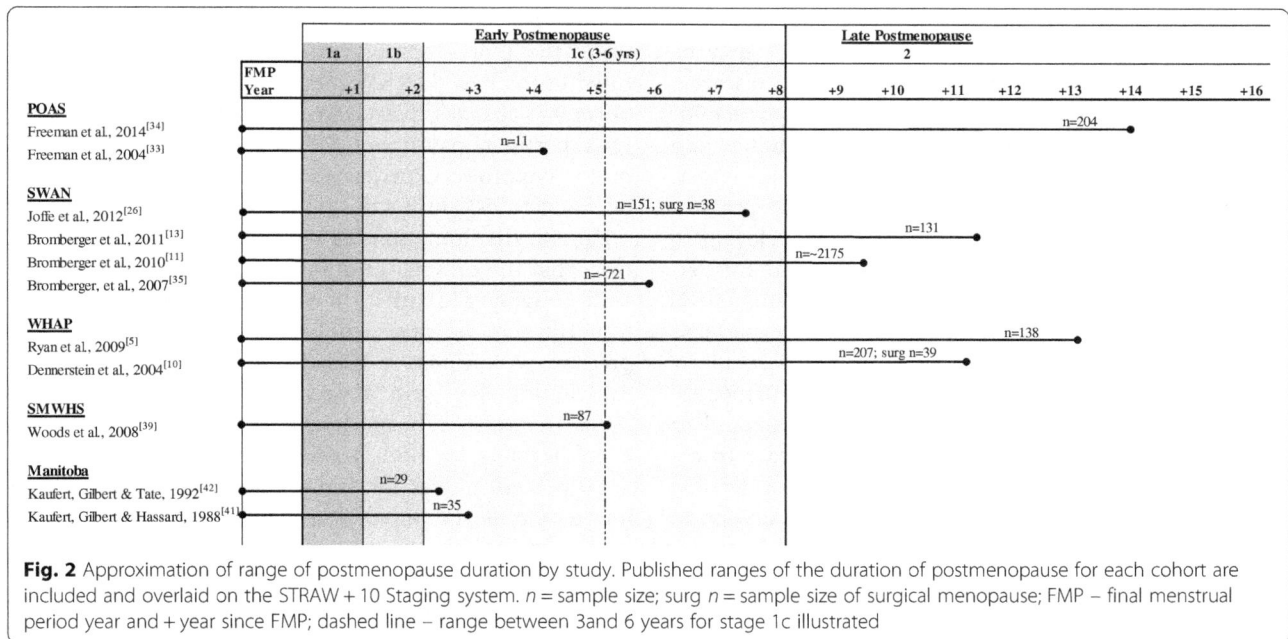

**Fig. 2** Approximation of range of postmenopause duration by study. Published ranges of the duration of postmenopause for each cohort are included and overlaid on the STRAW + 10 Staging system. *n* = sample size; surg *n* = sample size of surgical menopause; FMP – final menstrual period year and + year since FMP; dashed line – range between 3and 6 years for stage 1c illustrated

premenopause at 1.57 [30] and 1.79 [10]. For the surgical menopause group prevalence of depressive symptoms was 42 % for WHAP.

In considering clinical diagnoses, SWAN reported 42.4 % of participants met criteria for past or current depressive disorder and 9.8 % for major depressive episode. SWAN also described 31.6 % of the surgical postmenopause group as meeting criteria for past or current depressive disorder. The higher incidence rate is likely impacted by the inclusion of minor depression in the assessment criteria. EPOS reported <1 % Major Depressive Disorder in their postmenopausal sample but used a cut off of 11 or greater on the Edinburgh Depression Scale to determine presence of MDD rather than a clinical assessment.

The prevalence of depressive symptoms was relatively consistent across studies, with a range of 22 % to 25.7 %, (10, 18). Similarly, most studies demonstrated consistency in higher depressive symptom ratings for the surgical postmenopause group. The prevalence of depressive symptoms reported in these longitudinal studies were somewhat higher than those reported by the Women's Health Initiative Observation Study (WHI-OS), a large prospective study of postmenopausal women carried out in the United States [43]. Baseline characteristics of the 93, 676 multi-ethnic women in this study demonstrated depressive symptom levels at baseline as: 18.1 % for postmenopausal women aged 50–59; 14.8 % for women aged 60–69 and 14.5 % for those aged 70–79 years. Depressive symptoms were assessed using six items from the CESD and two items from the Diagnostic Interview Schedule [43]. The lower reports of depressive symptoms in this cohort may be due to the nature of the enrolment process, with participants representing a sample of convenience rather than being drawn from random population sampling. The prevalence of symptoms reported in this review were also slightly higher than estimates for community dwelling older adults of mixed gender which is thought to be approximately between 12 % and 20 % but varies greatly with prevalence between 0.4 % and 30 % reported in the literature [19, 44]. Studies of older adults or women in late-life cannot be used to generalize to the experiences of postmenopausal women. On average, women in the early postmenopause are aged between 51 and 56–59 years, at which time they enter late postmenopause. The definition of the age at which "late-life" begins is consistently reported as 60-65 years in the literature with "oldest old" age representing those 85 years or greater [19]. Studies that do describe prevalence of depressive symptoms and potential risk factors for women in late-life are greatly impacted by illness associated with old age as well as lifestyle factors unique to this age range such as hospitalisation, loss of loved ones and neurocognitive decline. Women in the postmenopause span mid-life, late life and the oldest old and are not necessarily "older" women as they may have been traditionally viewed.

This review includes data on prevalence reported by longitudinal epidemiological studies exploring mood and the menopausal transition. Any study that included prevalence rates of depressive symptoms or Major Depressive Disorder and reference to the postmenopause specifically were included. However, several of the studies that reported on the postmenopause did so in the context of examining the menopause in general and may not have focused in detail on the postmenopause. For this reason, sample sizes for these populations may be low as they were not the intended focus of the research. Similarly definitions of 'early' versus 'late' postmenopause may not have been relevant to these studies and as such this distinction was not made in many cases. Studies of ageing have reported prevalence of depressive symptoms by age group, including age ranges relevant to postmenopausal women [44, 45]. However, without definitional criteria relating to postmenopausal status one is unable to draw conclusions about prevalence patterns within the stages of postmenopause. This is particularly true for the first two substages of early postmenopause which may pose a period of vulnerability compared to other stages of the postmenopause [34]. In order to assess this distinct period of reproductive ageing a detailed assessment of the time of the final menstrual period needs to be included as a reference point for the onset of early postmenopause.

Differentiating between the effects of biological ageing and reproductive ageing on mood and depressive symptoms is most accurately captured using longitudinal assessment with repeated measures. Inconsistency in definitions and methodology used between, and even within, these studies highlights the need to apply standardised definitions and assessment tools. The STRAW criteria used in a majority of the studies described here was the gold standard staging system at the time. The updated STRAW + 10 system was developed based on our understanding of documented changes in menstrual, endocrine, and ovarian markers of reproductive aging [9, 16, 17]. Given the importance of the FMP in any examination of the climacteric, it would be beneficial for researchers to include specific information about this event in publications. Not only can it serve as a consistent frame of reference for reproductive age, but also as a means for comparing large data sets and conducting metanalyses regardless of the definition of menopausal status being used.

As our understanding of the postmenopause improves, the application of consistent measures and the use of definitions based on standardised criteria are both crucial to determine the prevalence of depressive symptoms across the postmenopausal transition.

## Conclusions

Prevalence of depressive symptoms in the postmenopause was most consistently reported to be between 22 % to 25 % however, wide variation in study design makes it difficult to accurately estimate the number of women at risk of experiencing depressive symptoms during this time. The term 'postmenopause' has been used to group both the early and late postmenopause. Based on recent research the early postmenopause may represent a

unique period of vulnerability and must be examined using the more thorough definitional parameters instituted in the new STRAW + 10 criteria. Given the distinct hormonal changes that occur during the substages of the early postmenopause and the higher likelihood of vasomotor symptoms experienced at this time, an assessment of changing risk during this time is essential.

Despite the limitations of currently available data, it is clear that the prevalence of depressive symptoms is high, with roughly a quarter of women experiencing symptoms during the postmenopause. The presence of depressive symptoms is associated with poorer overall functioning, [46] and a decreased quality of life [47]. While depression is the leading cause of neuropsychiatric disability for both sexes, the burden of depression is 50 percent higher for females [48]. Women are living longer and as the population of older women experiencing morbidity grows, it is crucial to identify modifiable risk factors which have the potential to improve mental health and quality of life in this population.

**Competing interests**
KEC and LD declare that they have no competing interests. Dr. Szoeke has provided clinical consultancy and been on scientific advisory committees for the Australian CSIRO, Alzheimer's Australia, University of Melbourne and other relationships which are subject to confidentiality clauses. She has been a Chief Investigator on investigator driven research projects in partnership with Pfizer, Merck, Vifor Pharma, Sisu Wellness, Bayer and GE. Her research program has received support from NHMRC, Alzheimer's Association, Collier Trust, Scobie and Claire McKinnon Foundation, JO and JR Wicking Trust, Shepherd Foundation, Brain Foundation, Mason Foundation, Ramaciotti Foundation, Alzheimer's Australia, and Royal Australian College of Physicians. She may accrue revenues from patent in pharmacogenomics prediction of seizure recurrence.

**Authors' contributions**
KEC carried out the literature review and drafted the manuscript. LD and CES edited the draft article and guided formatting and structure. KEC prepared the draft manuscript and finalised the changes. LD and CES edited the final manuscript. While LD and CES made a significant contribution KEC wrote a majority of the review. All authors read and approved the final manuscript.

**Acknowledgements**
The authors would like to thank the Department of Psychiatry at the University of Melbourne for providing funding and support to the PhD Candidate. She has been granted the Women's Healthy Ageing Project Scholarship as well as two trust scholarships from the Department of Medicine at the University of Melbourne: the Henry and Rachel Ackman Travelling Scholarship and the John and Allan Gilmour Research Award. A/Prof would like to acknowledge the ongoing support of the National Health and Medical Research Council.

**Author details**
[1]Department of Psychiatry, University of Melbourne, Victoria, Australia. [2]Department of Medicine, University of Melbourne, Victoria, Australia.

**References**
1. Kessler RC, McGonagle KA, Swartz M, Blazer DG, Nelson CB. Sex and depression in the National Comorbidity Survey I: lifetime prevalence, chronicity and recurrence. J Affect Disord. 1993;2:85–96.

2.  Lopez AD, Mathers CD. Measuring the global burden of disease and epidemiological transitions 2002–2030. Ann Trop Med Parasitol. 2006;100 (5–6):481–99.

3.  Panay N, Studd J. The psychotherapeutic effects of estrogens. Gynecol Endocrinol. 1998;12:353–65.

4.  Deecher D, Andree TH, Sloan D, Schechter LE. From menarche to menopause: exploring the underlying biology of depression in women experiencing hormonal changes. Psychoneuroendocrino. 2008;33:3–17.

5.  Ryan J, Burger H, Szoeke C, Lehert P, Ancelin ML, Dennerstein L. A prospective study of the association between endogenous hormones and depressive symptoms in postmenopausal women. Menopause. 2009;16:509–17.

6.  Soares CN, Zitek B. Reproductive hormone sensitivity and risk for depression across the female life cycle: a continuum of vulnerability? J Psychiatry Neurosci. 2008;33:331–43.

7.  Judd FK, Hickey M, Bryant C. Depression and midlife: are we overpathologising the menopause? J Affect Disord. 2012;136:199–211.

8.  Vesco KK, Haney EM, Humphrey L, Fu R, Nelson HD. Influence of menopause on mood: a systematic review of cohort studies. Climacteric. 2007;10:448–65.

9.  Harlow SD, Gass M, Hall JE, Lobo R, Maki P, Rebar RW, et al. Executive summary of the Stages of Reproductive Aging Workshop + 10: addressing the unfinished agenda of staging reproductive aging. Climacteric. 2012;15:105–14.

10. Dennerstein L, Guthrie J, Clark M, Lehert P, Henderson V. A population-based study of depressed mood in middle-aged, Australian-born women. Menopause. 2004;115:563–8.

11. Bromberger JT, Schott LL, Kravitz HM, Sowers M, Avis NE, Gold EB, et al. Longitudinal change in reproductive hormones and depressive symptoms across the menopausal transition: results from the Study of Women's Health across the Nation (SWAN). Arch Gen Psychiatry. 2010;67:598–607.

12. Woods NF, Mitchell ES, Percival DB, Smith-DiJulio K. Is the menopausal transition stressful? Observations of perceived stress from the Seattle Midlife Women's Health Study. Menopause. 2009;16:90–7.

13. Bromberger JT, Kravitz HM, Chang YF, Cyranowski JM, Brown C, Matthews KA. Major depression during and after the menopausal transition: Study of Women's Health Across the Nation (SWAN). Psychol Med. 2011;4:1879–88.

14. The World Bank: World Development Report 1993: investing in health. http://www.worldbank.org/en/publication/wdr/wdr-archive (2015). (Accessed 20 Feb 2015).

15. World Health Organization: World Health Statistics 2014. http://www.who.int/gho/publications/world_health_statistics/en/ (2015). (Accessed 02 Feb 2015).

16. Butler L, Santoro N. The reproductive endocrinology of the menopausal transition. Steroids. 2011;76(7):627–35.

17. Randolph JF, Zheng H, Sowers MFR, Crandall C, Crawford S, Gold E, et al. Change in follicle-stimulating hormone and estradiol across the menopausal transition: effect of age at the final menstrual period. J Clin Endocr Metab. 2011;96(3):746–54.

18. Maartens L, Knottnerus J, Pop V. Menopausal transition and increased depressive symptomatology: a community based prospective study. Maturitas. 2002;42:195–200.

19. Blazer DG. Depression in late life: review and commentary. J Gerontol A-Biol. 2003;58(3):249–65.

20. Turner MJ, Killian TS, Cain R. Life course transitions and depressive symptoms among women in midlife. Int J Aging Hum Dev. 2004;58(4):241–65.

21. World Health Organization: Research on the menopause in the 1990s: report of a WHO scientific group. http://apps.who.int/iris/handle/10665/41841 (2015). (Accessed 20 Nov 2014).

22. Soules MR, Sherman S, Parrott E, Rebar R, Santoro N, Utian W, et al. Executive summary: Stages of Reproductive Aging Workshop (STRAW). Climacteric. 2001;4(4):267–72.

23. Hunter M. The south-east England longitudinal study of the climacteric and postmenopause. Maturitas. 1992;14:117–26.

24. Freeman EW. Associations of depression with the transition to menopause. Menopause. 2010;17:823–7.

25. McKinlay JB, McKinlay SM, Brambilla D. The relative contributions of endocrine changes and social circumstances to depression in mid-aged women. J Health Soc Behav. 1987;28:345–63.

26. Joffe H, Chang YC, Dhaliwal S, Hess R, Thurston R, Gold E, et al. Lifetime history of depression and anxiety disorders as a predictor of quality of life in midlife women in the absence of current illness episodes. Arch Gen Psychiatry. 2012;69:484–92.

27. Lewinsohn PM, Seeley JR, Roberts RE, Allen NB. Center for Epidemiologic Studies Depression Scale (CES-D) as a screening instrument for depression among community-residing older adults. Psychol Aging. 1997;12(2):277.

28. Radloff LS. The CES-D scale. Appl Psych Meas. 1977;1(3):385–401.

29. Smarr KL, Keefer AL. Measures of depression and depressive symptoms: Beck Depression Inventory-II (BDI-II), Center for Epidemiologic Studies Depression Scale (CES-D), Geriatric Depression Scale (GDS), Hospital Anxiety and Depression Scale (HADS), and Patient Health Questionnaire-9 (PHQ-9). Arthrit Care Res. 2011;63(S11):S454–S66.

30. Cox JL, Chapman G, Murray D, Jones P. Validation of the Edinburgh Postnatal Depression Scale (EPDS) in non-postnatal women. J Affect Disorders. 1996;39(3):185–9.

31. First MB, Spitzer RL, Gibbon M, Williams JB. Structured Clinical Interview for DSM-IV Axis I Disorders, Clinician Version (SCID-CV). Washington: American Psychiatric Press, Inc; 1996.

32. Spitzer RL, Williams JB, Kroenke K, Linzer M, Verloin de Gruy F, Hahn SR, et al. Utility of a new procedure for diagnosing mental disorders in primary care: the PRIME-MD 1000 study. JAMA. 1994;272(22):1749–56.

33. Freeman EW, Sammel MD, Liu L, Gracia CR, Nelson DB, Hollander L. Hormones and menopausal status as predictors of depression in women in transition to menopause. Arch Gen Psychiatry. 2004;61:62–70.

34. Freeman EW, Sammel MD, Boorman DW, Zhang R. Longitudinal pattern of depressive symptoms around natural menopause. JAMA Psychiatry. 2014;71:36–43.

35. Bromberger JT, Matthews KA, Schott LL, Brockwell S, Avis NE, Kravitz HM, et al. Depressive symptoms during the menopausal transition: the Study of Women's Health Across the Nation (SWAN). J Affect Disord. 2007;103:267–72.

36. Bromberger JT, Lanza di Scalea T. Longitudinal associations between depression and functioning in midlife women. Maturitas. 2009;64(3):145–59.

37. Dennerstein L, Randolph J, Taffe J, Dudley E, Burger H. Hormones, mood, sexuality, and the menopausal transition. Fertil Steril. 2002;77 Suppl 4:42–8.

38. Szoeke CE, Robertson JS, Rowe CC, Yates P, Campbell K, Masters CL, et al. The Women's Healthy Ageing Project: fertile ground for investigation of healthy participants 'at risk' for dementia. Int Rev Psychiat. 2013;25:726–37.

39. Woods NF, Smith-DiJulio K, Percival DB, Tao EY, Mariella A, Mitchell ES. Depressed mood during the menopausal transition and early postmenopause: observations from the Seattle Midlife Women's Health Study. Menopause. 2008;15:223–32.

40. Murray L, Carothers AD. The validation of the Edinburgh Post-natal Depression Scale on a community sample. Br J Psychiatry. 1990;157:288–90.

41. Kaufert PA, Gilbert P, Hassard T. Researching the symptoms of menopause: an exercise in methodology. Maturitas. 1988;10:117–31.

42. Kaufert PA, Gilbert P, Tate R. The Manitoba Project: a re-examination of the link between menopause and depression. Maturitas. 1992;14(2):143–55.

43. Wassertheil-Smoller S, Shumaker S, Ockene J, Talavera GA, Greenland P, Cochrane B, et al. Depression and cardiovascular sequelae in postmenopausal women: the Women's Health Initiative (WHI). Arch Intern Med. 2004;164(3):289–98.

44. Beekman A, Copeland J, Prince MJ. Review of community prevalence of depression in later life. Brit J Psychiat. 1999;174(4):307–11.

45. Sonnenberg CM, Beekman AT, Deeg DJ, Tilburg WV. Sex differences in late-life depression. Acta Psychiat Scand. 2000;101(4):286–92.

46. Cole MG, Dendukuri N. Risk factors for depression among elderly community subjects: a systematic review and meta-analysis. Am J Psychiat. 2003;160(6):1147–56.

47. Dombrovski AY, Lenze EJ, Dew MA, Mulsant BH, Pollock BG, Houck PR, et al. Maintenance treatment for old-age depression preserves health-related quality of life: a randomized, controlled trial of paroxetine and interpersonal psychotherapy. J Am Geriatr Soc. 2007;55(9):1325–32.

48. Murray CJ, Jamison DT, Lopez AD, Ezzati M, Mathers CD. Global Burden of Disease and Risk Factors. Washington: World Bank and Oxford University Press; 2006.

# Permissions

All chapters in this book were first published in WMH, by BioMed Central; hereby published with permission under the Creative Commons Attribution License or equivalent. Every chapter published in this book has been scrutinized by our experts. Their significance has been extensively debated. The topics covered herein carry significant findings which will fuel the growth of the discipline. They may even be implemented as practical applications or may be referred to as a beginning point for another development.

The contributors of this book come from diverse backgrounds, making this book a truly international effort. This book will bring forth new frontiers with its revolutionizing research information and detailed analysis of the nascent developments around the world.

We would like to thank all the contributing authors for lending their expertise to make the book truly unique. They have played a crucial role in the development of this book. Without their invaluable contributions this book wouldn't have been possible. They have made vital efforts to compile up to date information on the varied aspects of this subject to make this book a valuable addition to the collection of many professionals and students.

This book was conceptualized with the vision of imparting up-to-date information and advanced data in this field. To ensure the same, a matchless editorial board was set up. Every individual on the board went through rigorous rounds of assessment to prove their worth. After which they invested a large part of their time researching and compiling the most relevant data for our readers.

The editorial board has been involved in producing this book since its inception. They have spent rigorous hours researching and exploring the diverse topics which have resulted in the successful publishing of this book. They have passed on their knowledge of decades through this book. To expedite this challenging task, the publisher supported the team at every step. A small team of assistant editors was also appointed to further simplify the editing procedure and attain best results for the readers.

Apart from the editorial board, the designing team has also invested a significant amount of their time in understanding the subject and creating the most relevant covers. They scrutinized every image to scout for the most suitable representation of the subject and create an appropriate cover for the book.

The publishing team has been an ardent support to the editorial, designing and production team. Their endless efforts to recruit the best for this project, has resulted in the accomplishment of this book. They are a veteran in the field of academics and their pool of knowledge is as vast as their experience in printing. Their expertise and guidance has proved useful at every step. Their uncompromising quality standards have made this book an exceptional effort. Their encouragement from time to time has been an inspiration for everyone.

The publisher and the editorial board hope that this book will prove to be a valuable piece of knowledge for researchers, students, practitioners and scholars across the globe.

# List of Contributors

**Ellen W. Freeman**
Department of Obstetrics/Gynecology and Department of Psychiatry, Perelman School of Medicine, University of Pennsylvania, 3701 Market Street, Suite 820 (Mudd Suite), Philadelphia, PA 19104, USA

**Carrie A. Karvonen-Gutierrez**
Department of Epidemiology, University of Michigan School of Public Health, 1415 Washington Heights, Room 6618, Ann Arbor, MI 48109, USA

**Wendy Marder**
Division of Rheumatology, Department of Internal Medicine, University of Michigan, Ann Arbor, MI, USA
Department of Obstetrics and Gynecology, University of Michigan, Ann Arbor, MI, USA

**Emily C. Somers**
Division of Rheumatology, Department of Internal Medicine, University of Michigan, Ann Arbor, MI, USA
Department of Obstetrics and Gynecology, University of Michigan, Ann Arbor, MI, USA
Department of Environmental Health Sciences, University of Michigan, 2800 Plymouth Rd, NCRC B14-G236, Ann Arbor, MI 48109-2800, USA

**Évelyne Vinet**
Division of Rheumatology, McGill University Health Centre, Montreal, Canada
Division of Clinical Epidemiology, McGill University Health Centre, Montreal, Canada

**Susanna D. Mitro and Siobán D. Harlow**
Department of Epidemiology, School of Public Health, 1415 Washington Heights, Ann Arbor, MI 48109, USA

**John F. Randolph and Barbara D. Reed**
School of Medicine, University of Michigan Ann Arbor, Ann Arbor, MI, USA

**Nancy Fugate Woods**
Department of Biobehavioral Nursing, University of Washington, Seattle, WA 98195, USA

**Ellen Sullivan Mitchell**
Department of Family and Child Nursing, University of Washington, Seattle, WA98195USA

**Siobán D. Harlow and Carrie Karvonen-Gutierrez**
Department of Epidemiology, School of Public Health, University of Michigan, 1415 Washington Heights, Suite 6610 SPH I, Ann Arbor, MI 48109-2029, USA

**Michael R. Elliott and Irina Bondarenko**
Department of Biostatistics, School of Public Health, University of Michigan, Ann Arbor, USA

**Nancy E. Avis**
Department of Social Sciences and Health Policy, Wake Forest School of Medicine, Winston-Salem, USA

**Joyce T. Bromberger**
Departments of Epidemiology and Psychiatry, University of Pittsburgh, Pittsburgh, USA

**Maria Mori Brooks**
Department of Epidemiology, University of Pittsburgh, Pittsburgh, USA.

**Janis M. Miller**
School of Nursing, University of Michigan, Ann Arbor, USA

**Barbara D. Reed**
Department of Family Medicine, University of Michigan School of Medicine, Ann Arbor, USA

**Catherine Kim**
Departments of Medicine and Obstetrics and Gynecology, University of Michigan, 2800 Plymouth Road, Building 16, Room 430W, Ann Arbor, MI 48109, USA

**Siobàn D. Harlow, Huiyong Zheng and Daniel S. McConnell**
Department of Epidemiology, University of Michigan, Ann Arbor, MI, USA.

**John F. Randolph Jr.**
Department of Obstetrics and Gynecology, University of Michigan, Ann Arbor, MI, USA

Chi-Son Kim, Deanna Tikhonov, Lena Merjanian and Adrian C. Balica
Department of Obstetrics, Gynecology and Reproductive Sciences, Rutgers Robert Wood Johnson Medical School, 125 Paterson Street, New Brunswick, NJ 08901, USA

Ellen Sullivan Mitchell
Family and Child Nursing, University of Washington, Seattle, USA

Nancy Fugate Woods
Biobehavioral Nursing and Health Informatics, University of Washington, Seattle, USA

Gita D. Mishra, Hsin-Fang Chung and Yalamzewod Assefa Gelaw
School of Public Health, The University of Queensland, Herston Road, Herston, Brisbane, QLD 4006, Australia

Deborah Loxton
Research Centre for Generational Health and Ageing, The University of Newcastle, Callaghan, NSW, Australia

Elizabeth Hedgeman, Carrie A. Karvonen-Gutierrez and Siobán D. Harlow
Department of Epidemiology, School of Public Health, University of Michigan, 6610B SPH I, 1415 Washington Heights, Ann Arbor, MI 48109-2029, USA

Rebecca E. Hasson
School of Kinesiology, School of Public Health, University of Michigan, Ann Arbor, USA

William H. Herman
Department of Internal Medicine, School of Public Health, University of Michigan, Ann Arbor, USA

Mags E. Beksinska and Jenni A. Smit
MatCH Research Unit [Maternal, Adolescent and Child Health Research Unit], Department of Obstetrics and Gynaecology, Faculty of Health Sciences, University of the Witwatersrand, 40 Dr AB Xuma Street, 11th floor, Suite 1108-9, Commercial City, Durban 4001, South Africa

Immo Kleinschmidt
London School of Hygiene and Tropical Medicine, Keppel Street, London WC1E, England

Claire Hardy, Eleanor Thorne and Myra S. Hunter
Department Psychology (at Guy's), Institute of Psychiatry, Psychology and Neuroscience, Kings College London, 5th Floor Bermondsey Wing, Guy's Campus, London SE1 9RT, UK

Amanda Griffiths
Division of Psychiatry and Applied Psychology, School of Medicine, University of Nottingham, Nottingham, UK

Lynnette Leidy Sievert
Department of Anthropology, Machmer Hall, 240 Hicks Way, UMass Amherst, Amherst, MA 01003-9278, USA

Laura Huicochea-Gómez and Diana Cahuich-Campos
Departamento de Sociedad y Cultura, El Colegio de la Frontera, ECOSUR, Campeche, México

Dana-Lynn Ko'omoa-Lange
Department of Pharmaceutical Science, University of Hawai'i at Hilo, Hilo, HI, USA

Daniel E. Brown
Department of Anthropology, University of Hawai'i at Hilo, Hilo, HI, USA

Annette Joan Thomas
College of Nursing, Seattle University, Seattle, Washington, USA

Ellen Sullivan Mitchell
Family and Child Nursing, University of Washington, Seattle, Washington, USA

Nancy Fugate Woods
Biobehavioral Nursing and Health Informatics, University of Washington, Seattle, Wahsington, USA

Linda M Gerber
Department of Healthcare Policy and Research, Division of Biostatistics and Epidemiology, Weill Cornell Medical College, 402 E. 67th St., LA-231, New York, NY 10065, USA
Department of Medicine, Division of Nephrology and Hypertension, Weill Cornell Medical College, New York City, NY, USA

Lynnette Leidy Sievert
Department of Anthropology, UMass Amherst, Amherst, MA, USA

**Kelley Pettee Gabriel and Jessica M. Mason**
Division of Epidemiology, Human Genetics and Environmental Sciences, University of Texas Health Science Center at Houston: School of Public Health–Austin Regional Campus, Austin, TX, USA
School of Public Health, Austin Regional Campus, 1616 Guadalupe Street, Suite 6.300, Austin, TX 78701, USA
Michael and Susan Dell Center for Healthy Living; University of Texas Health Science Center in Houston, Houston, TX, USA

**Barbara Sternfeld**
Division of Research, Kaiser Permanente Northern California, Oakland, CA 94612, USA

**Christine M. Chu, Lily A. Arya and Uduak U. Andy**
Division of Urogynecology, Department of Obstetrics and Gynecology, University of Pennsylvania School of Medicine, 3400 Spruce St., 1000 Courtyard Building, Philadelphia, PA 19104, USA

**Robert L. Reid and Bryden A. Magee**
Division of Reproductive Endocrinology and Infertility, Queen's University, Kingston, Ontario K7L 4 V1, Canada

**Katherine E Campbell and Lorraine Dennerstein**
Department of Psychiatry, University of Melbourne, Victoria, Australia

**Cassandra E. Szoeke**
Department of Medicine, University of Melbourne, Victoria, Australia

# Index

www.ingramcontent.com/pod-product-compliance
Lightning Source LLC
Chambersburg PA
CBHW061244190326
41458CB00011B/3574